Magnetic Resonance
of
Biomolecules

Magnetic Resonance of Biomolecules

An Introduction to the Theory and Practice of NMR and ESR in Biological Systems

P. F. Knowles
Biophysics Department, Leeds University

D. Marsh
Abteilung Spektroskopie, Max Planck Institut für Biophysikalische chemie, Göttingen

H. W. E. Rattle
Biophysical Laboratory, Portsmouth Polytechnic

A Wiley–Interscience Publication

JOHN WILEY & SONS

London · New York · Sydney · Toronto

Library of Congress Cataloging in Publication Data:

Knowles, P. F.
Magnetic resonance of biomolecules.

'A Wiley-Interscience publication.'
Includes bibliographical references and index.
1. Electron paramagnetic resonance. 2. Nuclear magnetic resonance. 3. Molecular biology—Technique. I. Marsh, Derek, joint author. II. Rattle, H. W. E., joint author. III. Title. [DNLM: 1. Electron spin resonance. 2. Nuclear magnet resonance. 3. Spectrum analysis. QC762 K73m]
QH324.9.E36K56 1976 574.8′8′0154308 75–4872

ISBN 0 471 49575 1 (cloth)
ISBN 0 471 01672 1 (pbk)

Typeset by Preface Ltd., Salisbury, Wiltshire and printed in Great Britain at The Pitman Press, Bath

Preface

Although magnetic resonance is now recognized as a very important tool in the study of biological molecules, its practical application still remains restricted to the relatively specialized user. The purpose of this book is to introduce magnetic resonance spectroscopy to biologists and biochemists, some of whom may have little knowledge of spectroscopy other than the straightforward application of ultraviolet and visible spectrophotometry. Our aim in this introduction is fourfold: firstly to give a feeling for the physical principles involved in magnetic resonance; secondly and thirdly to give an introduction to both the practical aspects of running a spectrum and the principles of spectral interpretation; and finally to give an appreciation of the scope of the biological applications of magnetic resonance. A particular feature of the approach is that practical aspects, spectral interpretation and applications are all treated with equal weight, although biological applications are used throughout the book to illustrate theoretical or practical points. The inclusion of both forms of magnetic resonance spectroscopy within the same volume is intended to illustrate the complementary nature of the information which can be obtained by the two methods. This is particularly so in the cases in which NMR is performed on a system containing a paramagnetic ion or spin label, and we believe that this reflects the growing trend among researchers to exploit both techniques in attacking their problems.

A parallel chapter layout has been adopted for both NMR and ESR, thus the reader primarily interested in NMR could first read Chapters 1, 2, 3, 4 and 5, whilst the reader interested in ESR would correspondingly read Chapters 1, 6, 7, 8 and 9. Chapter 1 consists of a brief introduction to the physical basis of spectroscopy, followed by an explanation of the physical origins of magnetic resonance and the principal features observed in ESR and NMR spectra. The biological examples are included in this chapter so that it could be read alone as an introduction for the student to the application of magnetic resonance to biological systems.

Chapters 2 and 6 contain the background needed for spectral interpretation, with the emphasis on the methods required in biological systems. Chapters 3 and 7 contain accounts of the practical aspects of the two methods, with special emphasis on sample handling and spectrometer operation. We have tried to give sufficient practical detail such that the reader can decide whether magnetic resonance would help him with his biological problem and, in particular, would indicate the amount and nature of sample he would need. Chapters 4 and 8 contain the biological applications of the two methods. Although other applications will be found throughout the book, in these two chapters we have chosen a few examples which are illustrative of the different types of applications and have considered them in some depth. In this way the discussions of Chapters 2 and 6 are reinforced and also some idea is gained of the variety of possible applications. Finally, Chapters 5 and 9 contain discussions of those methods which are of a more advanced nature, but are nevertheless of extreme importance in biological applications. These chapters contain an amalgam of both theory and practical details and contain a certain amount of material which might equally well have been included in the earlier chapters, but is included in these chapters so as not to overburden the former at a first reading. To ease the problems involved in mastering an interdisciplinary subject, we have included summaries at the end of each chapter highlighting the salient points and we have concluded the book with a glossary of key magnetic resonance, biological and chemical terms. We hope that these features will particularly appeal to the student.

In summary, we intend this book to be an introductory text which would either take a research biochemist or biologist to a level of knowledge where he could use magnetic resonance methods and begin to interpret his results, or could be used by a student as a first introduction to the applications of magnetic resonance to biological problems.

P.F.K. *Leeds*
D.M. *Göttingen*
H.W.E.R. *Portsmouth*

Acknowledgements

The authors would like to thank Drs R. C. Bray, G. Chapman, M. C. W. Evans and R. Jones for reading parts of the manuscript, Mr A. Watts for providing data and helping with the presentation of several figures in the ESR sections and the staff of P.C.M.U., Harwell, for running the spectra shown in Figures 2.21, 2.28, 3.6 and 3.11; we sincerely thank the typing staff of our various departments for patience during the development of the final manuscript and finally our wives for their forbearance.

Contents

Chapter 1
Magnetic Resonance

1.1 Introduction

Magnetic resonance is a form of spectroscopy well adapted to the study of molecular structure and dynamics. Application to biological molecules gives information on the chemical and structural changes involved in biochemical function. Protein conformational changes, the structure and reactivity of enzyme intermediates, the geometry and stereochemistry of ligand binding sites, redox changes in electron transfer components and the fluidity of membranes are all amenable to study by one or other of the two forms of magnetic resonance.

Electron spin resonance, ESR (also called electron paramagnetic resonance, EPR) requires unpaired (paramagnetic) electrons; it thus can be applied to paramagnetic metalloenzymes and other paramagnetic metalloproteins and to free radical intermediates in biochemical reactions. The method is extremely specific since there are unlikely to be many unpaired electrons in any one system. The range of applications can be extended by attaching stable, synthetic free radicals (spin labels) in a precise chemical and structural manner. An extremely important feature is the anisotropy of the spectrum with respect to the magnetic field orientation which can yield detailed structural information. The line splittings in the spectra are capable of yielding quantitative information on chemical bonding.

Nuclear magnetic resonance (NMR) can yield much more information since it is capable of looking at hydrogen nuclei (protons); in contrast hydrogen atoms are not easily observable by X-ray methods. This often means too much information, but progress is being made towards better resolution with higher-frequency spectrometers. The method can also be made more specific by using shift and broadening reagents, or by looking at other nuclei: carbon, phosphorus, nitrogen and sulphur and including isotopic substitution for protons. Molecular groups can be identified by line positions which also give information on the proximity of groups and chemical bonding. In smaller molecules conformational information is available from splittings in the lines, which are functions of the precise details of the molecular structure.

In this introductory chapter the general physical basis of magnetic resonance will be explained, including the basic spectral features observed in ESR and NMR. Thus the discussion starts with the spectroscopic transitions involved in magnetic resonance and goes on to the basic spectral features: *g*-values and chemical shifts, hyperfine and spin–spin splittings, linewidths and relaxation. Finally the chapter concludes with the discussion of several examples indicating the scope of application of NMR and ESR to biological systems.

1.2 Spectroscopic Transitions and the Electromagnetic Spectrum

Any form of absorption spectroscopy (of which magnetic resonance is an example) relies upon the fact that the absorption of radiation by a molecule involves an energy-level transition from its stable, ground state to an excited state of higher energy. Such a transition is indicated diagrammatically in Figure 1.1. For the transition to take place, the energy of the radiation quantum must match the energy difference, ΔE, between the ground and excited states. This equality is given by Planck's law

$$\bigstar \quad \Delta E = h\nu \tag{1.1}$$

where $h\nu$ is the energy of the radiation quantum, ν being the frequency of the radiation and h a universal constant called Planck's constant. Thus the spectrum of frequencies (or wavelengths) at which the molecule has strong absorptions gives a map of the energies of the excited states of the molecule. Different molecular groups have different excited energy levels, i.e. have absorptions at different parts of the spectrum, and thus their spectra can be used to identify groups and estimate molecular concentrations. Many readers will be familiar with the spectrophotometric determination of protein and nucleic acid concentrations using the ratio of the ultraviolet absorptions at wavelengths of 260 and 280 nm. The 260–280 nm method depends on the strong absorption by proteins at 280 nm and the strong absorption by nucleic acids at 260 nm. These absorptions both arise from transitions between the energy levels of the conjugated π-electrons (a glossary of commonly used chemical, biological and magnetic resonance terms will be found at the end of the book), those of the aromatic amino acids tryosine and tryptophan in the case of proteins and those of the purine and pyrimidine bases in the case of nucleic acids.

Magnetic resonance spectroscopy lies at the opposite end of the electromagnetic spectrum from ultraviolet spectroscopy, as shown in Figure 1.2. This is because the transition energies in magnetic resonance correspond to the weak interactions of an electron or nucleus with a magnetic field, whereas those in ultraviolet spectroscopy

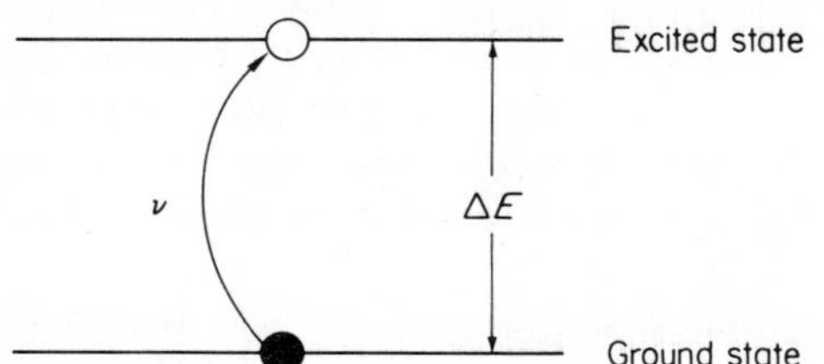

Figure 1.1 Spectroscopic transition involved in absorption spectroscopy

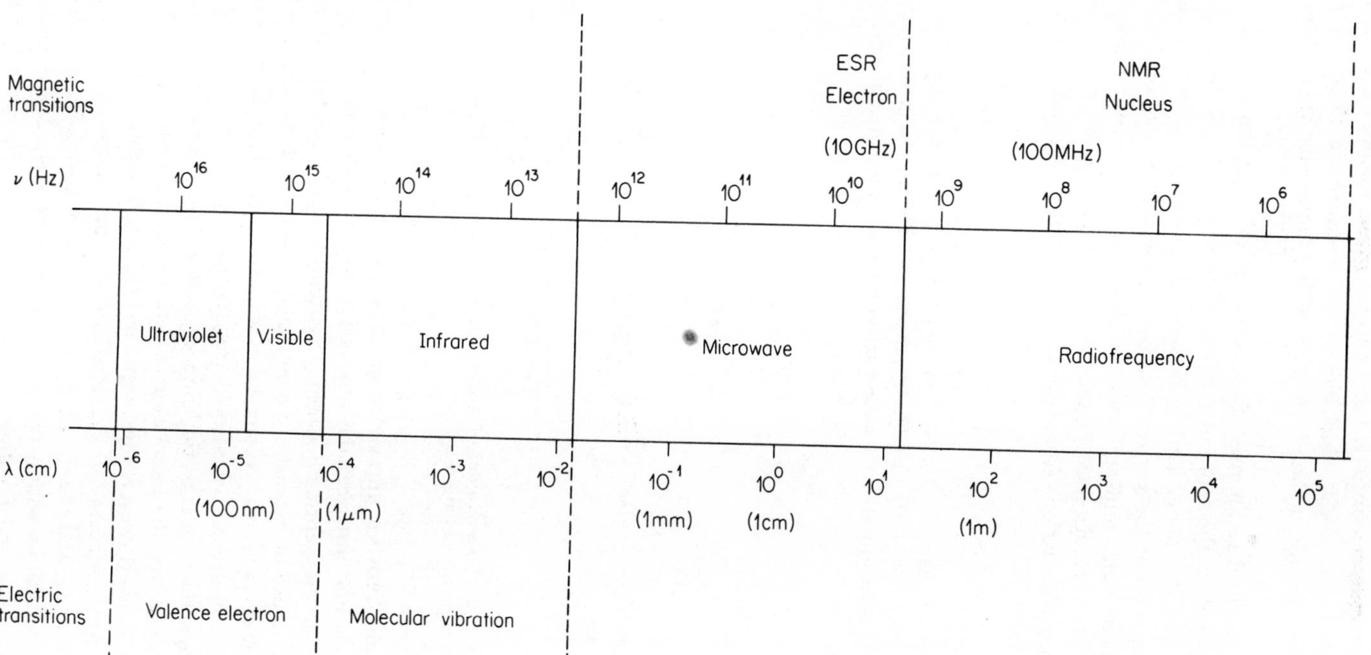

Figure 1.2 Spectral regions of the electromagnetic spectrum of interest in biological investigations

correspond to the strong electrostatic bond energies of the valence electrons of the molecule. Infrared spectroscopy, which lies in the intermediate frequency range, corresponds to the change in bond energies with atomic vibration within the molecule.

Although the practical techniques of spectroscopy differ in the various regions of the spectrum, as does the molecular information obtained, the basic spectroscopic principles are the same. This is because the essential nature of electromagnetic radiation remains the same; it consists of a wavelike variation of coupled electric and magnetic fields moving forward with the same velocity, c, irrespective of frequency (or wavelength) – see Figure 1.3. The frequency and wavelength are related by the familiar relation: (speed) = (distance)/(time), i.e. since frequency is 1/(time for one cycle)

$$c = \nu\lambda \tag{1.2}$$

c is the velocity of light, $= 3 \times 10^{10}$ cm/sec, thus the commonly used ESR microwave frequency of 9 GHz (1 GHz (gigahertz) = 10^9 Hz. Hertz is the unit one cycle per second), corresponds to a wavelength of 3 cm – the conventional X-band radar wavelength.

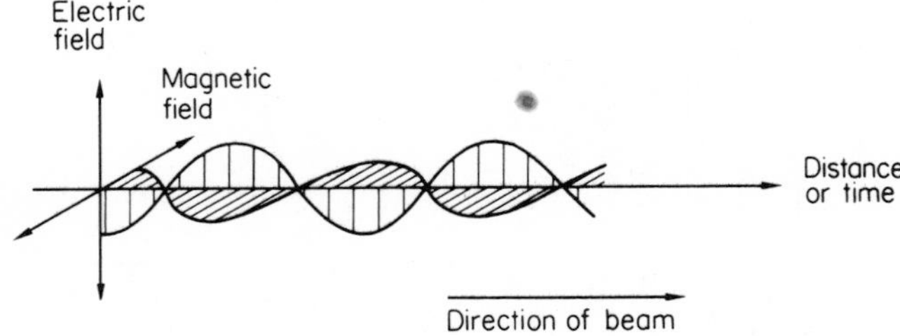

Figure 1.3 Wavemotion of the electric and magnetic fields of electromagnetic radiation

The connection between ultraviolet spectroscopy and molecular bonding and structure is clear. For instance, the absorption by the π-electrons of the single carbonyl groups of the peptide linkages in proteins occur in the far ultraviolet at 190 nm, whereas those of extensively conjugated systems such as carotene (which gives carrots their characteristic colour) lie in the visible region. Similarly in infrared spectroscopy, the molecular vibrational frequencies depend on bond angles and strengths. In magnetic resonance the connection is a little more subtle, since one is fundamentally measuring the interaction of a nuclear or electron magnetic moment with a magnetic field. However, this magnetic field interaction (i.e. the position at which the resonance occurs) is characteristic of the nature of the molecular structure and bonding, and the splittings in the spectrum arising from small electric and magnetic interactions within the molecule are sensitively dependent on both molecular arrangement and bonding. This is illustrated in Figures 1.4, 1.5 which

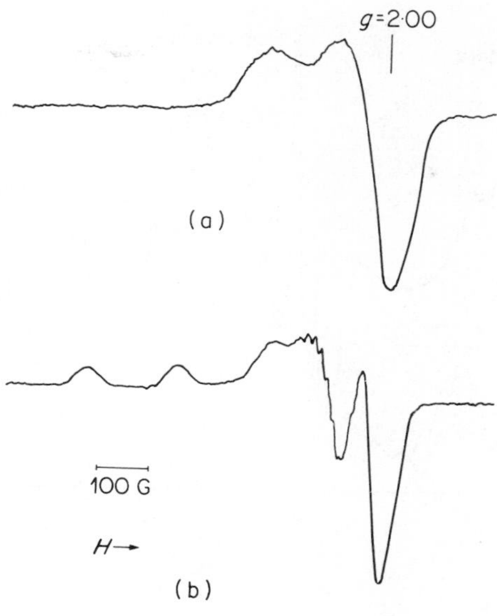

Figure 1.4 Copper ESR spectra of cytochrome-*c* oxidase: (a) native enzyme, 70 mg protein/ml; (b) denatured with 6.5 M urea, 25 mg/ml. (From Beinert, 1966. Reproduced by permission of Academic Press, Inc.)

compare the spectra of denatured (inactive) enzymes with those of the native (active) enzyme. In these cases, the ESR and the NMR spectra strongly reflect the chemical and structural changes which take place in the enzymes on denaturation.

On denaturation of cytochrome oxidase, weak binding sites are exposed for adventitious copper, possibly released from the active site. The ESR spectrum of the denatured enzyme not only shows the additional lines fron the adventitiously bound copper, but also an increase in the intensity of the signal from the strongly bound copper (compare protein concentrations in spectra (a) and (b), Figure 1.4). This clearly shows that some of the copper at the active site has undergone a valence change on denaturation from a diamagnetic to a paramagnetic state. The proton NMR spectrum of ribonuclease in its denatured or random coil form (Figure 1.5) is essentially a superposition of the resonances of the constituent amino acids. The side chains of the amino acid residues are largely unconstrained and thus their chemical shifts are almost independent of amino acid sequence. In the native, folded conformation, however, most of the side chains are closer together and are thus perturbed by their nearest neighbours, reflecting the protein sequence and tertiary structure. This is clearly seen in the low-field, 7 ppm, region of the spectra: the equivalence seen in the denatured protein between the protons of the aromatic residues is removed by the different nearest-neighbour interactions in the native protein.

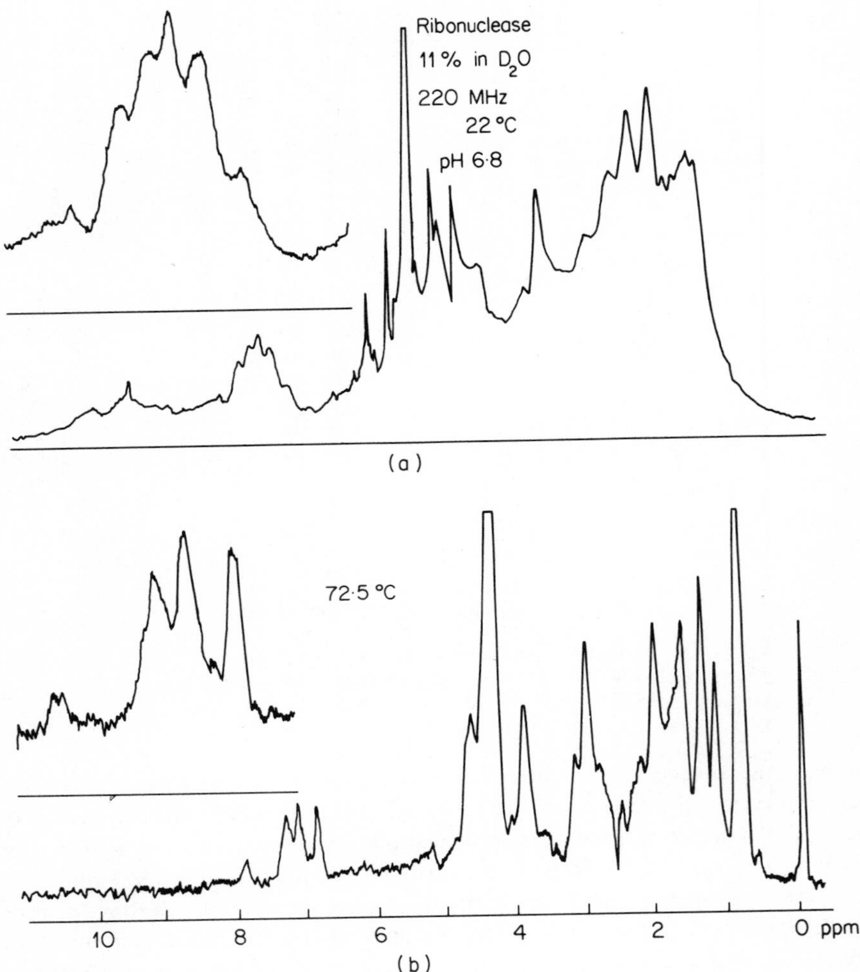

Figure 1.5 220 MHz proton NMR spectra of ribonuclease: (a) in its native conformation; (b) thermally denatured. (From Ferguson and Phillips, 1967. Reproduced by permission. Copyright 1967 by the American Association for the Advancement of Science)

1.3 Magnetic Moments and Magnetic Resonance (*g*-values and chemical shifts)

Magnetic resonance absorption can only be observed in those species which have a magnetic moment, since the prerequisite is that they should interact with a magnetic field in much the same way as does a simple bar magnet. Nuclei with an odd mass number have magnetic moments, as do atoms or molecules with an odd number of electrons. The electron pairing which causes effective cancellation of spins in chemical bonding means that transition-metal ions and free radicals are

Table 1.1
Magnetic species in biological systems

NMR	Abundance	
^{1}H, ^{13}C	100%, 1%	All
^{31}P	100%	Nucleotides, phospholipids, phosphorylated metabolites
^{14}N, ^{15}N, ^{33}S	99.6%, 0.4%, 0.7%	Amino acids, peptides, proteins
^{19}F, ^{2}H	100%, 0.2%	Isotopic label substituting for ^{1}H
ESR		
Transition metals		Metalloproteins, including metalloenzymes and haem proteins
Free radicals		Transient reaction intermediates, irradiated species
Stable free radicals		-Spin labels: covalently attached or intercalated

almost the only species with an electron magnetic moment. Nuclear binding is less exclusive and more nuclei have a magnetic moment, though the natural isotopic abundance is not always very high. The magnetic species which can be studied in biological magnetic resonance are given in Table 1.1.

If an electron cloud or a nucleus has a net magnetic moment, then its potential energy will be lower if the moment is pointing in the direction of the field than if it is pointing against it, just as a compass needle points north–south rather than south–north. The energy of the magnetic moment depends on its projection along the magnetic field (Figure 1.6)

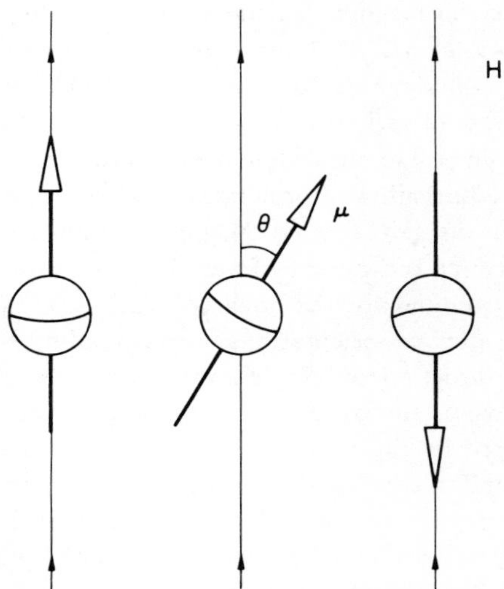

Figure 1.6 Magnetic moment, μ, in minimum, intermediate and maximum (left to right) energy orientations with respect to a magnetic field **H**

$$E = -\mu . \mathbf{H} \tag{1.3}$$

where μ is the magnetic moment and **H** the magnetic field. This commonly used vector notation (the scalar product) implies that the projection of μ along the direction of **H** is used in the product. In a quantum-mechanical description the magnetic moment of a nucleus or electron is related to its spin by

$$\mu = -g\beta\mathbf{S} \quad \text{for an electron}$$

and (1.4)

$$= g_n\beta_n\mathbf{I} \quad \text{for a nucleus}$$

where **S** and **I** are the electron and nuclear spins; β, β_n – the Bohr and nuclear magnetons respectively – are the natural units of electron and nuclear magnetic moments; and g, g_n are proportionality constants called the electron and nuclear g-values, respectively, whose value depends on the particular magnetic species under consideration. (The minus sign in the expression for the electron magnetic moment shows that the electron magnetic moment and spin are in opposite directions, whereas for a nucleus they are in the same direction. This has little practical importance, since magnetic resonance spectroscopy measures only the separation of the energy levels.) If m and M are the masses of the electron and the proton respectively ($M = 1836 \times m$) then

$$\beta = \frac{eh}{4\pi mc} \quad \text{and} \quad \beta_n = \frac{eh}{4\pi Mc} \tag{1.5}$$

which shows that the electron magnetic moments are about 2000 times larger than nuclear magnetic moments. $g_e = 2.0023$ for a free electron and $g_n = 5.5855$ for a free proton, though the values measured in ESR and NMR experiments may be appreciably different because of various environmental factors discussed below.

Electron and nuclear spins are quantized, in other words unlike a compass needle they can only take up certain allowed orientations relative to the magnetic field, each corresponding to a distinct energy. Magnetic resonance absorptions correspond to transitions between these energy levels. For a spin of a half, which is the case for an unpaired electron and for the nuclei of Table 1.1, except ^{14}N, ^{33}S and ^{2}H, there are only two allowed orientations, corresponding to spin projections along the magnetic field direction of: S_z (electron) or I_z (nucleus) = ± ½. These allowed projections, known as the parallel and antiparallel orientations or spin-up and spin-down, are depicted by the two outer spins of Figure 1.6. The energy-level diagram for a spin one-half system is shown in Figure 1.7. In the absence of a magnetic field, the single nucleus or unpaired electron can take up either of the two spin orientations, since these have equal energy as indicated by the two coincident energy levels. The application of a magnetic field causes the parallel orientation to have lower energy, hence this is the orientation which is preferred. The energy levels in a magnetic field are given by

$$E = +g\beta HS_z = \pm \tfrac{1}{2}g\beta H \tag{1.6}$$

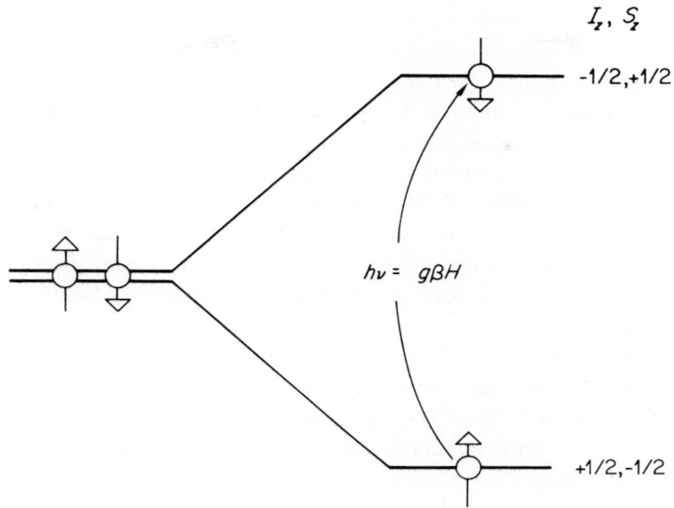

Figure 1.7 Energy-level splitting and magnetic resonance transition for an electron or nucleus, of a spin of one-half, in a magnetic field

Electromagnetic radiation can induce transitions, i.e. changes in spin orientation, from the lower- to the higher-energy spin orientation as indicated in Figure 1.7 and thus the condition for a spectroscopic transition, equation (1.1), is given by

★ $$h\nu = g\beta H \tag{1.7}$$

This equation holds equally well for NMR as for ESR, if the nuclear g-value and magneton are used. The angular frequency, $\omega = 2\pi\nu$, and the gyromagnetic ratio, $\gamma = g_n\beta_n$, are often used in NMR, giving the alternative form

★ $$\omega = \gamma H \tag{1.8}$$

The g-value thus specifies the position of the spectral absorption from a particular magnetic species and is characteristic of that species, e.g. protons or phosphorus nuclei. The position of the absorption also depends on the environment in which the magnetic species sits, though in a rather different way for NMR than for ESR. The magnetic moment of an electron depends not only on its spin, but also to a certain extent on its orbital motion within the atom. This orbital contribution depends on the neighbouring bonded atoms, in other words the electron g-value depends on its molecular environment. The gyromagnetic ratio of a nucleus is not affected in this direct way by its chemical environment, but the magnetic field which it sees is modified by a shielding effect of the surrounding electrons. The strength of the shielding depends on the local electron bonding and leads to NMR absorptions whose positions are also determined by the molecular environment. The environmental factor is emphasized in NMR by specifying the line positions of a particular species, e.g. protons, by a 'chemical shift' relative to a standard compound. The total spectral range is usually small compared with the absolute resonance frequency, e.g. electron g-values mostly only deviate by about ±0.2 from the free spin g-value of 2.0023 (with the important exception of Fe^{3+}) and proton chemical shifts are normally not more than 10 parts per million of the standard resonance frequency. Nevertheless the deviations are quite sufficient for significant resolution, as already indicated in Figures 1.4 and 1.5.

The resonance condition, equation (1.7), immediately enables one to calculate the fields required for an ESR or NMR experiment. For ESR at the normally used microwave frequencies of 9 GHz and 35GHz one requires fields in the region of 3.2 kG and 12.5 kG respectively, for $g = 2$. (The gauss (G) is the c.g.s. unit which is commonly used in ESR spectroscopy for expressing magnetic field strength and spectral splittings. 1 kG (kilogauss) = 10^3 G, and for those more familiar with SI units: 1 G = 10^{-4} Tesla.) Such fields are easily obtainable by normal electromagnets. For proton nuclear magnetic resonance at the commonly used radio frequencies of 60, 100 and 270 MHz, the fields required are 14.1, 23.5 and 63.4 kG, of which the latter is only attainable with a superconducting magnet. All other nuclei have smaller magnetic moments than protons and thus would require even larger fields. It is of advantage to operate one's spectrometer at a high frequency because this gives both better sensitivity and potentially better resolution, in the sense that overlapping spectra may become more spread-out. We see that NMR spectroscopy is confined to the radiofrequency region of the spectrum because of practical limitations of magnetic fields. Also ESR is largely confined to the lower half of the microwave range because of practical considerations of frequency sources. (Compare again Figure 1.2.)

There are two distinctive differences between magnetic resonance spectroscopy and the other forms of spectroscopy indicated in Figure 1.2, both of which arise from its magnetic nature. The first difference is that in scanning a spectrum it is usual, for technical reasons (compulsory for ESR), to sweep the magnetic field rather than the frequency. The magnetic resonance transition diagram of Figure 1.7 is thus more usually drawn as in Figure 1.8 in which a fixed frequency (indicated by the length of the vertical transition arrow) is matched to continuously variable magnetic field energy levels. The second difference is in the way the transitions are induced. In conventional ultraviolet, visible or infrared spectroscopy it is the electric field of the radiation (Figure 1.3) which interacts with the electric charge of the electron or polar molecular group. In magnetic resonance, however, it is the interaction of the magnetic field of the radiation with the magnetic moment of the nucleus or the electron, which induces the transitions. This has important practical considerations in the design of ESR and NMR spectrometers, but perhaps more important is the effect on which transitions are allowed and which are forbidden – that is, the selection rules. The selection rules arise from the fact that transitions between certain energy levels are forbidden by quantum mechanics. The selection rules for magnetic resonance are quite different from those for the other forms of spectroscopy mentioned; for instance a transition of the type depicted in Figure 1.7 is allowed in magnetic resonance spectroscopy, but not in ultraviolet, visible or infrared spectroscopy. The selection rules for magnetic resonance spectroscopy can be summarized as follows

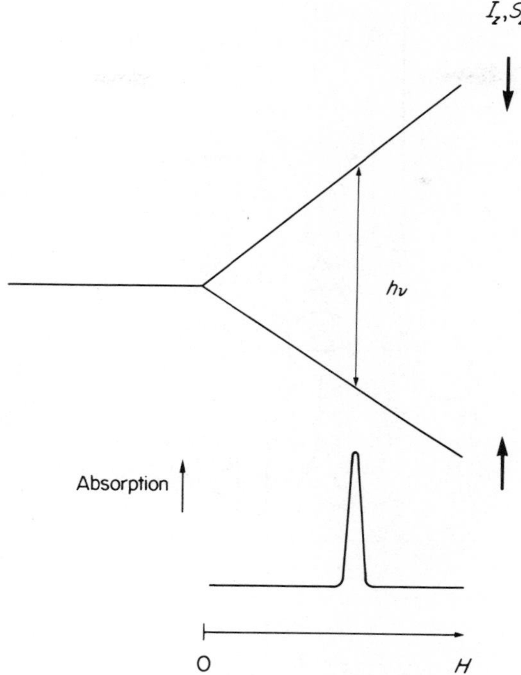

Figure 1.8 Electron or nuclear spin energy levels in an increasing magnetic field, H, and the constant frequency transition between them. (The arrows indicate the direction of the magnetic moment)

$$\star \quad \Delta S = 0, \quad \Delta S_z = \pm 1 \tag{1.9}$$

which means that the total spin S of the states between which the transition takes place remains the same and that the projection, S_z, of this spin along the magnetic field shall change by ± 1. Clearly this is the case for the system of Figure 1.7 in which $S = \frac{1}{2}$ for both states and S_z changes from $+\frac{1}{2}$ to $-\frac{1}{2}$. More complicated cases are considered in Chapter 6.

1.4 Hyperfine Structure and Spin–Spin Splittings

The two most important features of a spectrum are the points about which the lines are centred, specified by their g-values in ESR or chemical shifts in NMR, and the splittings of these lines – the hyperfine splittings in ESR or the spin–spin splittings in NMR.

Hyperfine and spin–spin splittings both arise from the interaction of the central magnetic moment (electron magnetic moment in ESR, nuclear magnetic moment in NMR), with the magnetic moments of the surrounding nuclei. The origin of the

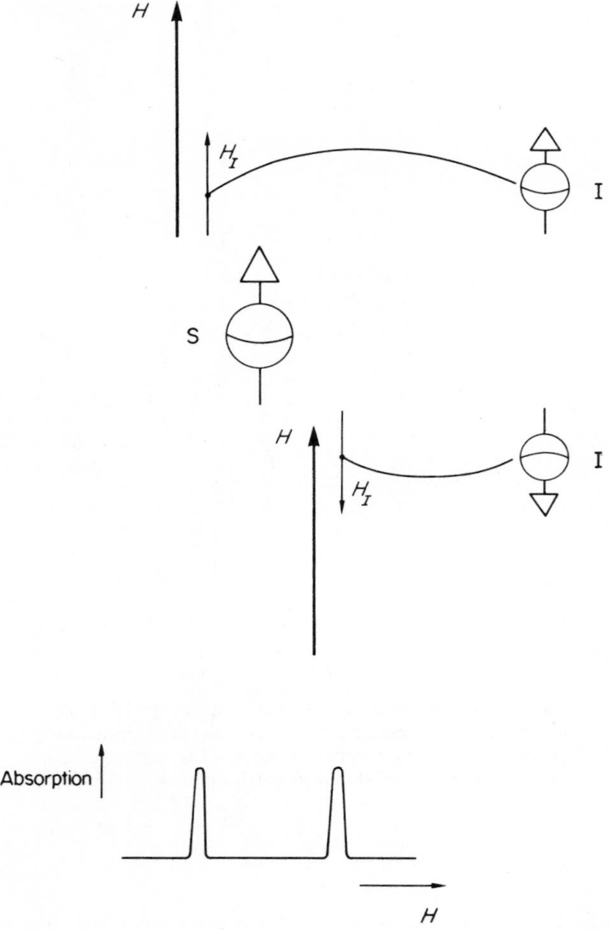

Figure 1.9 Hyperfine interaction of an electron spin, **S**, with different orientations of a nuclear spin, **I**

splitting of the central line by this interaction can be seen in Figure 1.9 for an electron interacting with a single nucleus. The electron spin, **S**, experiences a magnetic field, H_I, arising from the nuclear magnetic moment as well as the applied spectrometer field, H. The origin of this field from the nuclear moment is similar to that of the magnetic field associated with a bar magnet. The direction of the H_I field depends on the orientation of the nuclear spin; for $I = ½$ it can either oppose or reinforce the spectrometer field as indicated in the figure. The result is that the ESR line is split in two since the electron spin effectively experiences either of two different magnetic fields. The effect is exactly the same in NMR except that because the two nuclei influence each other a spin–spin splitting is produced in the NMR lines of both nuclei. The effect of the hyperfine interaction on the energy

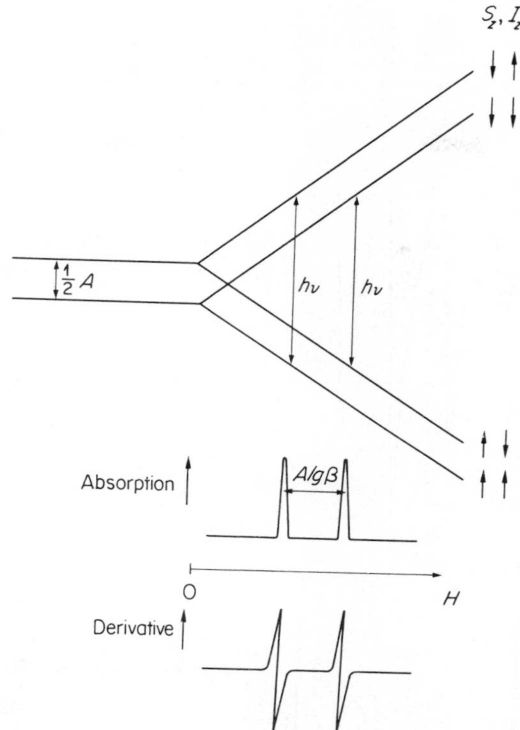

Figure 1.10 Hyperfine interaction: constant frequency transitions. A is the hyperfine splitting factor. (The arrows indicate the direction of the magnetic moments)

levels of an electron in a magnetic field is given in Figure 1.10. The transitions for a constant frequency, $h\nu$, are given using the selection rule $\Delta I_z = 0$ (since the nuclear-spin orientation is not changed in an ESR experiment). This clearly shows that the single transition is split into a doublet by the hyperfine interaction. In the figure, the magnetic resonance absorption is also displayed as its first derivative, i.e. the amplitude representing the slope of the absorption peaks. For practical reasons, this is the normal method of recording an ESR spectrum.

Clearly if more nuclei are present the splitting pattern becomes more complicated and is characteristic of the molecular arrangement experienced by the particular nucleus or paramagnetic electron. Examples of proton hyperfine structure and phosphorus spin–spin couplings are given in Figure 1.11. Figure 1.11(a) is the ESR spectrum of the benzosemiquinone, free radical intermediate produced in the oxidation of the hydroquinone substrate by the metalloenzyme laccase. The ESR spectrum arises from the unpaired electron of the free radical, and the characteristic hyperfine structure shows it to be completely delocalized, interacting equally with the four eqivalent protons of the aromatic ring. In Figure

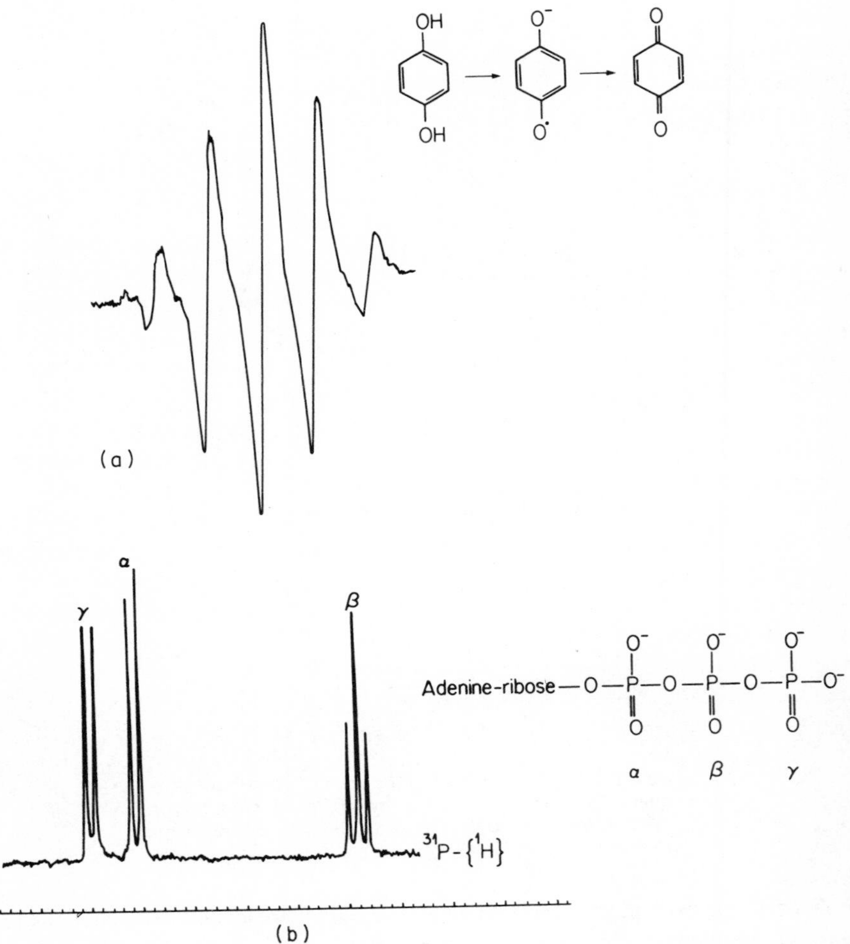

Figure 1.11 (a) Proton hyperfine structure in the ESR spectrum of benzosemiquinone free radical generated by enzymic oxidation. (From Nakamura, 1961. Reproduced by permission of Academic Press, Inc.) (b) Spin–spin splittings in the ^{31}P NMR spectrum of adenosine triphosphate. (Courtesy of JEOL Co. Ltd.)

1.11(b) is given the ^{31}P NMR spectrum of adenosine triphosphate. Three resonances are seen corresponding to the three phosphate groups. The β-phosphorus resonance is easily identified since its spin–spin splitting produces a triplet structure characteristic of the interaction with two other phosphorus nuclei – the α and the γ. The α- and γ-phosphorus nuclei interact only with the β-phosphorus and thus have only doublet splitting. The fact that all the splittings are equal shows that the α- and γ-phosphorus atoms are conformationally equivalent with respect to the β-phosphorus. The magnitudes of the hyperfine or spin–spin splittings clearly depend on the molecular geometry and bonding. Spin–spin splittings are often determined by bond angles and are used in conformational analysis. Hyperfine splittings are a measure of the covalent bonding in the molecule or electron densities in free radicals, and are used to infer chemical reactivities of molecules and energy levels of liganded transition-metal ions.

1.5 Thermal Equilibrium and Spin—Lattice Relaxation

Having formed a simple static picture of the magnetic resonance absorption we will now go on to look at the dynamic effects. These have both important practical consequences and extremely useful applications in probing molecular environments. As will be seen below, the possible practical consequences are a decrease in signal intensity (or the actual disappearance of lines) due to saturation or an increase in linewidth due to relaxation time broadening. The applications involve either the direct measurement of relaxation times or the investigation of saturation characteristics, to determine the strength of the interaction between the magnetic electron or nucleus and its surroundings.

The picture given so far in Figure 1.7 has depicted the resonance absorption as a spin transition from the low-energy parallel orientation to the higher-energy antiparallel orientation. Unfortunately electromagnetic radiation is just as effective in causing spin flip transitions in the opposite direction involving the emission of radiation of the same frequency. To discover whether there will be any detectable magnetic resonance absorption it is thus necessary to consider not just a single spin but the whole collection of spins. Thus there will be a net absorption of radiation only if there are initially fewer spins in the upper than in the lower state.

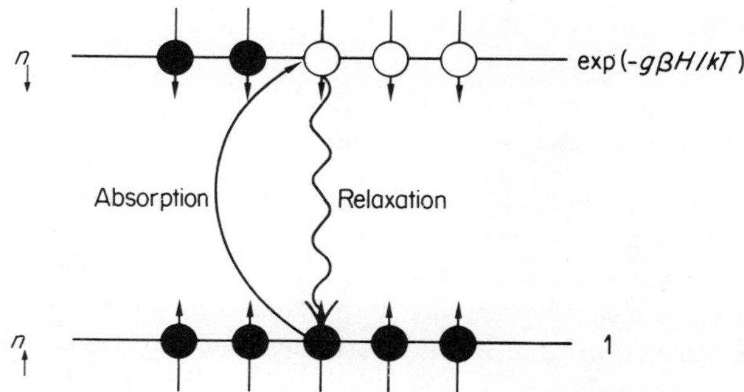

Figure 1.12 Thermal populations of energy levels and spin—lattice relaxation from the excited energy level

This is always the case when the spins are in thermal equilibrium because it is energetically more favourable for a spin to be in the lower energy level as depicted in Figure 1.12. Not all spins will be in the lower state since the thermal (heat) energy of some will be sufficient to excite them into the higher level. The ratio of the number of spins in the two levels depends on the relative values of the average thermal energy, kT, and the energy gap, $g\beta H$, between states, and is given by the

Boltzman distribution

★ $$\frac{n_\downarrow}{n_\uparrow} = \exp(-g\beta H/kT) \tag{1.10}$$

In fact the energy splitting $g\beta H$ is so small that this ratio is almost unity at room temperatures, especially for NMR. This means that one requires very sensitive detection systems. In the absence of undesirable side-effects (such as line-broadening which is frequently the case) there will thus always be a gain in sensitivity by cooling the sample to lower temperatures.

However, when the system is undergoing electromagnetic transitions it is no longer necessarily in thermal equilibrium. The populations in upper and lower levels will soon become equalized, unless the excess spins in the upper state are able to lose energy by some external means and drop down into the lower state thus maintaining the thermal equilibrium Boltzman distribution as illustrated in Figure 1.12. The process by which the spins in the upper state lose energy externally is known as spin–lattice relaxation and the speed with which they do this is characterized by the spin–lattice relaxation time, T_1. For a solid material, spin–lattice relaxation involves literally that: the loss of energy from the spins to the crystal lattice (i.e. the atoms in the crystal), which involves a heating of the whole crystal instead of a local departure from thermal equilibrium in the spin system. In liquid systems, the 'lattice' refers to the thermal motions of the liquid molecules which provide a similar, but less effective thermal sink. A system which affords extremely effective spin–lattice relaxation of nuclei is the magnetic interaction with a paramagnetic ion. This has very useful application in the study of ion binding with biological molecules, as illustrated by the Mn^{2+}–ATP system discussed in the final section of this chapter.

1.6 Relaxation time broadening and Saturation

The spin–lattice relaxation time depends on the molecular environment, i.e. how strongly the spin is 'coupled' to the lattice. Relaxation times are thus short in solids or systems with paramagnetic ions (fast relaxation), but relatively long in liquids (slow relaxation). This has two very important practical effects. On the one hand if the spin–lattice relaxation time is too short the lines may be broadened out so much as to be undetectable, or on the other hand if it is too long, the radiation power may be so high that the signal saturates because the radiation-induced transitions take place too quickly for the relaxation process to be effective.

The origin of relaxation time broadening can be easily visualized in terms of the Heisenberg Uncertainty Principle, which is one of the important consequences of the wavelike nature of matter. The Uncertainty relation implies that if a system exists in a certain energy state for only a short time duration, then the energy of the state is not well-defined. The possible energy range, ΔE, of the state is related to its lifetime, τ, by

$$\Delta E \cdot \tau \approx h \tag{1.11}$$

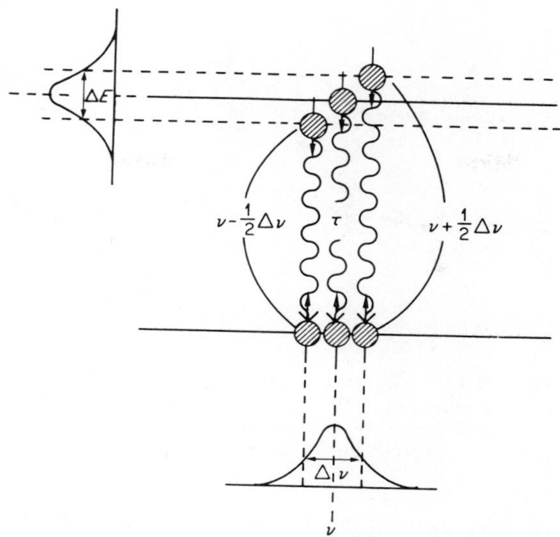

Figure 1.13 Lifetime broadening of a spectral line, as a result of the Uncertainty Principle

This causes a corresponding broadening in the spectral transition as indicated in Figure 1.13, the linewidth being given by Planck's relation

$$h\Delta\nu \cdot \tau \approx h$$

i.e.

★ $$\Delta\nu \approx \frac{1}{\tau} \tag{1.12}$$

For a transition in which the magnetic field is swept instead of the frequency, the corresponding linewidth is given, from equation (1.7) by

$$\Delta H \approx \frac{h}{g\beta} \cdot \Delta\nu = \frac{h}{g\beta} \cdot \frac{1}{\tau} \tag{1.13}$$

Lifetime broadening is often encountered in the ESR of transition-metal ions which are strongly coupled to the molecular lattice, and the remedy is to cool the sample to lower temperatures at which the relaxation times are longer, e.g. Fe^{3+} in haem proteins. In nuclear resonance relaxation times are generally much longer and disappearance of lines due to relaxation time broadening is only encountered in systems which are strongly paramagnetic, undergoing slow chemical exchange (although strictly speaking this is a T_2-process not a T_1-process – see Chapter 2), or contain quadrupolar nuclei such as ^{14}N or ^{35}Cl. Chemical exchange causes the disappearance of the peaks from –OH protons in D_2O solutions, and broadening of $-NH_2$ proton peaks is a result of quadrupolar relaxation by the ^{14}N nucleus.

Saturation occurs if the radiation power is so high that the relaxation

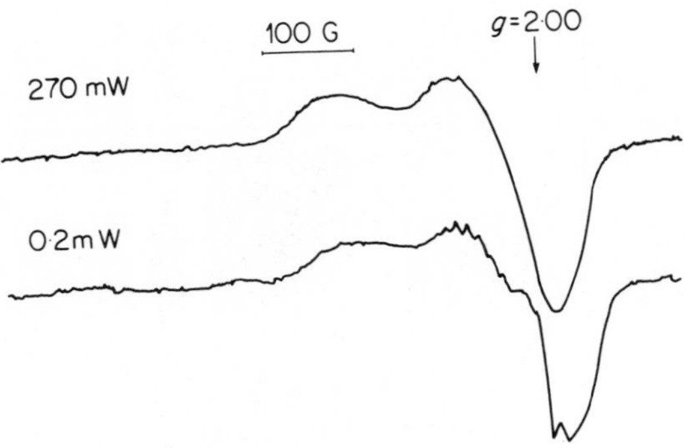

Figure 1.14 Copper ESR spectrum of cytochrome-*c* oxidase recorded with high (upper) and low (lower) microwave power. (From Beinert, 1966. Reproduced by permission of Academic Press, Inc.)

mechanisms cannot keep up with the transitions induced by it. The relaxation then becomes so ineffective that it might as well not be there. One is back at the situation described at the beginning of the previous section, in which the radiation-induced transitions equalize the number of spins in the two levels and the signal disappears. The characteristics of saturation are thus a broadening and eventual disappearance of the line with progressively increasing radiation power. Clearly under normal circumstances, saturation is to be guarded against by examining the spectrum at different powers. The saturation characteristics of a line depend on the environment in which the spin sits, since it is determined by the spin–lattice relaxation time. This can be put to good use in probing molecular environment: an example is afforded by the ESR spectrum of cytochrome oxidase discussed previously. Figure 1.14 shows the copper spectrum recorded under conditions of both high and low microwave power. The sample consisted of the active enzyme which had a small amount of bound adventitious copper. Clearly at high powers the adventitious copper signal saturates, whereas the signal from the copper bound at the active site does not. This indeed formed the basis for the identification of the adventitious copper: because it is only weakly bound its spin–lattice relaxation time is long and it saturates easily. The copper at the active site is strongly bound and has a short spin–lattice relaxation time (requiring low temperatures to observe an unbroadened spectrum).

Strong environmental effects on relaxation are observed in NMR. In fact, investigations have been taken to a much more sophisticated level at which relaxation times are measured directly. The Mn^{2+}-ATP system quoted at the end of the chapter is a good illustration of this.

1.7 Spin–Spin Relaxation and Linewidths

It was said above that the magnetic interaction between nuclei and paramagnetic electrons (the so-called magnetic dipole–dipole interaction) is an extremely

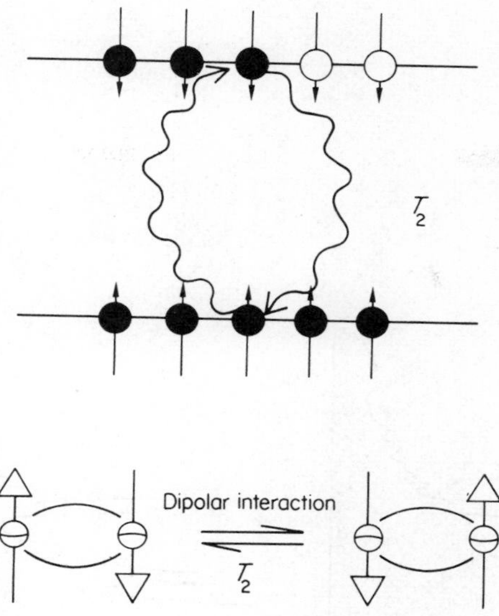

Figure 1.15 Dipolar spin flips and spin–spin relaxation

efficient means of relaxing nuclei from their upper spin state. What then is the effect of the magnetic interactions between the nuclei themselves in NMR or between one electron magnetic moment and another in ESR? In solids the static dipolar interaction can lead to extremely broad lines which is the reason why NMR is usually performed in liquids and ESR on magnetically dilute samples. One of the dynamic effects of the dipolar interaction between like spins is to cause mutual spin flips as illustrated in Figure 1.15. This process limits the lifetime of a spin in the upper state, as shown in Figure 1.15, without changing the total number of spins in the state. This spin–spin relaxation, unlike spin–lattice relaxation is unable to alleviate saturation but contributes to the lifetime broadening of the line. Often it is the spin–spin relaxation time, T_2, which limits the observed linewidth, thus from equation (1.12)

★ $$\Delta\nu \approx \frac{1}{T_2} \tag{1.14}$$

This is the common situation in NMR and in the ESR of free radicals in solution; the lineshape is then Lorentzian. At this point it should be emphasized that, under normal circumstances, it is T_2 and not T_1 which determines the intrinsic linewidth. For ESR in solids, observed linewidths are much broader than predicted by equation (1.14), being a superposition of lines arising from slight crystal imperfections, unresolved ligand hyperfine structure and static dipolar interactions. In such cases the lineshapes are usually Gaussian, characteristic of a random spread of superimposed lines.

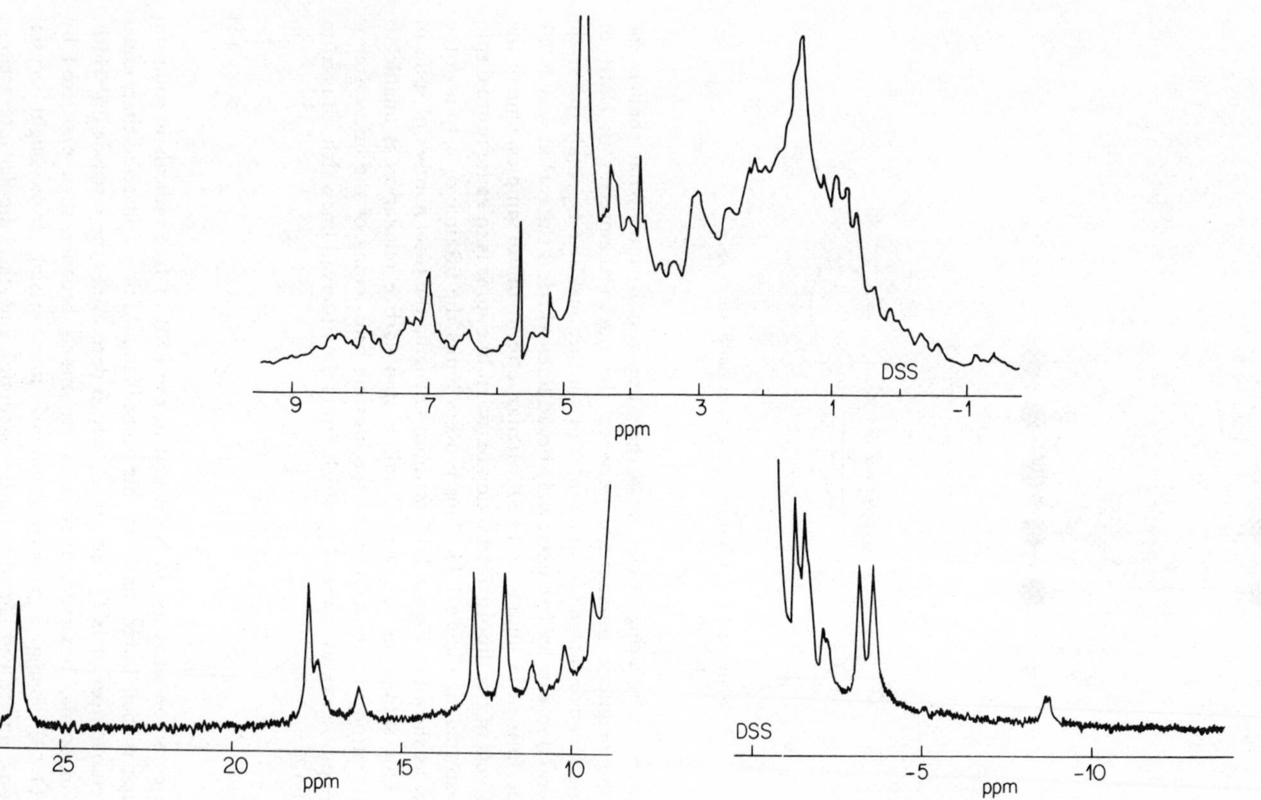

Figure 1.16 220 MHz proton NMR spectrum of aqueous (D_1O) myoglobin cyanide. (From Wüthrich *et al.*, 1970. Reproduced by permission of the American Society of Biological Chemists, Inc.)

1.8 Scope of Magnetic Resonance in Biological Systems

We finish this chapter with a few examples indicating the scope of the magnetic resonance technique applied to biological systems. The examples are chosen to contrast the applications of ESR and NMR and illustrate the different types of information which are available from the two spectroscopic methods.

The first example is the application of ESR and NMR to the study of the haem protein myoglobin. This both contrasts the specificity of ESR with the universality of proton NMR and also illustrates the complementary nature of the information which can be obtained by the two methods. Figure 1.16 gives the 220 MHz proton NMR spectrum of aqueous (D_2O) myoglobin. Contrast this wealth of spectral lines with the single doublet ESR line obtained from an oriented single crystal of myoglobin fluoride in Figure 1.17. The difference is very well illustrated by the molecular model of myoglobin in Figure 1.18. The ESR spectrum arises from the single electron magnetic moment in the molecule, that of the haem iron atom, and thus reflects only the orientation of the haem plane and the nature of the haem group ligands. On the other hand, the NMR spectrum arises from the protons of the amino acid residues of the entire polypeptide chain. The proton NMR spectrum provides information about the entire molecule, whereas the ESR spectrum furnishes specific information about the prosthetic group of the molecule.

The myoglobin molecule acts physiologically as an oxygen store in muscle; the oxygen molecule is taken up in the sixth coordination position of the haem iron atom (the other five coordination positions are occupied by nitrogen ligands, four

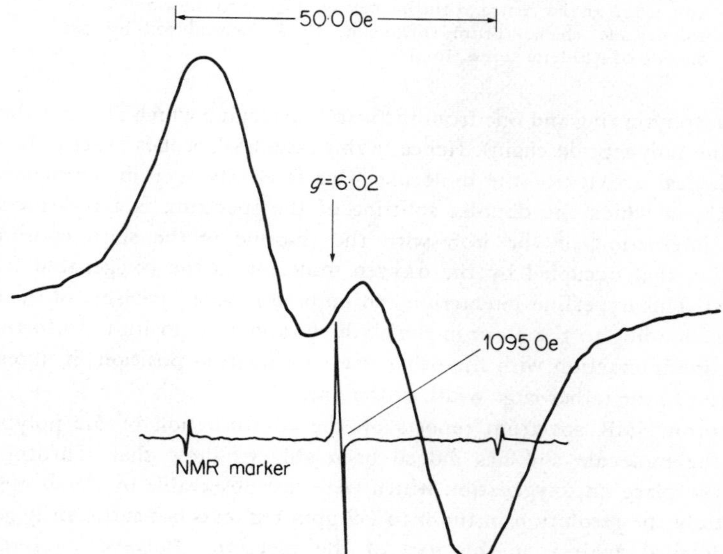

Figure 1.17 Fe^{3+} ESR spectrum of an oriented single crystal of myoglobin fluoride. (From Kotani and Morimoto, 1967. Reproduced by permission of Pergamon Press, Ltd)

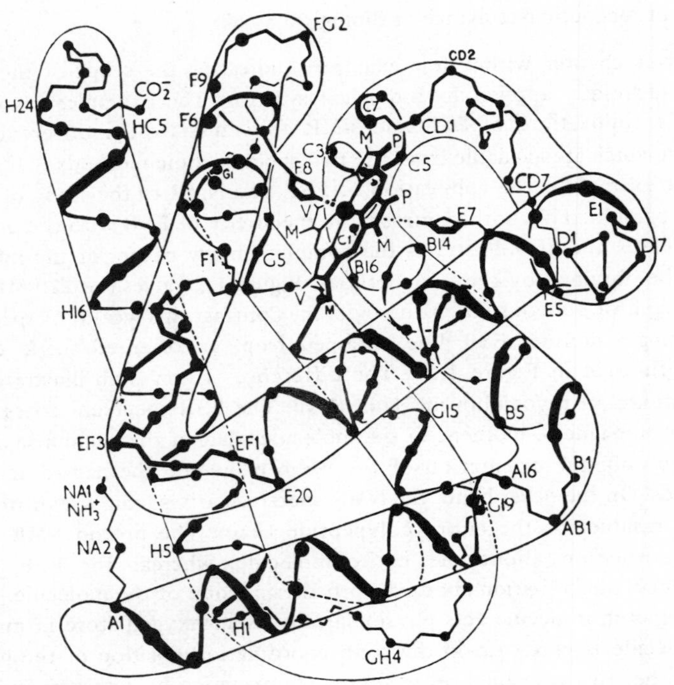

Figure 1.18 Myoglobin molecule, indicating the position of the iron atom, at the centre of the haem ring, relative to the whole of the polypeptide chain. (From Dickerson, 1964. Reproduced by permission of Academic Press, Inc.)

from the porphyrin ring and one from the histidine residue which attaches the haem group to the polypeptide chain). Hence in this case, ESR probes exactly the centre of physiological activity of the molecule. This is clearly seen in the spectrum of Figure 1.17, in which the doublet splitting of the spectrum is a measure of the hyperfine interaction of the iron with the fluorine in the sixth coordination position (i.e. that occupied by the oxygen molecule in the oxygenated form of myoglobin). This hyperfine interaction can be used to give a measure of the degree of covalent bonding to the atom in the sixth coordination position. Unfortunately the hyperfine interaction with the other five coordination positions is unresolved, but gives rise to the rather large width of the lines.

The proton NMR spectrum reports on the conformation of the polypeptide chain of the molecule and has indeed been able to show that conformational changes take place on oxygenation which were not observable by X-ray methods. Unfortunately the resolution in the 0 to −9 ppm region is not sufficiently good to make a detailed analysis in this part of the spectrum. However, well-resolved resonances are observed in the outer regions of the spectrum from −9 to −30 ppm and 0 to +10 ppm. Such resonances are characteristic of a system in which both ESR and NMR are observable; for example, the proton NMR spectra of ribonuclease, which contains no magnetic electrons, has resonances only in the central region 0 to −9 ppm as shown in Figure 1.5. (Such a system with its wealth of NMR absorptions has no ESR spectrum at all.) The myoglobin proton resonances in the outer regions are shifted out from the central region by paramagnetic interactions with the haem iron electron spin. One can thus immediately say that they arise from amino acid residues which lie in close proximity to the haem group. The specificity of ESR is passed on to NMR enabling one to obtain precise information not just about the haem group itself but also about the regions of the polypeptide chain which approach close to it in the tertiary structure of the protein. This is a clear example of the complementary nature of the ESR and NMR methods.

The second pair of examples contrasts different applications of the two methods. One of the major advantages ESR has over other methods of spectroscopy is its ability to resolve differently orientated centres. This arises from the anisotropy of the spectrum with respect to the orientation of the magnetic field. Experiments which determine the angular variation of the ESR spectrum with respect to the orientation of the magnetic field relative to single crystal axes can be used to determine the symmetry of the site in which the paramagnetic species is situated. The angular variation of the spectrum in Figure 1.17 has been used, for instance, to show that the haem iron of myoglobin is in a site of axial symmetry, and to determine the orientation of the haem planes with respect to the crystal axes. The anisotropy of the ESR spectrum can also be utilized in dynamic studies. This method has, to date, been most frequently used with spin labelled proteins or membrane structures. If the spin-labelled molecule is rotating rapidly and randomly in its environment, then all anisotropy is averaged out and a sharp (three-line) spectrum is obtained. If the molecule is rotating more slowly, then the spectra are increasingly broadened corresponding to incomplete averaging of the anisotropy, until the molecules are stationary and there is no averaging at all. Protein molecules rotate so slowly in aqueous solution that they can be considered to be essentially stationary on an ESR time scale; the spin label spectrum then reflects the motional freedom of the spin label with respect to the protein. This motional mobility is determined by the method of attachment and the protein conformation in the region of attachment. The method is illustrated in Figure 1.19. The spectrum of the spin–labelled stearic acid in chloroform is characteristic of a rapidly, isotropically tumbling molecule, whereas that of the stearic acid bound to aqueous bovine serum albumen is characteristic of a strongly bound, almost completely immobilized molecule. This is in line with the function of bovine serum albumen as a fatty acid transporting protein.

Though in principle the application would be just the same, spectral anisotropy is not usually exploited in NMR. This is because the resulting greater intricacy of the spectrum results in so many spectral overlaps that nothing at all is resolved in the case of proton NMR spectra. Instead solutions are used in which the spectral anisotropy is averaged out ('isotropic averaging'), giving rise to a less complicated spectrum. Structural information is then available from isotropic splittings as explained previously.

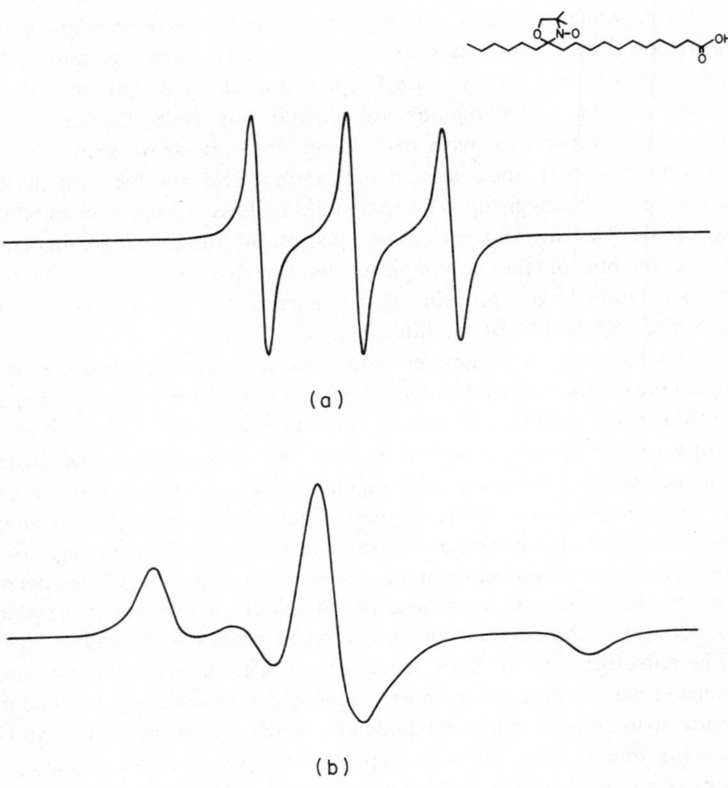

Figure 1.19 ESR spectrum of a spin-labelled stearic acid molecule: (a) dissolved in chloroform; (b) bound to bovine serum albumen in aqueous solution

Since practically complete motional averaging of spectral anisotropy is required for good resolution in NMR, partial motional averaging is thus (unlike ESR) little used for obtaining dynamic information; relaxation measurements are used instead. Relaxation time measurement is relatively little developed in ESR, on the other hand, because ESR relaxation times are on the whole much faster and thus practically more difficult to determine. Nuclear relaxation times are determined by the strength and nature of the interaction of the nucleus with its environment. Thus they are capable of giving two types of dynamic information either about molecular motion, if the relaxation time is limited by the rate of motion, or about chemical equilibria, if the relaxation time is limited by the rate of chemical exchange. In chemical equilibria involving the binding of paramagnetic ions, distances of approach may also be derived. An example of the latter is given by the ^{31}P NMR of manganese-bound ATP illustrated in Figure 1.20. Divalent metal ions are essential in the enzymatic reactions involving this high-energy adenine nucleotide, e.g. as the metal-complex substrate in the kinase hydrolysis of ATP.

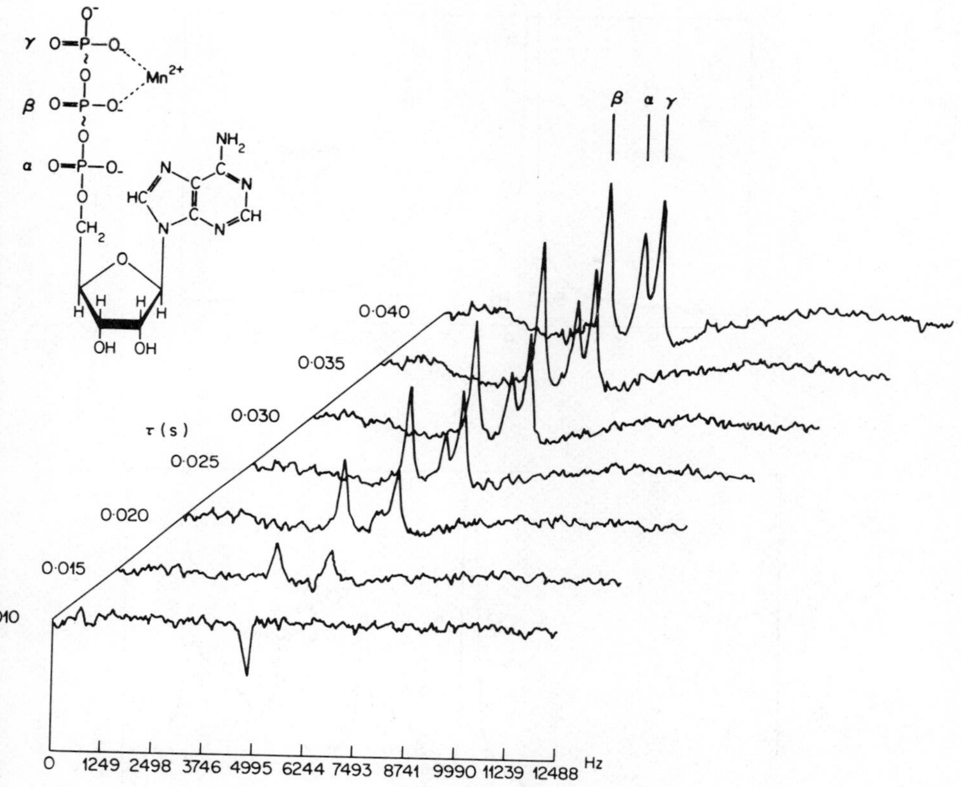

Figure 1.20 ^{31}P NMR spectrum of ATP. Perspective of the $180°-\tau-90°$ RF pulse sequence used in determining the spin–lattice relaxation time, T_1. (Courtesy of Dr F. F. Brown)

The spectra of Figure 1.20 represent the measurement of T_1, the spin–lattice relaxation time, for the three phosphorus nuclei of ATP. A pulse Fourier-transform method is used in which the nuclear moment is inverted, but for the time being (see later Chapters 2 and 5) the diagram may be considered to represent the state of recovery of the NMR signal at various times, τ, after complete saturation. The γ and β resonances recover at the same rate (i.e. have the same T_1) which is considerably faster than the rate for the α-resonance. This shows that the Mn^{2+} ion binds more closely to the β- and γ-phosphates causing more efficient relaxation (shorter T_1), in fact distances of closest approach of the Mn^{2+} ion to the phosphorus nuclei can be calculated from the measured values of T_1. Proton NMR data on the adenine ring have shown that the Mn^{2+} ion also binds to the N_7 position of the five-membered ring, whereas other divalent metal ions are only bound to the pyrophosphate groups. This may explain the metal-ion specificity in certain enzymatic hydrolysis and phosphorylation reactions of ATP.

As a final example we consider the application of magnetic resonance spectroscopy to whole biological tissues. The obvious problem with nuclear

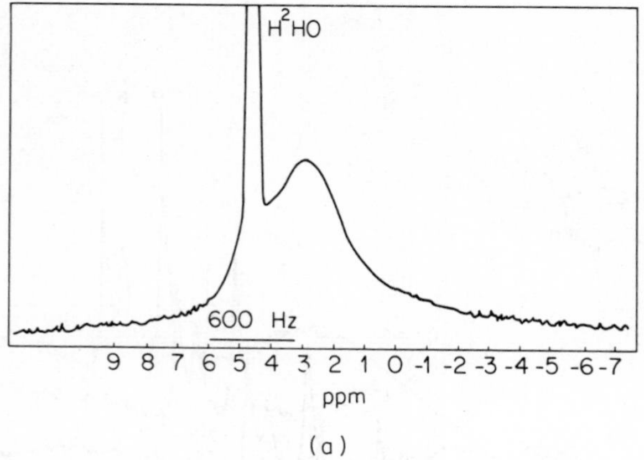

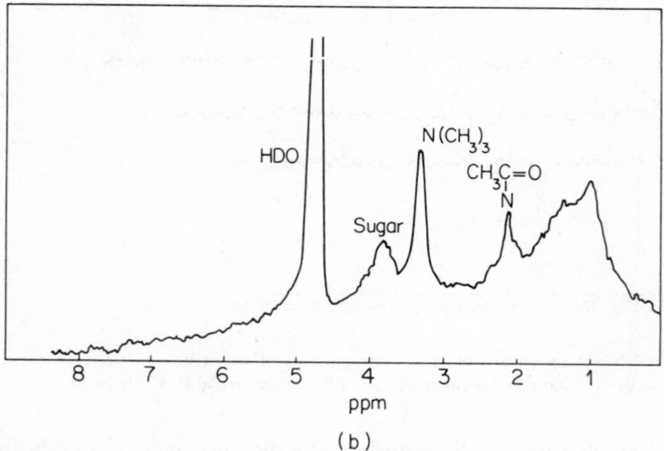

Figure 1.21 60 MHz proton NMR spectrum of (a) whole, and (b) sonicated erythrocyte membranes. (From Chapman and Kamat, 1968a,b. Reproduced by permission of ASP Biological and Medical Press)

magnetic resonance of whole tissues is one of resolution. Because of the vast numbers of nuclei with a very large range of environments and mutual interactions, multiple overlapping of spectral lines is inevitable. Added to this is the problem of line broadening due to immobilization of the molecular groupings in the tissue. The situation is illustrated in Figure 1.21, by the 60 MHz proton NMR spectrum of intact erythrocyte membrane, one of the few tissues to have been studied by high-resolution proton NMR. All the proton resonances merge into one broad, structureless line. A considerable improvement in resolution is obtained on sonicating the membrane which homogenizes the tissue suspension and increases the mobility of certain molecular groups. Peaks are observed in the sonicated membrane spectrum characteristic of the sugar residues of the glycoprotein coat, of the $N^+(CH_3)_3$ protons in the choline headgroup of the membrane phospholipids, and of the *N*-acetyl groups of sugars and protein. The broad absorption around 8.5 ppm arises, at least in part, from the immobilized hydrocarbon chains of the phospholipids. It is clear that improved resolution is required if information is to be obtained from whole tissues. This can be achieved by going to higher frequencies

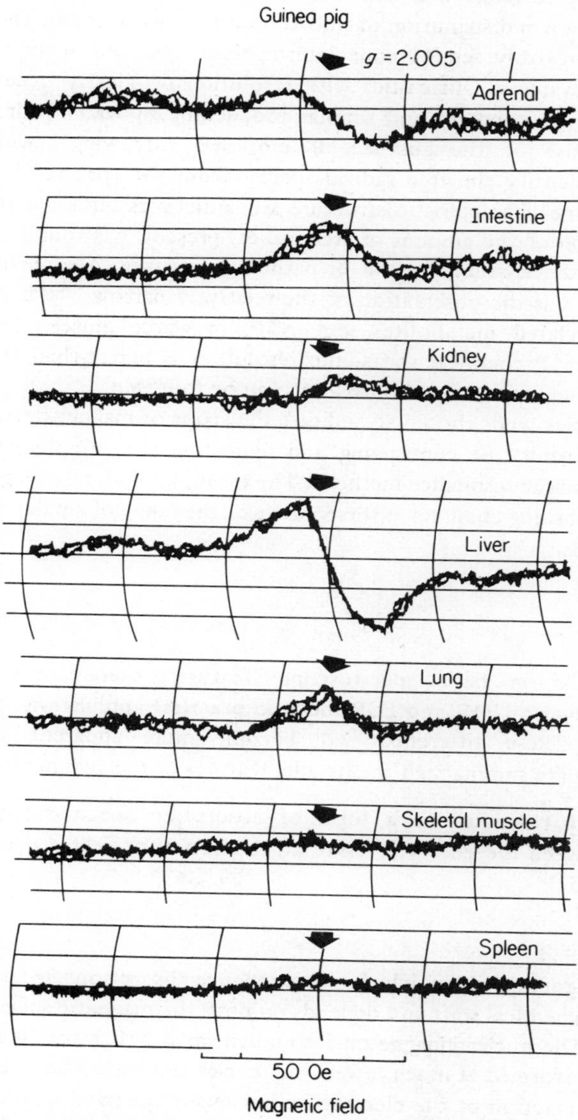

Figure 1.22 ESR spectra of surviving tissue from various guinea pig organs. (From Commoner and Ternberg, 1961)

and indeed it is possible to resolve some of the proton resonances from intact erythrocyte membrane at 220 MHz.

The problems involved in ESR of whole tissues are less acute, since the numbers of paramagnetic species are much smaller. The observation of any ESR spectrum at all is a significant result. Figure 1.22 gives the ESR spectra of surviving tissue from various guinea pig organs. The spectra arise from free radicals and their relative intensities mostly correlate well with the metabolic activities of the corresponding organs and the known distribution of mitochondria between them. The free radicals are thus most probably semiquinone intermediates involved in the mitochondrial redox enzyme systems. Difficulties with resolution do clearly occur, because of distributions of environment and dipolar broadening by water protons (which is important because of the absence of motional narrowing), which makes it impossible to identify the free radical species from the spectra alone. However, spectra with some characteristic structure are sometimes obtained and this, along with quantitation of the amount of free radical present, has found useful medical applications in the characterization of pathological tissue. A somewhat analogous situation in NMR is the observation of the relatively narrow ^{31}P NMR resonances from phosphorylated metabolites, e.g. ATP, in whole muscle. Because of the relatively large ^{31}P chemical shifts, the resolution is better than in ESR and the time course of the various metabolite levels can be followed.

These examples were chosen to indicate the scope of magnetic resonance and to take the opportunity of contrasting and indicating the complementarity of the electron and nuclear resonance methods. The examples will, of course, be discussed further in the ensuing chapters in the context of the range of similar applications of the two methods.

1.9 Summary

Although similar in basic spectroscopic features, there are very important distinctions between NMR and ESR; both in practical applications and in spectral interpretation. These differences will become more apparent in the ensuing chapters; below are summarized the parallel features of the two methods.

(1) Magnetic resonance is a form of absorption spectroscopy arising from transitions between the energy levels of an electron or nuclear magnetic moment in a magnetic field

$$h\nu = g\beta H$$

(2) The magnetic field at which the resonance absorptions occur is specified by the *g*-value or chemical shift and depends on both the magnetic species itself and its environment. The nuclear magneton is so much smaller than the electron magneton that NMR is performed at much lower frequencies and higher fields than ESR.

(3) The interaction of the electron or nucleus in question with the other nuclei in the molecule causes hyperfine splittings of ESR lines and spin–spin splittings of NMR lines. The splitting patterns are characteristic of the number of nuclei

involved and the magnitude of the splitting gives covalent bonding parameters in ESR or bond angles in NMR.

(4) Spin–lattice relaxation causes line broadening and disappearance of the resonance if the relaxation time is too short, or saturation at high power if it is too long.

(5) Spin–spin relaxation normally determines the linewidth in liquids when the lineshape is Lorentzian. In solids linewidths are usually much larger and lineshapes Gaussian.

References

Beinert, H. (1966). In *The Biochemistry of Copper*, Peisach, J., Aisen, P., and Blumberg, W. E. (Eds.), Academic Press, New York.

Chapman, D., and Kamat, V. B. (1968a). *Biochim. Biophys. Acta,* **163**, 411.

Chapman, D., and Kamat, V. B. (1968b). In *Regulatory Functions of Biological Membranes*, Järnefelt, J. (Ed.), B.B.A. Library Vol. 11, Elsevier, Amsterdam.

Commoner, B., and Ternberg, J. L. (1961). *Proc. Natl. Acad. Sci. U.S.A.*, **47**, 1374.

Dickerson, R. E. (1964). In *The Proteins*, Vol. II, Ch. 11, Neurath, H. (Ed.), Academic Press, New York.

Ferguson, R. C., and Phillips, W. D. (1967). *Science*, **157**, 257.

Kotani, M., and Morimoto, H. (1967). In *Magnetic Resonance in Biological Systems*, Ehrenberg, A., Malström, B. G., and Vänngard, T. (Eds.), Pergamon Press, Oxford.

Nakamura, T. (1961). In *Free Radicals in Biological Systems*, Blois, M. S., Brown, H. W., Lemmon, R. M., Lindblom, R. O., and Weissbluth, M. (Eds.), Academic Press, New York.

Wüthrich, K., Shulman, R. G., Yamane, T., Wyluda, B., Hugli, T. E., and Gurd, F.R.N., (1970). *J. Biol. Chem.*, **245**, 1947.

Chapter 2
The NMR Spectrum

2.1 Introduction

Features of the spectrum

Like all the other spectral techniques, nuclear magnetic resonance finds its main usefulness in making available details of structures and phenomena at a molecular level. A 'normal' NMR spectrum is characterized by several parameters; the positions, widths, intensities and multiplicities of its lines are the main ones. Each of these parameters can give information on a different aspect of molecular structure and motion, so that a single spectrum can sometimes give all the information required to solve the structure of a small molecule. In addition, special techniques, including the use of variable temperatures, pulse methods and spin decoupling, can add further data to make NMR an extremely powerful tool in the investigation of molecules. We shall begin with a simple consideration of the main features of an NMR spectrum, and then continue with an explanation of the physical phenomena underlying them.

Figure 2.1 (a) shows a proton resonance spectrum, at fairly low resolution, of the amino acid valine, an important constituent of many proteins. As can be seen, it consists of a number of resonance lines of different areas spread out along a frequency scale. Each of these lines represents the protons which are the nuclei of a particular group of hydrogen atoms within the molecule; the integrated area under the line is proportional to the number of protons in the group (so that, for example, the area of the line representing the $-(CH_3)_2$ grouping is six times that of the $-CH$) and the position of the line on the scale is characteristic of the particular molecular environment in which the group of protons finds itself. Thus this spectrum tells us: (a) how many different groups of protons are present, (b) the relative numbers of protons in each group and (c) something about the molecular environment in which these groups are found.

Figure 2.1 (b) shows the same spectrum, but at an improved resolution. A new feature now appears: some of the lines are split into multiplets. This phenomenon is caused by the magnetic interactions between a group of protons and its neighbouring groups; in general, if the neighbouring group contains n hydrogen nuclei, the line under consideration is split into $(n + 1)$ components. The line due to a proton on a carbon atom adjacent to a $-CH_3$ group will thus be split into four

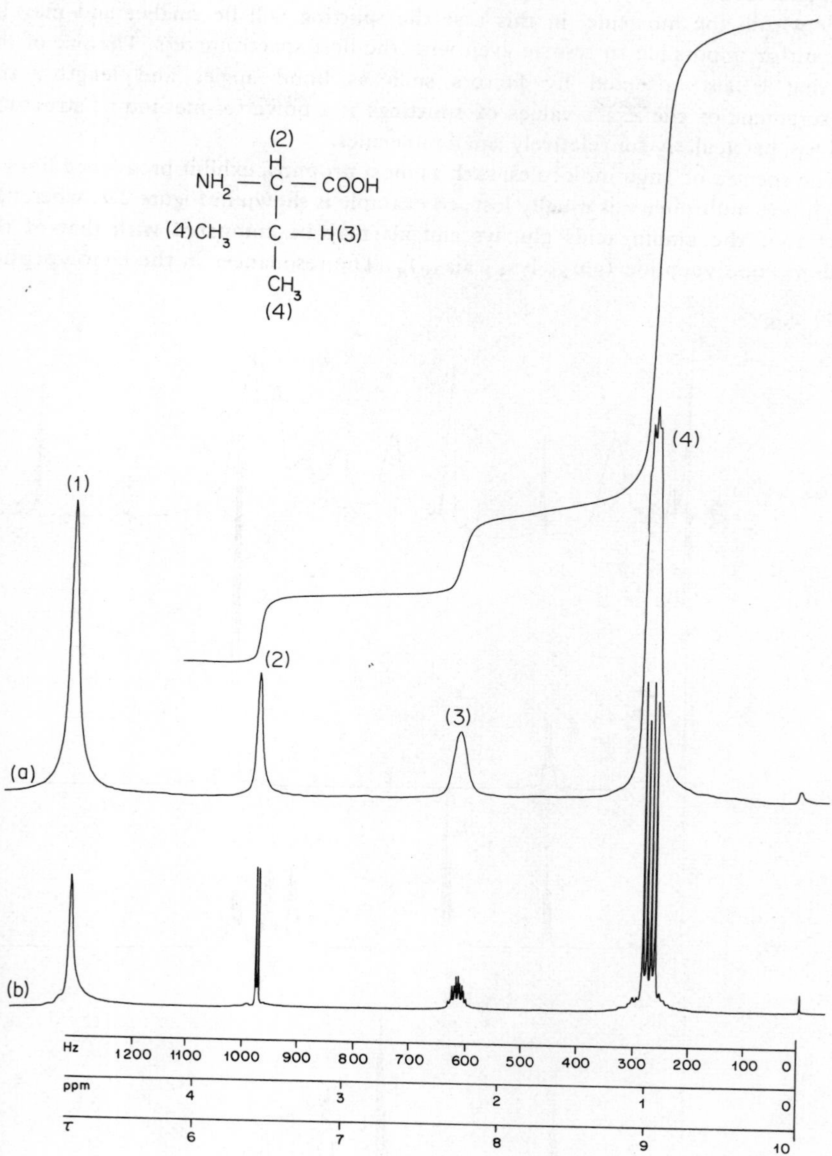

Figure 2.1 Proton magnetic resonance spectrum of valine (a) at low resolution and (b) at higher resolution. The numbers by each resonance peak correspond to the numbers on the molecular formula. Peak (1) respresents residual protons in the deuterium oxide (D_2O) solvent. Resonances from the $-COOH$ and $-NH_2$ groups are not visible as these groups have become deuterated

components. Splittings may also be caused by hydrogen nuclei at greater distances away within the molecule; in this case the splitting will be smaller and may be difficult or impossible to resolve even with the best spectrometers. The size of the splitting is also affected by factors such as bond angles and lengths, and measurement of the exact values of splittings is a powerful method of structural analysis, particularly for relatively small molecules.

The spectra of large molecules, such as most proteins, exhibit broadened lines in which line multiplicity is usually lost; an example is shown in Figure 2.2, where the spectra of the amino acids glu, lys and ala may be compared with that of the random copolypeptide $(glu_{28}\ lys_{42}\ ala_{30})_n$. The resonances in the copolypeptide

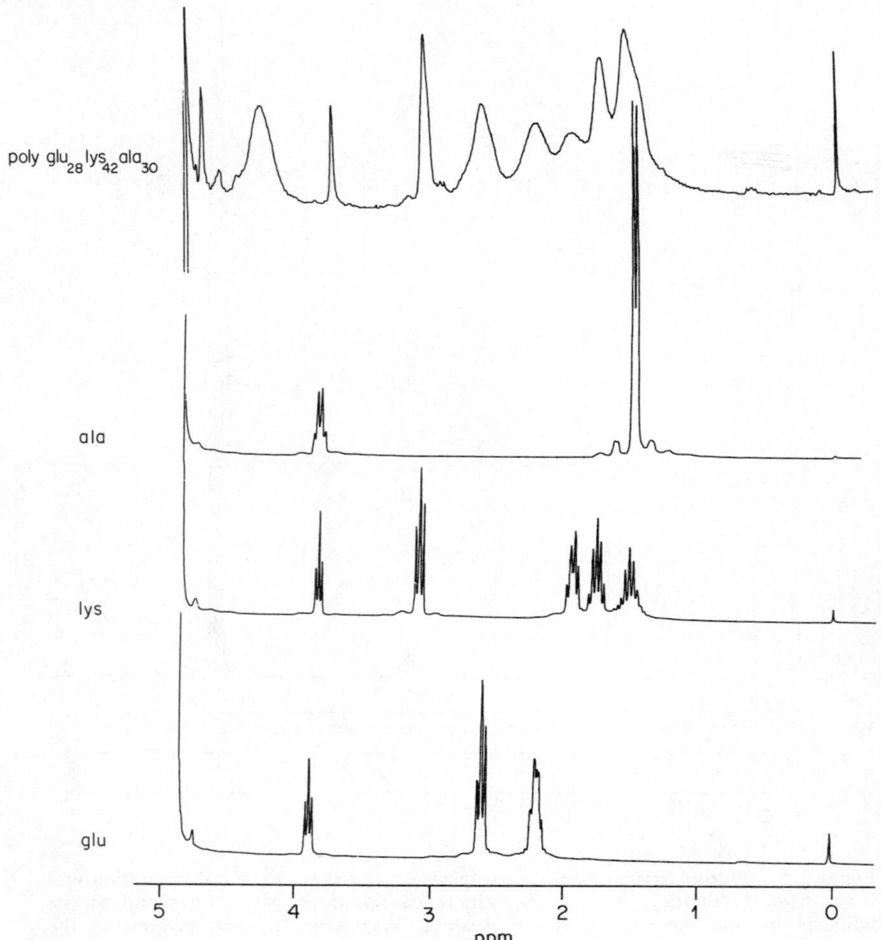

Figure 2.2 Proton spectra at 270 MHz of glutamic acid, lysine, alanine and the random copolypeptide $(glu_{28}\,lys_{42}\,ala_{30})_n$ all in D_2O

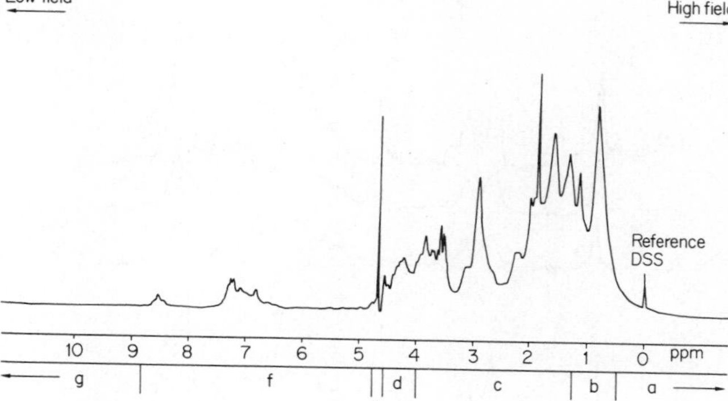

Figure 2.3 A 'typical' protein proton spectrum. The 270 MHz NMR spectrum of denatured bull-sperm ribonuclease, showing the main regions of the spectrum. (a) Ring-current shifted resonances, or resonances shifted by paramagnetic effects. (b) Methyl (CH_3) group resonances. (c) Methylene (CH_2) group resonances. As a general rule, the nearer the methylene group is to an electronegative (e.g. oxygen, nitrogen, sulphur) atom, the lower the field at which the resonance occurs. (d) α-CH resonances. (e) Residual solvent water peak. The water resonance in this spectrum has been reduced to about one-tenth of its normal size by a gated decoupling method (see Chapter 5). (f) Aromatic group resonances (tyrosine, histidine, phenylalanine and trytophan). NH resonances also occur in this region but here have been fully deuterated by exchange with the solvent and so do not appear. (g) Region where resonances highly perturbed by a powerful ring-current or paramagnetic effect may appear. (Spectrum by courtesy of Dr L. Paolillo)

are clearly identifiable by their chemical shift, but the splittings are completely masked by the line broadening. For this reason, splittings are usually only of use for proteins below a total of about 20 amino acids, although if splittings *can* be resolved for larger molecules they are of course very useful.

In fact, the linewidth of a large-molecule spectrum may itself be a useful probe of structure. In general, linewidths increase with the size and rigidity of the molecule, so that transitions from a denatured to a rigid native structure or association of several molecules into an aggregate cause increases in the linewidths of the resonances from the part of the molecule involved. The spectra of Figure 2.4 are those of histone fraction H4 (a) in D_2O and then (b,c) in solutions containing increasing amounts of sodium chloride. It can clearly be seen that as the salt concentration increases certain peaks of the spectrum fall in intensity relative to the others; a careful analysis of the changes can lead to the conclusion that so many lysines, so many arginines etc., appear to be involved in a rigid structure, as their peaks effectively disappear. From a knowledge of the sequence of amino acids in the H4 molecule it is then possible to locate the section of the molecule which is taking part in the interaction, in this case the section from residues 33–102 of the 102–residue molecule. The assignment of the broadening to this part of the

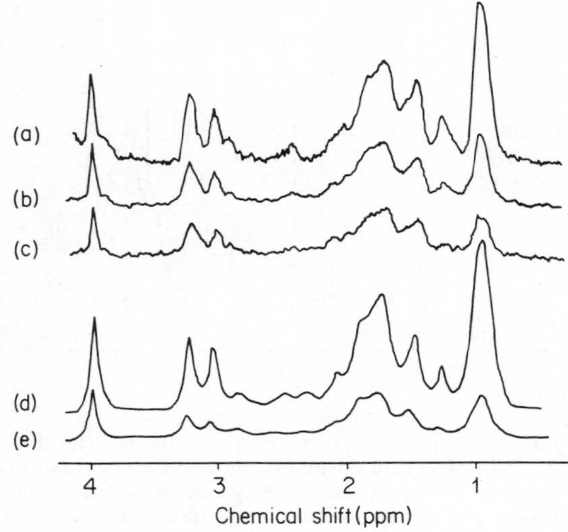

Figure 2.4 Observed 220 MHz upfield spectra of histone H4 in (a) ^2H_2O, (b) 0.1 M NaCl/^2H_2O and (c) 0.2 M NaCl/^2H_2O; simulated spectra of (d) the random-coil form of H4 and (e) that obtained by broadening resonances from segment 33 to 102. (From Bradbury and Rattle, 1972. Reproduced by permission of the Federation of European Biochemical Societies)

molecule was assisted by the simulated spectra of Figure 2.4 (d) and(e) which were simply drawn from a knowledge of the amino acid composition and sequence of the molecule, using a computer to speed the process.

Overlapping information and spectrometer frequency

A second major obstacle to the analysis of the structure of large molecules by NMR is that any spectrum with a large number of peaks suffers from peak overlap. This is already becoming apparent in Figure 2.2, where, even with only three different amino acids in the polypeptide chain, the peaks at about 1.5 ppm due to the alanine CH_3 and lysine α–CH_2 are not resolved. Peak overlap of this kind is perhaps the greatest difficulty in the NMR of biomolecules and especially in proton magnetic resonance: it must often be sidestepped by concentrating on peaks which lie away from the main spectrum, by using a different nucleus such as ^{13}C where the problem is less marked because of greater inherent peak separations or by using various probe techniques to be detailed later. Ultimately, the problem can only be overcome by increasing the operating frequency of the spectrometer, since peak separation is proportional to this frequency. Figure 2.5 shows spectra of the same molecule, a lysine rich histone, at 60 MHz and 270 MHz. It is clear that the 4½-fold increase in frequency (coupled with a tenfold increase in the cost of the spectrometer!) vastly increases the amount of information available.

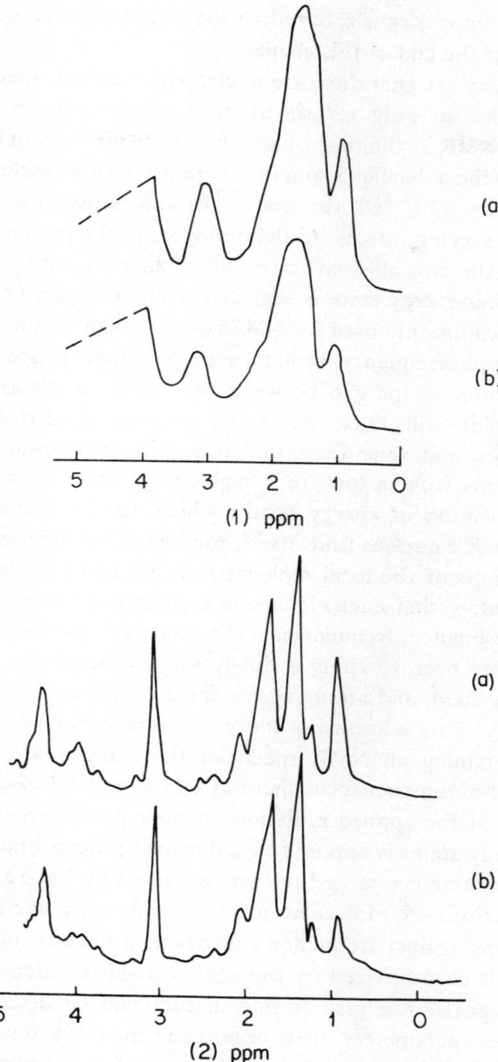

Figure 2.5 Histone fraction H1 spectra in (a) D_2O and (b) D_2O/1 M NaCl solution. Spectra obtained at frequencies of (1) 60 MHz and (2) 270 MHz

Origins of the spectrum

Before going on to a more detailed consideration of the various parameters to be obtained from NMR, how they arise and how they may be used by the researcher, it may be of use here to summarize briefly the main ideas behind the NMR method as described in Chapter 1. For a more detailed explanation of the physical mechanism of NMR, the reader is referred to the excellent reference texts given in the short reading list at the end of this chapter.

Briefly, then, we may say that there are nuclei which exhibit space quantization, that is they may take up only certain allowed orientations in space. For the purposes of practical NMR at the time of writing, those nuclei which have only two allowed orientations (those having a spin of ½) are used; these include the nuclei of hydrogen (^{1}H), carbon–13 (^{13}C), fluorine (^{19}F) and phosphorus (^{31}P), together with many others of varying interest to the biologist. In the presence of a magnetic field, the energies of the two allowed states differ slightly, and in consequence the population of the lower-energy state is slightly (by about 1 part in 10^7 for protons at the field strengths commonly used for NMR) greater than that of the upper state. The application of radiofrequency radiation of the appropriate frequency (this being a direct function of the gap between the energy levels and hence of the applied magnetic field) will cause nuclei to undergo transitions between the available energy states, and since the population difference ensures that there are rather more transitions from a low- to a high-energy state than in the opposite direction, a net absorption of energy results which may be detected. The precise magnetic field in which a nucleus finds itself, and hence the precise frequency of its resonance, are functions of the local molecular environment at the nucleus as well as of the applied field, so that nuclei in chemical groups of different kinds will have slightly different resonance frequencies. The practical method of obtaining a spectrum has therefore been to apply a slowly varying frequency of radiation to a sample in a magnetic field, and arranging for the absorption maxima to be plotted against the frequency. This is known as the 'continuous-wave' method, and was the only method of obtaining an NMR spectrum for many years. It is now being superseded by the Fourier-transform method which will be described later. The disturbing influence of the applied radiation on the equilibrium of the populations of the different energy states is opposed by a dynamic process known as relaxation, in which the original state is regained at a rate governed by 'relaxation times' which are themselves functions of molecular motions and other factors. The plot of resonance absorptions against frequency constitutes a nuclear magnetic resonance spectrum, and this is characterized by the chemical shifts, intensities, multiplicity and width of the signals. The rest of this chapter will be devoted to a detailed consideration of these parameters, their origins and the ways in which they may be applied. Chapter 4 contains examples of the use of the various parameters as applied to the investigation of biological molecules.

2.2 The Chemical Shift

Units and measurements

As has just been stated, the resonance frequency of a given nucleus is directly proportional to the magnetic field which it experiences. In all NMR experiments, the major contribution to this field comes from the magnet in which the sample is placed (the 'applied field' H_0), but this may be modified by many factors arising from the nature of the molecule in which the nucleus is located. The resultant field at a particular nucleus may be termed the local field, or H_{loc}, and the alteration in resonance frequency consequent upon this modification of the applied field is called the 'chemical shift'. The modification is never very large, at least in the high-resolution spectra which are the subject of this discussion; variations in the chemical shift for protons of thirty parts per million (ppm) of applied field or frequency would be considered very large. Chemical shifts for other nuclei are frequently much larger; for example, a ^{13}C spectrum is found spread over a range of 200 ppm or more.

It is technically possible to measure the exact frequency for a given field corresponding to each resonance in a spectrum; however, this would be very difficult and is normally unnecessary, since a resonance frequency may be measured relative to that of a reference compound. This may be mixed directly with the sample (internal referencing), or, when there is a danger of chemical interaction with the sample or it is particularly important that the sample remains unadulterated, may be placed in a separate container within the sample tube (external referencing). The reference compound should ideally be a compound which gives a single sharp resonance, well clear of the region where the majority of peaks are to be found. In proton and ^{13}C resonance spectroscopy, frequent use is made of one of a family of compounds which have several CH_3 groups bound to a silicon atom, the simplest of which is tetramethyl silane, usually abbreviated to TMS. The protons and ^{13}C nuclei of this compound are very highly shielded from H_0, so that their resonances appear at the extreme right-hand (high-field) end of a normal spectrum, clear of most other resonances. A water-soluble derivative of TMS is also commonly used; its name (2,2 dimethylsilapentane 5-sulphonic acid) is commonly abbreviated to DSS.

Having specified the reference compound used in a spectrum, the positions of all the other peaks may be related to it. These positions may be given in frequency units, but a major disadvantage of this method is that, just as absolute resonance frequencies vary with H_0, so do relative frequencies. Thus a chemical shift value given in Hz is meaningless unless the main measuring frequency is also stated. A peak appearing 250 Hz away from a reference peak when run on a 100 MHz spectrometer would be 500 Hz away on a 200 MHz spectrum. To overcome this difficulty, which makes it awkward to compare, say, a 220 MHz spectrum with a 270 MHz one, the chemical shifts are usually given in parts per million (ppm)

$$\text{Chemical shift (ppm)} = \frac{\text{sample frequency} - \text{reference frequency}}{\text{reference frequency}} \times 10^6$$

A resonance appearing 250 Hz from a reference in a 100 MHz spectrum would thus be 2.5 ppm away; the same resonance in a 220 MHz spectrum would be 550 Hz from the reference, but this would still be 2.5 ppm.

The TMS family of references give a signal at the upper (conventionally the right-hand) end of the spectrum. Peaks downfield (to the left) of this are normally assigned positive shift values, and those to the right negative values. An exception to this is found in publications which make use of the 'τ-scale' in which the signal of TMS is assigned a chemical shift value of 10 and counting, in units of 1 ppm, is from left to right. A chemical shift of 2.5 ppm relative to TMS may therefore be written as 7.5τ. Both conventions appear in the literature. For comparison purposes, the scales of Figure 2.1 are written in terms of Hz, ppm and τ; otherwise proton NMR spectra in this book will employ a ppm scale unless taken from a publication which uses τ. Further details of the practical aspects of referencing appear in Chapter 3.

Physical mechanisms underlying chemical shifts

The applied field H_0 may be modified at any nucleus by several mechanisms. In each case the local field at the nucleus, H_{loc}, may be expressed as a function of H_0 and a 'shielding factor', σ, such that $H_{loc} = H_0(1 - \sigma)$. The effects may be roughly divided into intramolecular, intermolecular and paramagnetic effects.

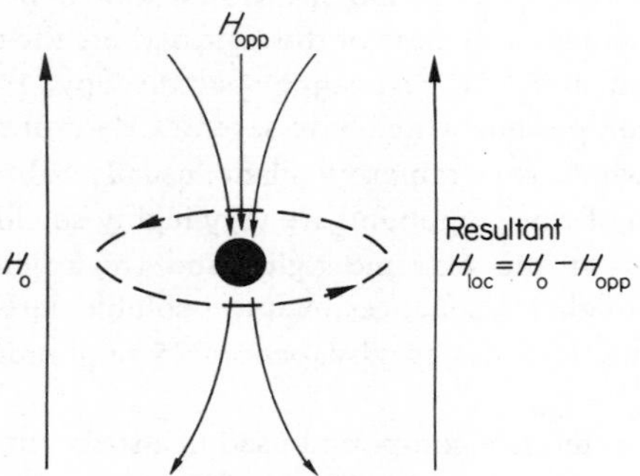

Figure 2.6 Shielding effect on a nucleus due to applied field H_0. ---> represents the electron motion induced by H_0; the net field at the nucleus is $H_{loc} = H_0(1-\sigma)$, where σ is the shielding factor

(a) Intramolecular diamagnetic effect. The nucleus is surrounded by a moving electron cloud which it shares with the nuclei of other atoms to which it is chemically bonded. The application of H_0 modifies the motion of the electrons, in such a way that their new motion produces a field to oppose H_0. H_{loc} is thus smaller than H_0; the nucleus is shielded (Figure 2.6). The effect is proportional to the strength of H_0 and also to the density of the electron cloud around the nucleus. Thus a proton or other nucleus with a dense cloud of electrons round it (e.g. the protons of $-CH_3$ group) is more highly shielded than one with a thin cloud (e.g. the proton of a –C–O–H group) and will thus appear nearer the high-field end of the spectrum. This effect is normally the main contributor to the chemical shifts observed in NMR spectra.

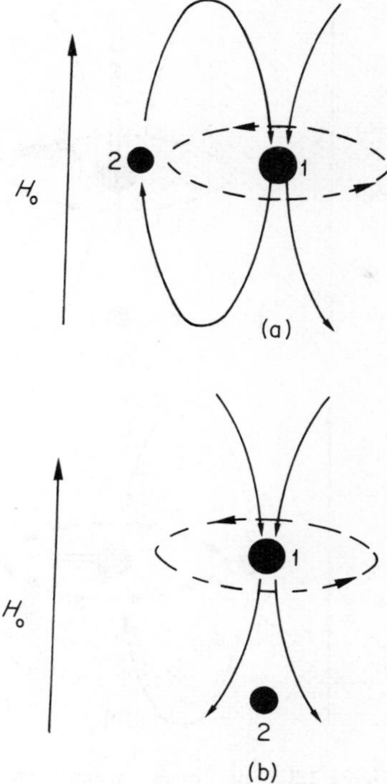

Figure 2.7 Effect of the electron cloud of a neighbouring nucleus. In (a) the electron cloud surrounding nucleus 1 produces a deshielding effect at 2; In (b) the effect is in the opposite direction. Whether the effect cancels to zero over all orientations of the molecule depends on the configuration of the electron cloud round 1

(b) Neighbour diamagnetic effect (Figure 2.7). Just as the electron cloud directly round a given nucleus is caused by H_0 to produce a field opposing H_0, those round neighbouring atoms are similarly affected; the resulting opposing fields may either add to H_0 (Figure 2.7a), or subtract from it (Figure 2.7b) at the nucleus under consideration, according the orientation of the molecule relative to H_0. When taken over all possible orientations of the molecule, the resultant value of σ will depend on the relative strengths of the two effects. In some cases the effect may account for chemical shifts of up to 0.4 ppm for protons.

(c) Neighbour paramagnetic effect (Figure 2.8). In some types of molecular structure, in which the charge distribution about the direction of H_0 is not symmetrical, the application of H_0 may cause an additional effect which does not

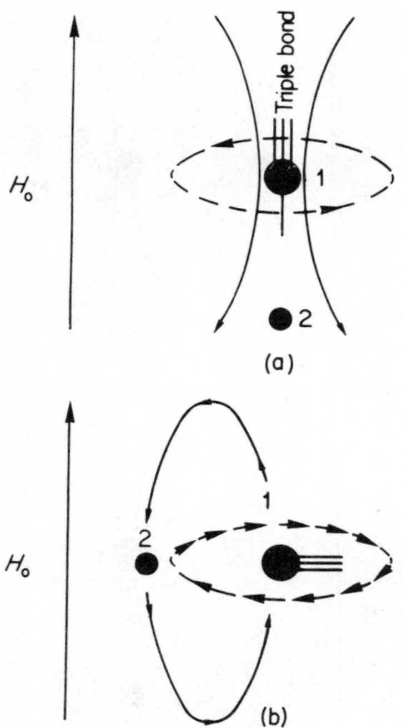

Figure 2.8 In cases where the electron cloud of 1 is highly asymmetric, e.g. the carbons of acetylene, the presence of an applied field H_0 perpendicular to the bond axis may cause a paramagnetic effect, increasing the shielding of 2. The effect is not present in (a) when the bond axis is parallel to the field, so that there is a net shielding of 2 in all orientations of the molecule

tend to cancel over all orientations of the molecule. The effect may be quite marked in the case of carbon atoms, where the hybrid electron orbitals may be modified by H_0 to the extent of causing a change of energy state. The result may be quite a large magnetic field parallel to H_0 at the carbon atom, and a resultant shielding effect at a neighbouring atom. The effect is normally of little importance, but appears in molecules with a more complex bonding structure, e.g. acetylene HC≡CH. In Figure 2.8 the hydrogen atom (2) is deshielded for all orientations of the molecule.

The above three effects are the major contributors to the chemical shift structure of a normal NMR spectrum; they can be considered as always present. It is possible to generalize from them and from data measured from real spectra, and to produce indications of where particular chemical groupings may be expected to fall in a spectrum. Figure 2.9–2.11 and Table 2.1 show the regions of the NMR

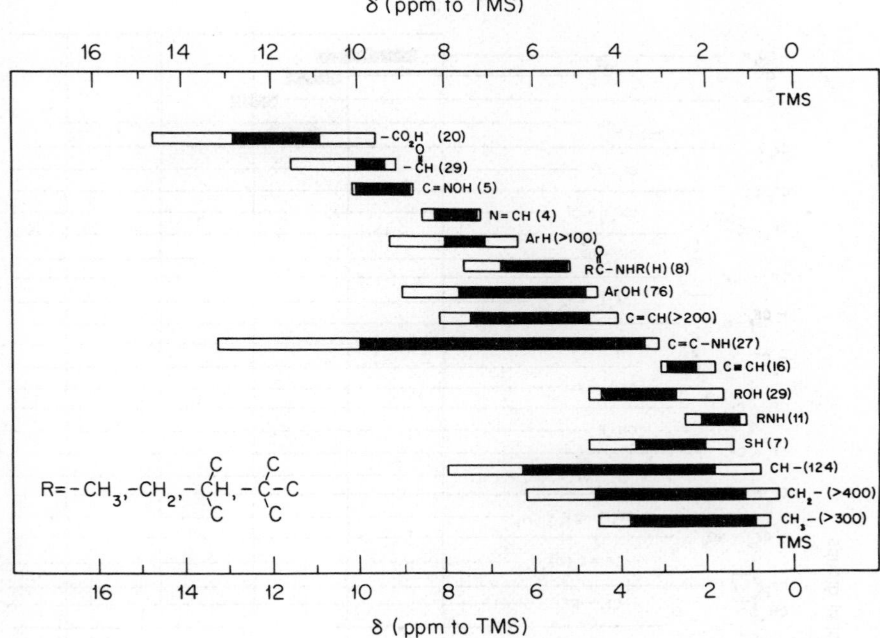

Figure 2.9 Structure correlation chart of proton chemical shifts for main proton groups. Open bar denotes extreme 10% of data

spectrum in which various common groupings involving ^{1}H, ^{13}C, ^{19}F and ^{31}P nuclei may be expected to fall. As a further aid in the interpretation of the proton magnetic resonance spectra of proteins, Table 2.2 gives chemical shift values, relative to the reference DSS, obtained for amino acids incorporated in proteins.

Chemical shift perturbations

(a) Ring-current effects. Just as the application of H_0 to a small system of electrons circulating round a single nucleus causes an opposing field H_{opp}, so its application to the much larger system of circulating electrons found in aromatic ring structures such as the phenolic ring of tyrosine, the rings of phenylalanine and tryptophan, the porphyrin ring of the haem group and others may cause a much larger H_{opp}. This H_{opp} will oppose H_0 within the ring and reinforce it outside, but in the plane of the ring (Figure 2.12). Figure 2.13 shows a haem group; the chemical shift difference between a shielded proton within the ring and a deshielded proton outside it may be as great as 12 ppm. The upfield-shifting effect of ring-current shifts is probably of greatest importance for biological NMR; the CH_3 group at position A of Figure 2.12 will be shielded and will appear at a chemical shift value up to 1 or 2 ppm higher than it would have in the absence of the tyrosine, thus appearing in the otherwise clear region of the

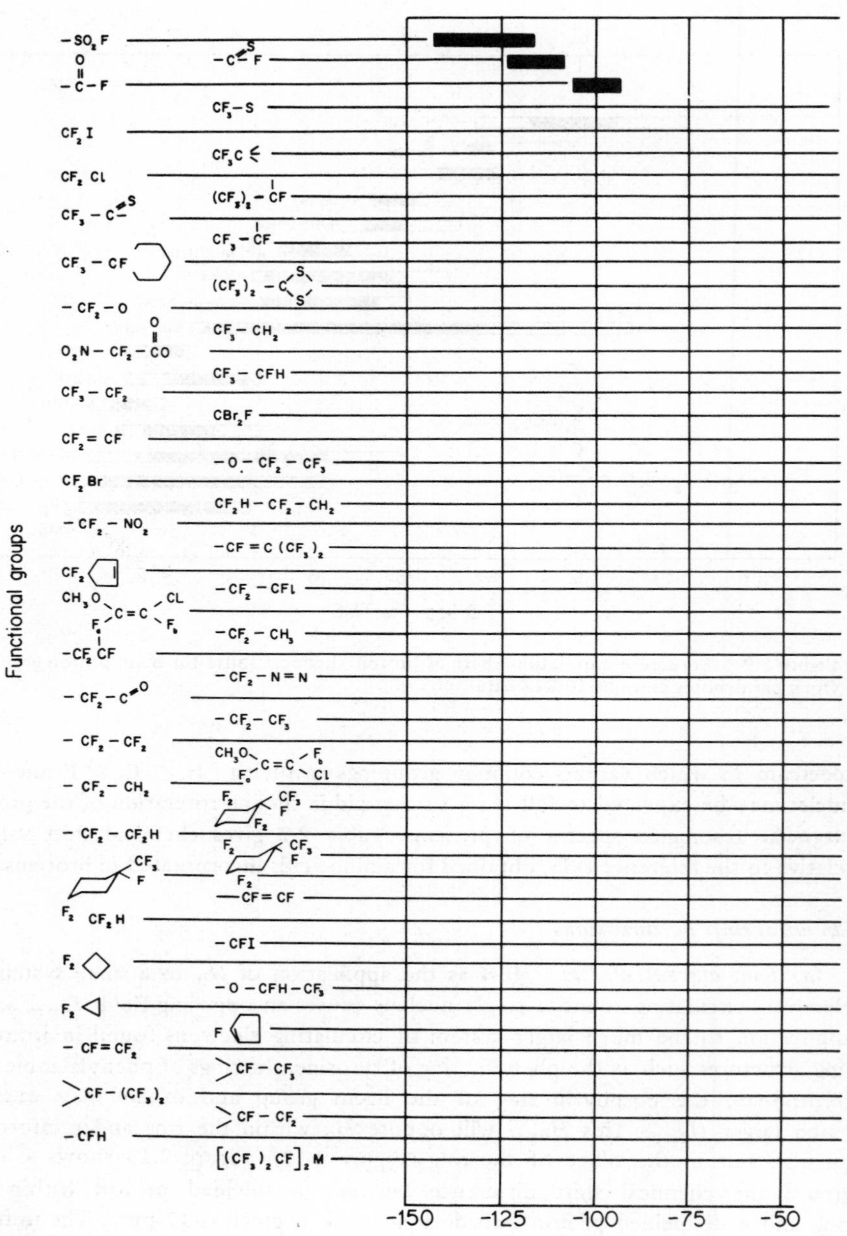

Figure 2.10 [19]F Chemical shift values for various fluorine-containing chemical groups. (Reprinted with permission from Brame, E. G. (1962). *Anal. Chem.*, 34, 591. Copyright by the American Chemical Society)

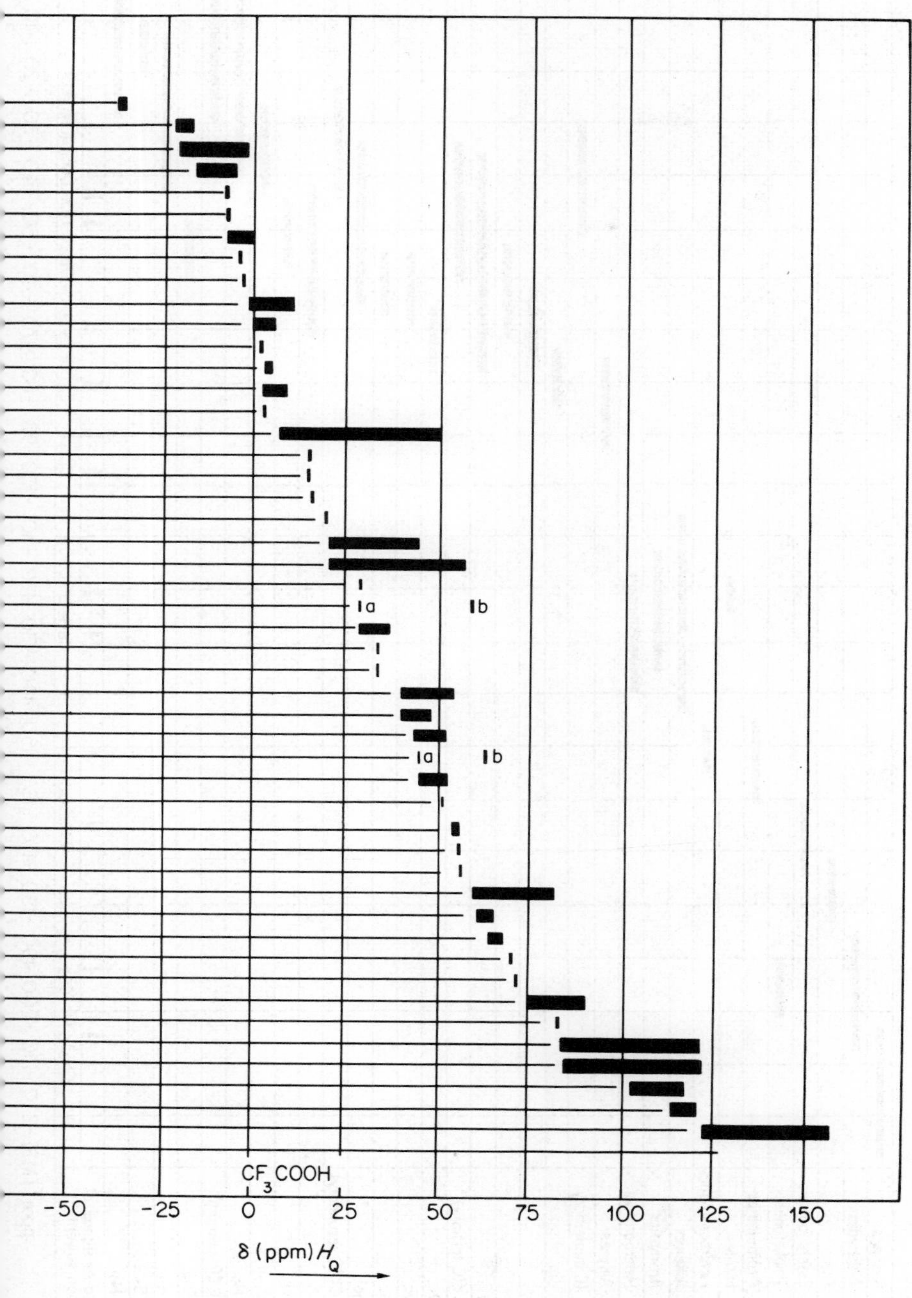
a
b
a
b
CF3COOH
-50
-25
0
25
50
75
100
125
150
δ (ppm) HQ

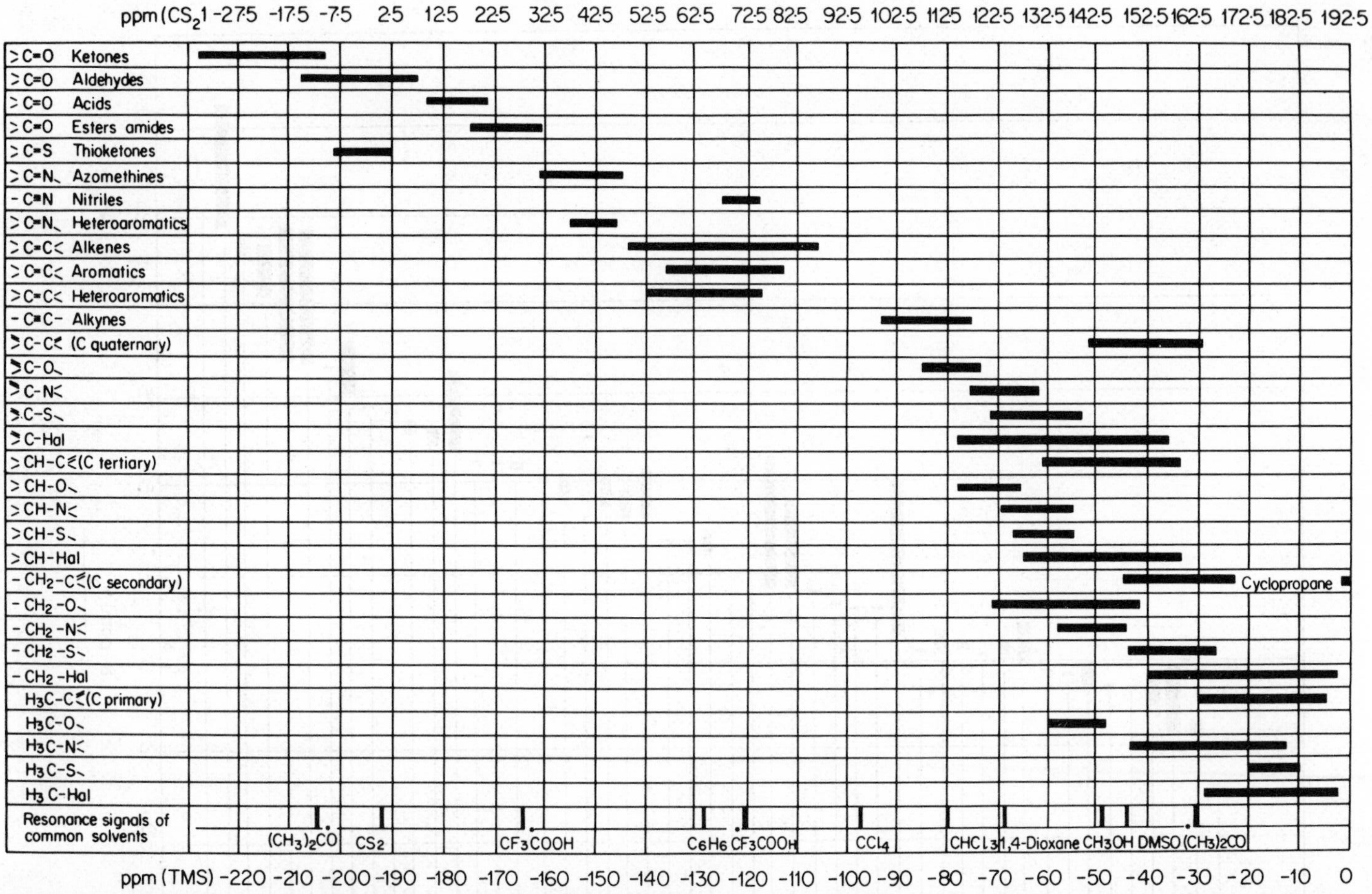

ppm (CS_2) -27·5 -17·5 -7·5 2·5 12·5 22·5 32·5 42·5 52·5 62·5 72·5 82·5 92·5 102·5 112·5 122·5 132·5 142·5 152·5 162·5 172·5 182·5 192·5

>C=O Ketones
>C=O Aldehydes
>C=O Acids
>C=O Esters amides
>C=S Thioketones
>C=N< Azomethines
-C≡N Nitriles
>C=N< Heteroaromatics
>C=C< Alkenes
>C=C< Aromatics
>C=C< Heteroaromatics
-C≡C- Alkynes
>C-C< (C quaternary)
>C-O<
>C-N<
>C-S<
>C-Hal
>CH-C< (C tertiary)
>CH-O<
>CH-N<
>CH-S<
>CH-Hal
$-CH_2-C$< (C secondary) Cyclopropane
$-CH_2-O$<
$-CH_2-N$<
$-CH_2-S$<
$-CH_2-Hal$
H_3C-C< (C primary)
H_3C-O<
H_3C-N<
H_3C-S<
H_3C-Hal
Resonance signals of common solvents: $(CH_3)_2CO$ CS_2 CF_3COOH C_6H_6 CF_3COOH CCl_4 $CHCl_3$ 1,4-Dioxane CH_3OH DMSO $(CH_3)_2CO$

ppm (TMS) -220 -210 -200 -190 -180 -170 -160 -150 -140 -130 -120 -110 -100 -90 -80 -70 -60 -50 -40 -30 -20 -10 0

Table 2.1

Table of phosphorus-31 chemical shift values for various compounds. (Reprinted with permission from Dietrich, M. W., and Keller, R. E. (1964) *Anal. Chem.*, **36**, 258. Copyright by the American Chemical Society.)

Compound type	Specifications	δ	No. of different compounds examined
$R(R'O)_2P$	(a) R, R′ = aliph. higher than CH_3	−183 ± 1	2
	(b) $R = CH_3 \neq R'$	−175 ± 2	7
$R(R'S)_2P$	(a) $R = CH_3$ R′ = aliph. higher than CH_3	−69.4 ± 0.7	2
	(b) $R = CH_2$ R′ = aromatic	−84.5	1
$(RO)_3P$ symmetrical	(a) R = aliph. higher than CH_3	−138 ± 1	10
	(b) $R = CH_3$	−139	1
	(c) R = aromatic	−127 ± 1	2
$(RS)_3P$ symmetrical	R = aliph. higher than CH_3	−117 ± 1	2
$R_3P(O)$ symmetrical	(a) R = aliph. higher than CH_3	−46.0 ± 2.5	2
	(b) R = aromatic	−23.0	1
$R(R')(R''O)P(O)$	(a) R, R′, R″ = aliph. higher than CH_3, R = R′	−54.9 ± 0.2	1
	(b) $R = R' = CH_3$ R″ = aliph. higher than CH_3	−49.5 ± −49.5 ± 0.5	2
	(c) $R = CH_3$, R′, R″ = aliph. higher than CH_3	−53.0 ± 1.0	2
$R(R'O)_2P(O)$	(a) R, R′ = aliph. higher than CH_3	−32.8 ± 1.5	5
	(b) $R = CH_3$, R′ = aliph. higher than CH_3	−28.4 ± 0.9	5
	(c) R = aliph. higher than CH_3, $R' = CH_3$	−35.0	1
$R(R'O)(R''S)P(O)$	(a) R, R′, R″ = aliph. higher than CH_3	−56.5 ± 0.8	2
	(b) $R = CH_3$ R′, R″ = aliph. higher than CH_3	−50.5 ± 1.4	9
$R(R'S)_2P(O)$	$R = CH_3$ R′ = aliph. higher than CH_3	−55.8	1
$(RO)_3P(O)$ symmetrical	(a) R = aliph. higher than CH_3	+1.07 ± 1.00	5
	(b) R = aromatic	+17.4 ± 0.3	4
$(RO)(R'O)_2P(O)$	R = aliph. higher than CH_3 R′ = aromatic	+12.0	1

Table 2.1 (continued)

Compound type	Specifications	δ	No. of different compounds examined
$(RO)_2(R'S)P(O)$	(a) R, R′ = aliph. higher than CH_3	−26.5 ± 0.3	6
	(b) R = aliph. higher than CH_3 R′ = CH_3	−28.4	
	(c) R = aliph. higher than CH_3 R′ = aromatic	−21.5 ± 0.5	2
$(RS)_3P(O)$ symmetrical	R = aliph. higher than CH_3	−61.3	1
$R_3P(S)$ symmetrical	R = aliph. higher than CH_3	−51.0 ± 3.0	2
$R(R'O)_2P(S)$	(a) R, R′ = aliph. higher than CH_3	−101.7	1
	(b) R′ = aliph. higher than CH_3 R = CH_3	−94.5 ± 0.9	8
$R(R'S)_2P(S)$	R = CH_3 R′ = aliph. higher than CH_3	−74.0 ± 3.0	2
$(RO)_3P(S)$	(a) R = aliph. higher than CH_3	−68.1 ± 1.2	11
	(b) R = CH_3	−73.0	1
$(RO)_2(RS)P(S)$	R = aliph. higher than CH_3	−94.9	1
$(RS)_3P(S)$ symmetrical	R = aliph. higher than CH_3	−92.9	1
$(R_2N)_3P$ symmetrical	(a) R = aliph. higher than CH_3	−118	1
	(b) R = CH_3	−122	1
$(R_2N)_3P(O)$ symmetrical	(a) R = aliph. higher than CH_3	−23.0	1
	(b) R = CH_3	−23.4	1
$(R_2N)_2P(O)OR'$	R′ = aliph higher than CH_3, R = CH_3	−16.3	1
$(R_2N)_3P(S)$ symmetrical	R = aliph. higher than CH_3	−76.0 ± 1.0	2
$(R_2N)_2P(O)R'$	R = R′ = CH_3	−38.0	1
$(R_2N)P(O)(OR')_2$	R′ = aliph. higher than CH_3, R = CH_3	−35.0	1
$(R_2N)P(S)(OR')_2$	R, R = aliph. higher than CH_3	−75.0	1

Table 2.2
Proton chemical shift assignments for amino acid residues –NH–CHR–CO– incorporated in random-coil proteins. The values given represent the centres of multiplet peaks. Full details of the multiplet structure may be found in Roberts and Jardetzky (1970)

Name (abbreviation)	Side-chain (R) group	Assignments: Group	Shift (ppm from DSS)
Alanine (ALA)	$-\beta CH_3$	αCH βCH_3	4.35* 1.42
Arginine (ARG)	$-\beta CH_2-\gamma CH_2-\delta CH_2-\overset{H}{N}-NH_2$	αCH βCH_2 γCH_2 δCH_2	4.35* 1.83* 1.67* 3.23*
Asparagine (ASN)	$-\beta CH_2-CONH_2$	αCH βCH_2	– 2.79
Aspartic acid (ASP)	$-\beta CH_2-COOH$	αCH βCH_2 (pH 3) βCH_2 (pH 7)	– 2.84 2.68
Cysteine (CYS)	$-\beta CH_2-SH$	αCH βCH_2	– 3.05
Glutamine (GLN)	$-\beta CH_2-\gamma CH_2-CONH_2$	αCH βCH_2 γCH_2	– 2.05 2.42
Glutamic acid (GLU)	$-\beta CH_2-\gamma CH_2-COOH$	αCH βCH_2 (pH 3) βCH_2 (pH 7) γCH_2 (pH 3) γCH_2 (pH 7)	– 2.10 2.01 2.51 2.31
Glycine (GLY)	$-\alpha CH_2$	αCH_2	4.00
Histidine (HIS)	(C–4)HC–NH–CH(C–2)=N–C(–βCH_2–)=C (imidazole ring)	C–2H (acid pH) C–4H (acid pH) βCH_2 αCH	8.64 7.19 3.15 –
Isoleucine (ILE)	$-\beta\overset{H}{C}(\gamma' CH_3)-\gamma CH_2-\delta CH_3$	αCH βCH $\gamma' CH_3$ γCH_2 δCH_3	4.13* 2.06* 0.99* 1.18* 0.88*

Notes:
(1) Figures marked * are recent determinations by spin-decoupling on protamine and histone samples.

Table 2.2 (continued)

Name (abbreviation)	Side-chain (R) group	Assignments	
		Group	Shift (ppm from DSS)
Leucine (LEU)	$-\beta CH_2-\gamma CH\langle^{\delta CH_3}_{\delta CH_3}$	αCH βCH_2 γCH $\delta(CH_3)_3$	4.17* 2.10* 1.63* 0.98*
Lysine (LYS)	$-\beta CH_2-\gamma CH_2-\delta CH_2-\epsilon CH_2-NH_2$	αCH βCH_2 γCH_2 δCH_2 ϵCH_2	4.35* 1.80* 1.49* 1.73* 3.03*
Methionine (MET)	$-\beta CH_2-\gamma CH_2-S-\epsilon CH_3$	αCH βCH_2 γCH_2 ϵCH_3	— 2.27 2.70 2.12
Phenylalanine (PHE)	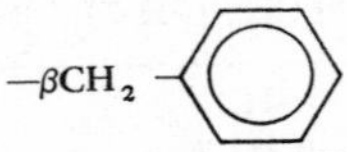 $-\beta CH_2-$ (phenyl ring)	αCH βCH_2 ϕ	— 3.13 7.27 (complex)
Proline (PRO)	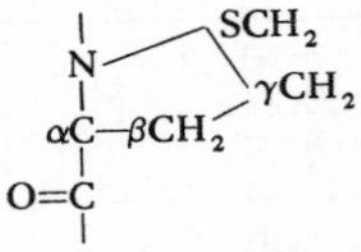 N, δCH_2, γCH_2, $\alpha C-\beta CH_2$, $O=C$ (ring)	αCH βCH_2 γCH_2 δCH_2	 3.67*
Serine (SER)	$-\beta CH_2-OH$	αCH βCH_2	4.48* 3.89*
Threonine (THR)	$-\beta CH(OH)-\gamma CH_3$	αCH βCH γCH_3	— 4.20* 1.24*
Tryptophan (TRP)	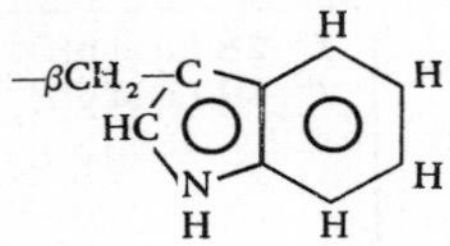 $-\beta CH_2-C$, HC, N–H (indole ring, H, H, H, H)	βCH_2 Ring protons	3.38 7.32 7.28 7.20 7.54 7.68
Tyrosine (TYR)	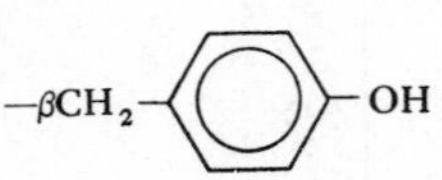 $-\beta CH_2-$ (phenyl ring) $-OH$	αCH βCH_2 ϕ 3, 5 H ϕ2,6H	 3.00 6.82 7.12
Valine (VAL)	$-\beta CH\langle^{\gamma CH_3}_{\gamma CH_3}$	αCH βCH $\gamma(CH_3)_2$	4.17* 2.11* 0.96*

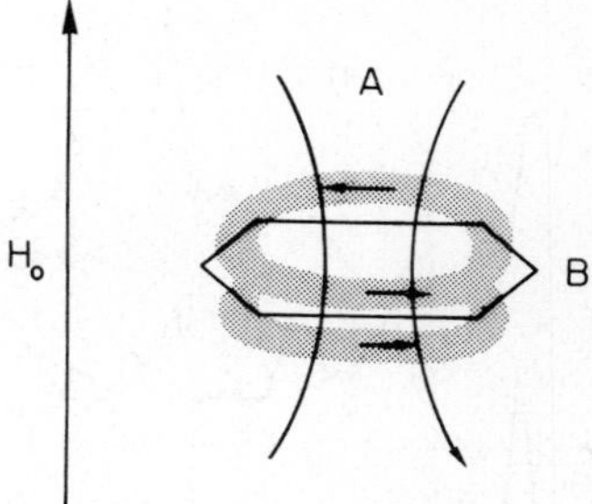

Figure 2.12 Strong diamagnetic effect of the motion of electrons in a π-system on application of field H_0. A methyl group at position A will be strongly shielded by the ring-current effect; its resonance will shift upfield by up to 2 ppm

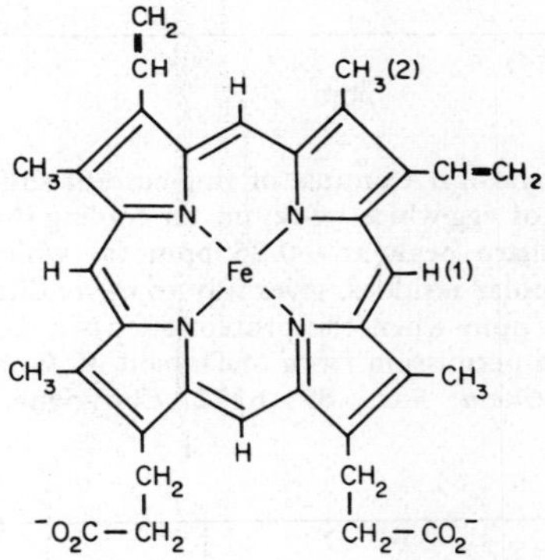

Figure 2.13 A haem group. The protons and groups outside the π-system will be strongly deshielded by the ring currents induced in the system by an applied field perpendicular to the plane of the molecule. To these effects must be added the paramagnetic shifts due to the iron atom, which will depend on its spin state

spectrum around 0 ppm. The precise value of this alteration in chemical shift will depend in a very sensitive way on the relative positions and orientations of the ring and the methyl, thus providing an accurate measure of their relation in space. Further, any changes in their relative positions will be readily monitored from changes in the chemical shift of the methyl group. Figure 2.14 shows the high-field spectrum of lysozyme in its denatured state and in the native state in which several

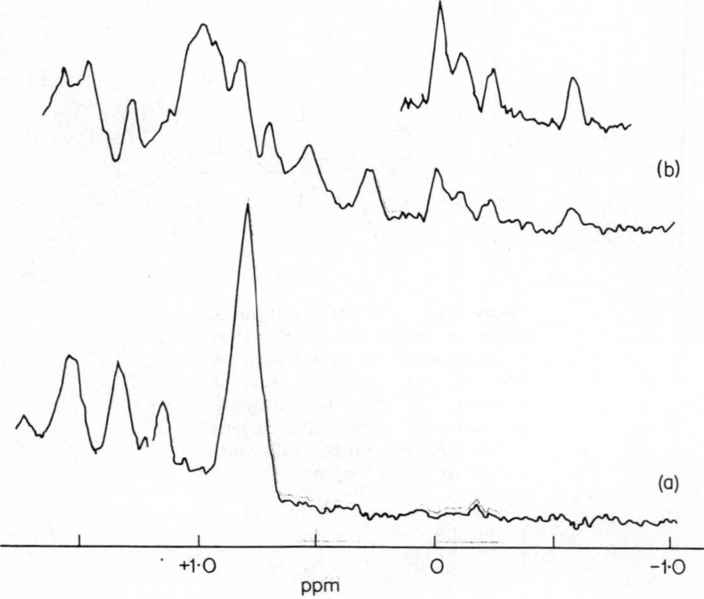

Figure 2.14 The classical example of ring-current shifts: changes in the 220 MHz spectrum of egg-white lysozyme on cooling through its refolding temperature. The sharp peak at −0.85 ppm (a) which is attributed to methyl groups of apolar residues, gives way to many different peaks in the range −0.7 to +0.7 ppm when the protein adopts a native conformation (b). (Reprinted with permission from McDonald, C. C., and Phillips, W. D. (1967). *J. Amer. Chem. Soc.*, **89**, 6332. Copyright by the American Chemical Society)

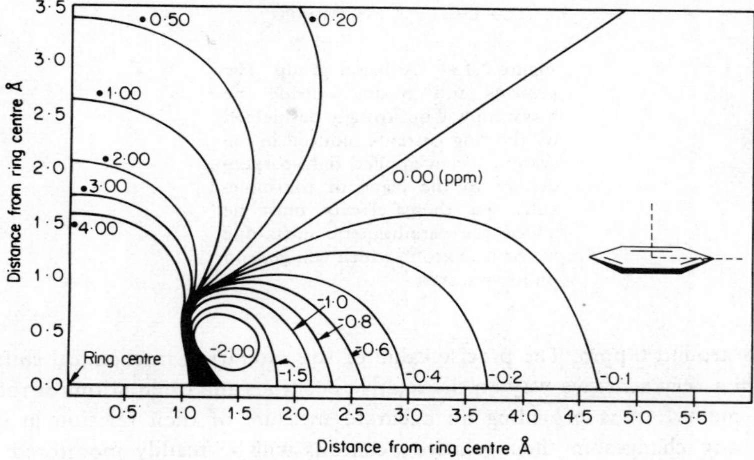

Figure 2.15 Chart of chemical shift changes induced in protons in various positions relative to benzene ring. (After Johnson and Bovey 1958)

rings and methyl groups come into the right sort of spatial conjunction for ring-current shifts to occur. Of course, the effect also causes *downfield* shifts of the resonances of groups in the plane of the ring but outside it (position B of Figure 2.12) but since this moves the peaks into the main body of the spectrum, they disappear from view and are of little or no use analytically. A quantitative expression of the shifts is given in Figure 2.15 (Johnson and Bovey, 1958).

(b) The effects of paramagnetic ions. As was mentioned in Chapter 1, the magnetic moment of an electron is very much greater than that of the magnetic nuclei used in NMR. Normally in chemical bonding the electrons in the molecule are arranged in such a way that their magnetic moments cancel out (diamagnetic molecules); in some molecules and ions, however, notably the transition-metal ions such as iron, cobalt, copper and nickel, the cancellation is incomplete so that these ions have a magnetic moment. The presence of such a paramagnetic ion in a molecule not only means that it will have an ESR spectrum, but also may have a profound effect upon its nuclear resonance spectrum; apart from effects on the relaxation times (and resultant resonance linewidths) of the nuclei, large chemical shift changes may be induced. As discussed in the chapters on ESR, many biologically active molecules already contain paramagnetic ions, examples being haemoglobin (iron), azurin (copper) and enolase (manganese), while the introduction of a paramagnetic ion as a perturbing factor into a normally diamagnetic molecule may also produce shift changes. The shifts involved can be very large: 80 ppm and more has been reported, although smaller shifts are more common. Peaks shifted by the presence of a paramagnetic ion may be distinguished from those affected by ring currents by the fact that their shifts are temperature-dependent while ring-current shifts in general are not. The shifts induced by paramagnetic ions are variously referred to as scalar shifts, isotropic hyperfine shifts or contact shifts and an alternative means of interaction, termed pseudo-contact interaction, is also invoked by some workers as a mechanism which may sometimes contribute to the changes in the spectrum. In each case the effects may be thought of as simply the effect on H_{loc} of the presence of a magnetic moment, that of the paramagnetic ion, within the molecule. This picture, while simple, is inadequate for quantitative use since the phenomenon may only be described and analysed properly in quantum-mechanical terms. When this is done, a considerable amount of information may be obtained about the precise electronic state of the region of the molecule around the paramagnetic site. Since this is frequently the active site of the molecule, it is clear that such analyses may be of considerable value in elucidating the way that a metallo enzyme 'works'. Similarly, the use of paramagnetic ions as probes in otherwise diamagnetic molecules is an analytical tool of considerable power. Examples of the use of such techniques may be found in Chapter 4, and more detail on the analysis of their effects in Chapter 5.

(c) Titration effects on chemical shift. In amino acids which still contain ionizable groups after incorporation into protein chains, the electronic structure

and thus the chemical shifts of the resonances are functions of the ionization state of the residue. The changes in chemical shift observed in titration may be quite large, up to 1 ppm or more. The residues particularly of interest in protein NMR are aspartic acid, glutamic acid and histidine, the resonances most affected being the βCH_2 of aspartic acid, the γCH_2 of glutamic acid, and the C-2H and C-4H resonances from the imidazole ring of histidine.

Aspartic acid	Glutamic acid	Histidine
–N(H)–αC(H)–C(=O)–	–N(H)–αC(H)–C(=O)–	–N(H)–C(H)–C(=O)–
βCH_2	βCH_2	CH_2
C=O	γCH_2	H–C$_4$=C–N=CH(C–2)–N (imidazole ring)
OH	C=O	
	OH	
pKα ~ 4.6	pKα ~ 4.6	pKα ~ 6.8

In each case, the titration may be followed and the pK of the residue determined; histidine is particularly useful in this respect as not only are histidines frequently found at the active sites of proteins, but the histidine C-2H resonance lies between 7 and 8.3 ppm in the protein spectrum, a region which is almost entirely free of other resonances. An example of the application of this method to staphylococcal nuclease is given in Figure 2.16, where the individual pK values of the four histidine residues are determined. Naturally, this experiment would have to be preceded by a series in which the four resonances were assigned to the individual histidines in the sequence if the biological significance of the different pK values was to be determined.

2.3 Line multiplicity in NMR

When the molecules under investigation are small enough or flexible enough for line multiplicities not to be blurred out, they offer a very powerful method of structural analysis. Not only do the patterns of splittings afford information on which groups are neighbours, but the size of the splittings is dependent on bond lengths and angles, so that a great deal of useful structural data may be obtained.

Origins of line multiplicity

The local field at any nucleus is a function not only of the effects described in the preceding section, but also of the fields produced by other magnetic nuclei in its vicinity. These fields may be experienced directly by the nucleus in question, or may be transmitted indirectly to it from magnetic nuclei in the same molecule by way of the electron clouds surrounding them. Of the two effects, the direct one

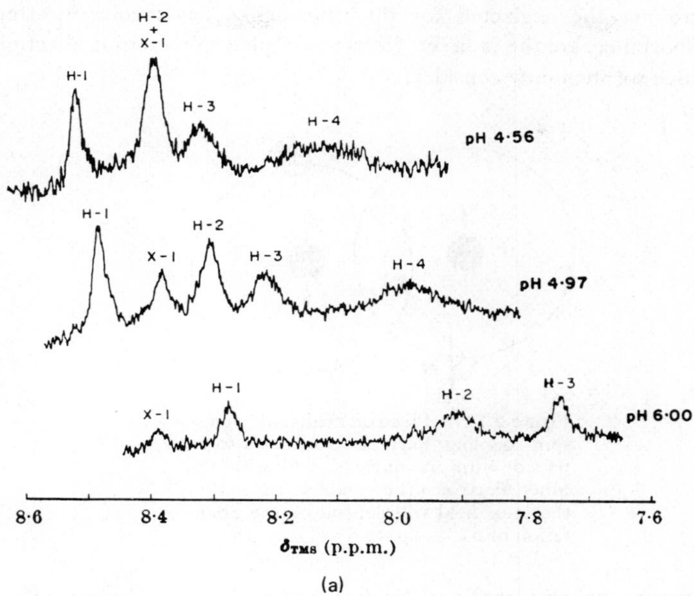

(a)

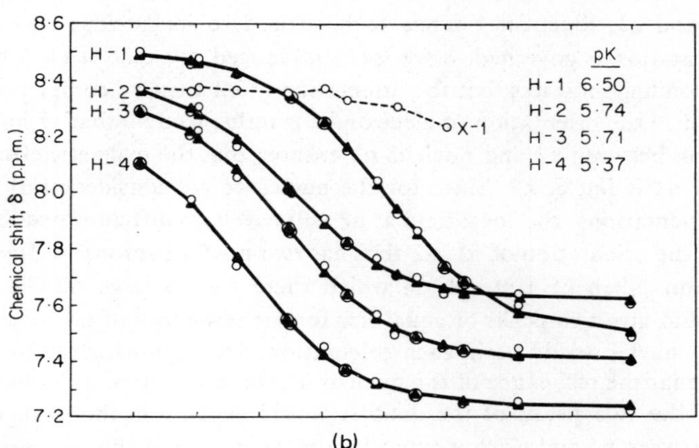

(b)

Figure 2.16 Example of investigation of pK values for the different histidine residues of a protein. (a) Spectra of low-field resonances of staphylococcal nuclease at pH 4.56, pH 4.97 and pH 6.00; (b) titration curves for the four histidine resonances visible. (From Cohen *et al.*, 1970. Reproduced by permission of Macmillan (Journals) Ltd) (dipolar effect) is capable of exerting relatively very large fields, corresponding to chemical shifts of ppm, on the nucleus; however, in the liquid samples which we are discussing these effects are averaged to zero by the tumbling motion of the molecules, except in the case of very large slow-moving molecules or highly viscous solutions, and may be neglected for the time being. Far smaller in effect, but greater in importance, are the indirect, electron-coupled spin–spin interactions, and it is these which we shall now consider.

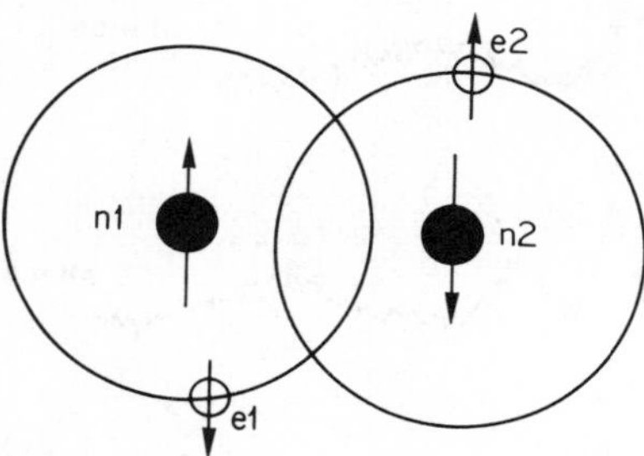

Figure 2.17 Electron-mediated spin–spin coupling. Each electron tends to be paired with its nucleus, and with the other electron. The result at n2 is that the local field will depend on the orientation of n1

The mechanism whereby the local field at one nucleus is indirectly affected by the presence of another is easy to grasp in a qualitative way. Consider the sketch of Figure 2.17 which shows two atoms 1 and 2 bonded by the sharing of two electrons e1 and e2. Electron 1 tends to be paired to its nucleus n1 – in other words its orientation is governed, or at least influenced, by that of nl. A basic rule of chemical bonding indicates that the orientation of e2 must be complementary to that of e1, and so the orientation of electron e2 is influenced by that of nucleus n1. The interaction between e2 and nucleus n2 ensures that the magnetic effect of the orientation of n1 is felt at n2. Since for the nuclei we are considering n1 can have one of two orientations, the local field at n2 will have two different possible values depending on the orientation of n1. n2 thus has two possible resonance frequencies, and a spectrum taken of a sample in which there were a large number of 1–2 molecules would give two peaks of equal size for the resonance of n2, since roughly half of the n1 nuclei would be in each orientation. The argument can be reversed, of course, so that the resonance of the nucleus n1 will also appear as a doublet. The separation of the two peaks of the doublet would depend on the strength of the interaction between n1 and n2, but typically the separation of the two peaks would range from a fraction of a Hz to perhaps 10 Hz for proton–proton coupling, with larger values in general for couplings between other nuclei. The magnitude of the splitting is termed the 'coupling constant' for the interaction and is given by the symbol J. Note that the field produced at 1 by 2 is independent of H_0, so that J, measured in Hz, has the same value for a given pair of nuclei at any value of the measuring frequency.

If there is more than one n-type nucleus, the number of possible variations of field at n2 is multiplied accordingly. Two spins, with four possible combinations of orientations give rise to a triplet having relative intensities 1:2:1 (Figure 2.18). Three give a quartet of intensities 1:3:3:1, and so forth. The relative intensities of the lines of the multiplet depend on the number of possible ways of orientating the spins doing the splitting.

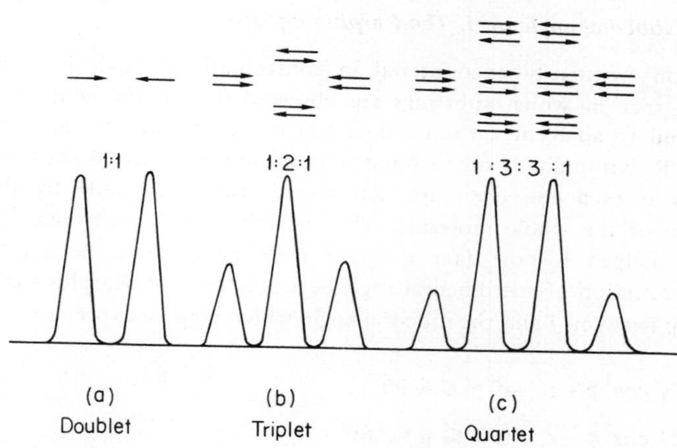

Figure 2.18 Simple (first-order) AX, AX_2 and AX_3 spectra: multiplet patterns observed when neighbouring group as (a) 1 spin, (b) 2 equivalent spins, (c) 3 equivalent spins

In our consideration of the mechanism of spin–spin splitting, it is evident that nucleus n1 must maintain its orientation during the whole time taken by n2 to undergo a transition, so that n2 sees a steady field; if this is not the case, then the interaction clearly becomes more complex. In the limiting case, where n1 is actually undergoing its transition at the same time as n2 (or in other words, if n1 and n2 have the same resonance frequency) the effects of n1 on n2 will average out completely and there will be no splitting of n2's peak. In this case n1 and n2 are said to be members of an 'equivalent set'; a typical example will be found in the case of the three protons of a CH_3 group. Thus when the NMR frequencies of two nuclei are very different ($J \ll \delta$, the difference between their resonant frequencies) we get a splitting which may be described simply in terms of the orientations of spins; such spectra are often described as first order. When $J \gg \delta$, the case of an equivalent set, there is no splitting. The intermediate case, $J \approx \delta$, is far more complex and only the simpler aspects of its analysis will be dealt with in this book.

Two points are worthy of note before continuing, however:

(a) The condition $J \approx \delta$ may be altered to $J < \delta$ by raising δ – in other words by raising the measuring frequency so that a given chemical shift difference in ppm increases in terms of Hz. Hence the interest of many research workers concerned with spin–spin splittings in spectrometers operating at 220 MHz, 300 MHz or even higher frequencies: spectra can be very much simpler to analyse at these frequencies. (b) Computer programs are available for calculating and analysing spin–spin interactions. Details may be obtained from the NMR spectrometer manufacturers.

The effect of dihedral angle on J. The Karphus equation

A situation frequently encountered in conformational analysis of biological molecules is that in which splittings are observed due to the coupling between protons bound to adjacent carbon atoms which are attached to each other by a single bond. Rotation about such a bond is free, and the relative orientations of the C–H groups at each end of it are determined stereochemically by the overall conformation of the whole molecule. The analysis of this conformation may be considerably helped by the fact that the coupling constant between the two protons is a function of the dihedral angle between them. M. Karplus has proposed a relationship between J and the dihedral angle which may be expressed as

$$J_1 = K_1 \cos^2\phi + c \quad (0 \leqslant \phi \leqslant 90^\circ)$$

$$J_2 = K_2 \cos^2\phi + c \quad (90^\circ \leqslant \phi \leqslant 180^\circ)$$

where K_1 and K_2 are constants depending on the other substituents on the HC–CH fragment, and c is another constant which is frequently very small or zero, Dihedral angle ϕ is as defined in Figure 2.19, which also shows graphically the form of the Karplus equation. A revised form of the Karplus equation for $HC_\alpha{-}C_\beta H$ proton coupling in amino acids has been given by Kopple *et al.* (1973) as

$$J = 11.0 \cos^2\phi - 1.4 \cos\phi + 1.6 \sin^2\phi$$

Analysis of spin systems

Before going on to further consideration of the analysis of spin–spin interactions, it is necessary to introduce the standard notation. It is usual to refer to nuclei which are not members of an equivalent set but whose relative chemical shifts are of the same order as their spin–spin coupling constants by the letters A, B, . . ., while nuclei whose signals are far from the A, B, . . . signals are referred to by the symbols X, Y, ... Thus the spectrum of an ethyl group $-CH_2-CH_3$, where the chemical shift difference of about 2 ppm (200 Hz at 100 MHz measuring frequency) between the two equivalent sets of protons may be considered large relative to the coupling

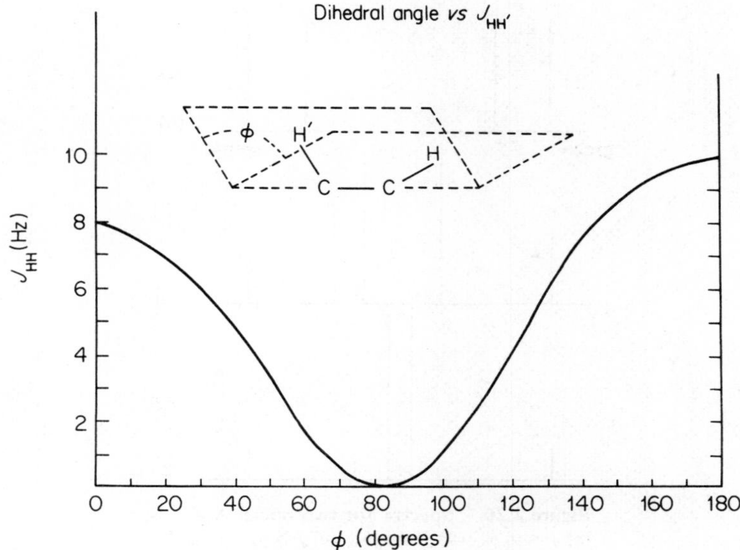

Figure 2.19 The form of the Karplus equation which relates dihedral angle ϕ to coupling constant $J_{HH'}$

constant J of about 7 Hz between them, may be referred to as an A_2X_3 (or A_3X_2) type. If the spectrum of the same group were run at a very low frequency of, say, 5 MHz, 2 ppm would become 10 Hz, J would still be 7 Hz, so $\delta \approx J$ and the spectrum would be an A_2B_3 (or A_3B_2) type. A classification of this type is valuable since it permits general discussion of multiplet phenomena to a very high level under a few simple headings.

The remarks that follow refer only to the simplest two-and three-spin systems, since these are the ones most applicable to the standard investigation of biological molecules, which is our subject. Several excellent textbooks which cover more complex spin systems in depth are included in the reading list at the end of the chapter.

The AX spectrum. This is the simplest of all, and simply consists of a pair of doublets, the components of each doublet being of equal intensity and each doublet being split by the same amount J_{AX}. The chemical shift difference between the doublets is, of course, large compared with J_{AX}. (Figure 2.20a.)

The AB spectrum. As the chemical shift difference between the components of an AX spectrum is reduced, changes in the relative intensities of the components of each doublet appear, with the inner members of the doublets increasing in intensity at the expense of the outer members (Figure 2.20 b,c.) The reason for this is that interaction between the nuclei causes a change in the probabilities of the various transitions between spin states of the nuclei – a phenomenon only properly

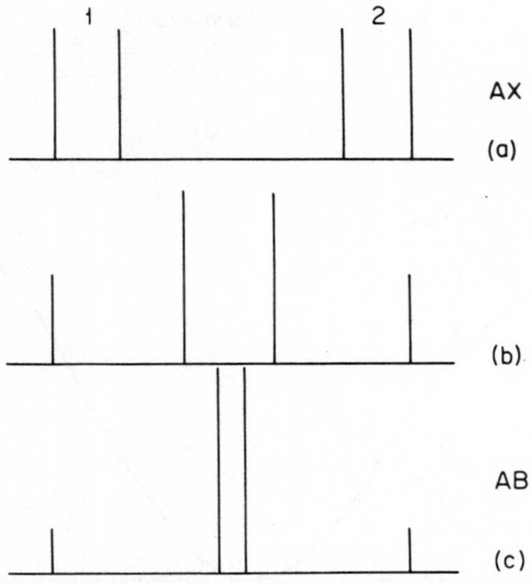

Figure 2.20 Spectra for two nuclei A and B. (a) $J \ll \nu_0\delta$, (b) $J \approx \nu_0\delta$, (c) $J > \nu_0\delta$.δ and J assumed positive, δ in ppm, so $\nu_0\delta$ is in Hz.

described by the use of the wavefunctions of the states. The more closely δ_{AB} approaches zero, the larger the inner peaks become, until in the limiting case of $\delta_{AB} = 0$ (an equivalent set) only a single peak is left, the inner peaks having merged and the outer ones diminished to zero.

The AX_2, AX_3, A_2X_2, A_2X_3 systems. These very simple first-order spectra are quite common, and may be recognized by their characteristic patterns; in each case there will be two multiplets in the spectrum having the same value of J, and the number of protons causing the multiplet splitting may be determined by subtracting 1 from the number of peaks in the multiplet (for example, a quartet is caused by a neighbouring group containing 3 protons). In addition, the total integrated areas of the multiplets will be in direct ratio to the number of protons in them. Simple examples may be seen in the spectrum of lysine in Figure 2.21. The αCH peak and the ϵCH_2 peak are both adjacent to single CH_2 groups, so that each is a triplet, the ϵCH_2 triplet having twice the total area of the αCH triplet.

The AMX spectrum. A typical example of this type, in which a group is subjected to splitting by two other, non-equivalent groups is to be found in the αCH of almost any residue in a protein chain. It is spin-coupled both to the proton of the N—H group and to the protons of the β-carbon. In Figure 2.21 the spectrum of lysine shows how the triplet caused by the splitting of the βCH_2 by the γCH_2 is split again by the αCH. Some of the central peaks overlap as the J-values for the two splittings are almost equal, and the result is a multiplet which is not easy to analyse. There is, however, a technique, which is of considerable help in such

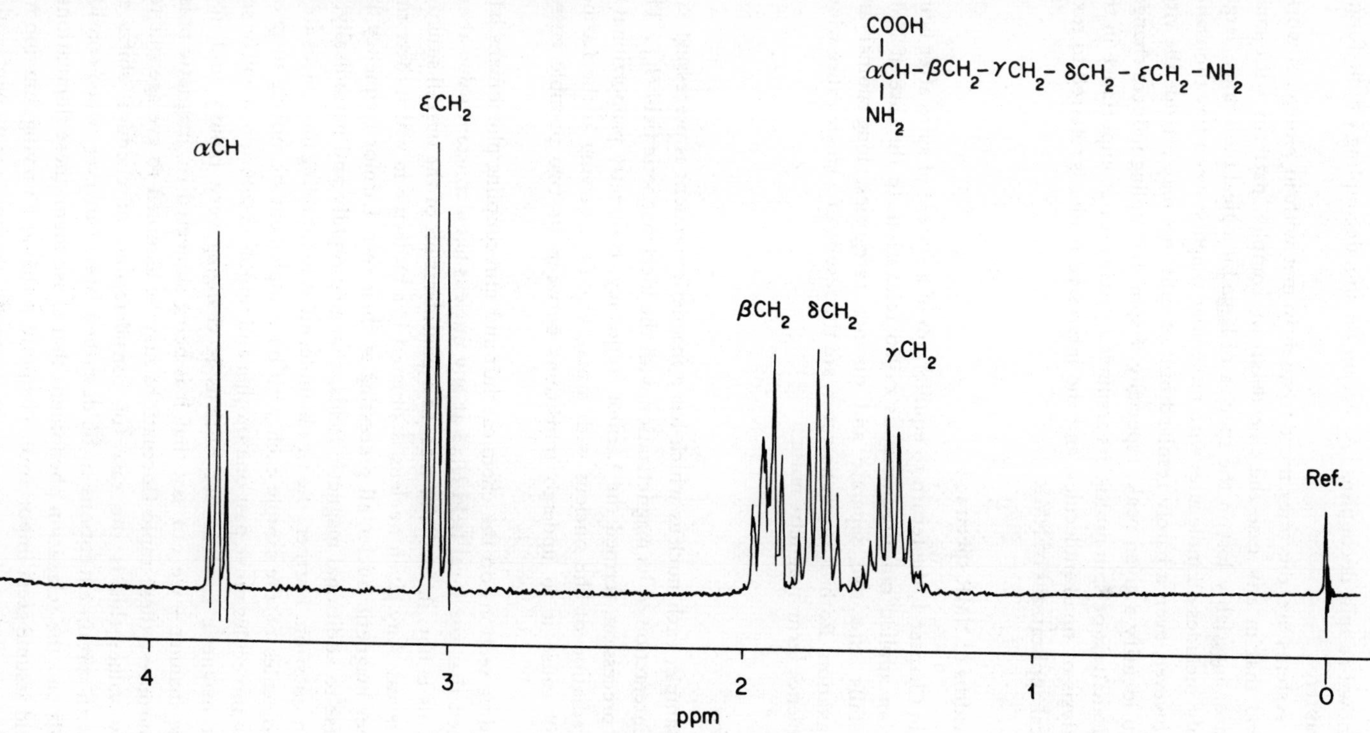

Figure 2.21 Proton spectrum of lysine at 220 MHz

cases and is known as spin decoupling. A section on spin decoupling will be found later in the chapter.

The above systems are the ones most frequently met with in biological work, bearing in mind that in any case the fine detail of complex patterns with small J-values is almost invariably lost in the spectra of large biological molecules; 'large' in this certainly includes all molecules with molecular weights over a few thousand. Sometimes, however, even a barely resolved hint of splittings may provide the vital clue needed to identify a given peak, especially if spin decoupling induces changes in it. Detailed analysis of spin multiplets assumes a vastly greater importance in the structural analysis of small molecules, and the interested reader is referred to texts on the chemical applications of NMR.

2.4 The linewidths of NMR spectra

As described in Chapter 1, the return to equilibrium of a system of spins after being perturbed by an applied radiofrequency is called relaxation. In the case of NMR this process falls into two separate and distinct categories, longitudinal and transverse relaxation. Both of them, however, are the results of a single cause which we for convenience term 'magnetic noise'.

'Magnetic Noïse'

In an NMR sample, each nucleus which has a magnetic moment is precessing as a result of the interaction of its magnetization with the local magnetic field H_{loc}. The frequency of precession, termed the Larmor frequency, is directly proportional to H_{loc}, and irradiation of the nucleus with a magnetic field varying at the Larmor frequency will cause it to undergo transitions between its two possible energy states.

The preceding sections on the chemical shift and spin-coupling phenomena have tacitly assumed that the local field H_{loc} at any nucleus has a constant value at any given time. This is not, in fact, the case, as a consideration of the overall situation will quickly reveal. Any given nucleus is situated in a molecule in which there may be many other magnetic nuclei, all precessing at their own Larmor frequency and thus giving rise to additional magnetic fields, changing rapidly and periodically, at the nucleus in question. Further, the whole molecule is in tumbling motion, as are all the other molecules of the sample each with its complement of moving magnetic nuclei. As the molecules move past one another and tumble in solution, it will be seen that the net magnetic field at our nucleus is changing very rapidly and in an unpredictable manner – we can say that it is being subjected to 'magnetic noise'. For many purposes, these rapid fluctuations may be assumed to average out to a single steady value; this is the case for considerations of chemical shifts and multiplets, with certain exceptions to be described later. However, when considering linewidths and the relaxation phenomena that cause them, these fluctuations in magnetic field assume great importance. The point is that any varying function may be assumed to consist of a number of regularly varying components added together; in the case of the magnetic noise these components will have many frequencies, among them the Larmor frequency of the nucleus which we are considering. The randomly varying magnetic field thus contains components which will be able to cause spin-state transitions in the nucleus, and it is these transitions, tending as they do to restore the equilibrium state which has been disturbed by our applied radiofrequency radiation, which are the mechanisms for the relaxation of the nuclei.

The Bloch formulation

While the mechanisms of relaxation are best understood with reference to the behaviour of individual nuclei, the ideas of the overall effects of relaxation on line shape and width and of the difference between longitudinal and transverse relaxation are most easily approached from considerations of the collective behaviour of the nuclei. In particular it is easiest to consider the resultant vectors arising from a summation of the magnetic moments of all the nuclei of a given species and Larmor frequency in the sample. Normally, all of the precessing nuclei are at different stages of their precession about the direction of H_0, i.e. they are all out of phase with each other (Figure 2.22a,b) and so, if H_0 is taken in the z-direction, all of the x- and y-components of the vectors cancel out, and there is no net magnetic resultant M_{xy}. There is, however, a net resultant magnetic moment M_z since more of the spins are aligned in the direction of H_0 than against it so that their z-components do not cancel out completely. This is the equilibrium state of affairs, with a finite value of M_z and no M_{xy}, as shown diagrammatically in Figure 2.22(b). Application of the transition-inducing radiofrequency radiation during an NMR experiment has two effects; firstly, since transitions are induced in nuclei aligned in both allowed directions, the equilibrium distribution which ensured an excess of nuclei aligned along H_0 is disturbed and the population difference between the two states reduced; M_z is thus also reduced. Secondly, after undergoing transitions the precessing spins tend to be in phase with each other (Figure 2.22 c) so that their x- and y-components no longer cancel and we now have a resultant M_{xy} which is itself moving around the z-direction with the Larmor frequency. The restoration of the original state of affairs is the relaxation process, and it can take place both by reestablishment of the full value of M_z, the component along H_0 (the process known as longitudinal relaxation) and, separately, by the loss of phase coherence between the spins and the consequent decay of M_{xy} to zero (since M_{xy} lies transversely to the direction of H_0 this process is known as tranverse relaxation). In theory at least, these two processes are independent.

A very important, though basically simple, mathematical treatment of resonance and relaxation phenomena was first proposed by Bloch. His basic assumption was that return to equilibrium of M_z would be exponential with a characteristic time T_1 (the longitudinal relaxation time) and that relaxation of M_{xy} to zero would similarly be exponential with characteristic time T_2, the transverse relaxation time.

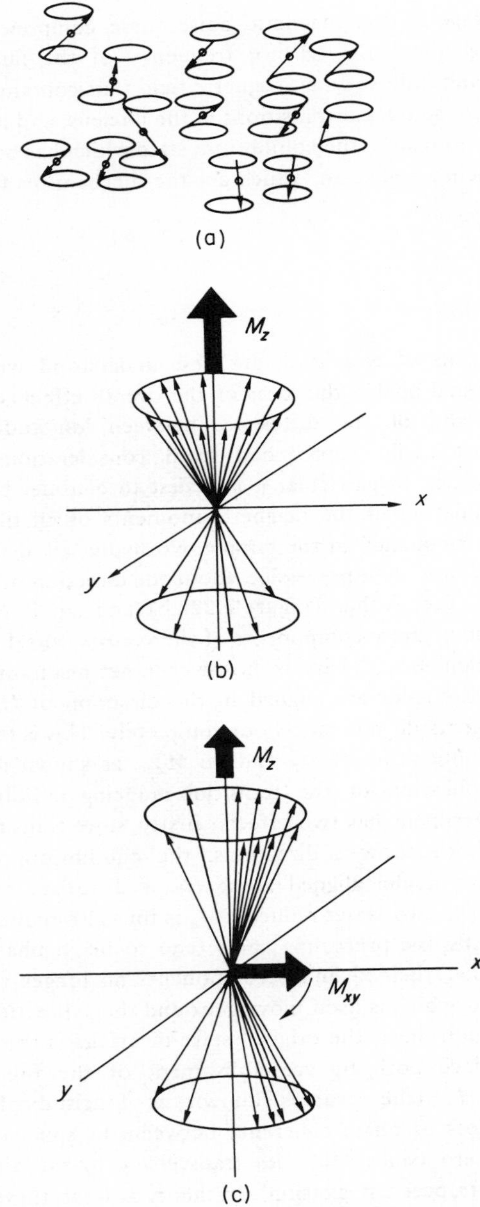

Figure 2.22 The many precessing spins (a) in a sample may conveniently be represented by bringing them to a common origin, (b). This shows the equilibrium condition in which an excess of spins points in the positive z-direction, producing a resultant M_z, but there is no phase coherence and thus no resultant in x- or y-directions. (c) Shows the situation during irradiation with a varying field at the Larmor frequency. The population excess in the z-direction (and thus M_z) is reduced, but the spins are now in phase, producing a new field M_{xy} in the xy plane

From this simple basic assumption, equations for the lineshape of NMR resonances in both absorption and dispersion modes are derived. In its simplest form, the equation for normal absorption mode NMR peaks which results from this treatment may be expressed as

★ $$g(\nu) = \frac{2T_2}{1 + T_2^2(\omega_0 - \omega)^2} \qquad (2.1)$$

In this expression $g(\nu)$ is a measure of the intensity of resonance at a frequency ω, when the actual Larmor frequency of the resonating nuclei is ω_0. The whole expression defines the *shape* of the nuclear resonance line; it is known as a Lorentzian lineshape. Our resonance lines are not, as has been made clear from the diagrams of spectra shown earlier, infinitely sharp lines at precise frequencies ω_0, but do have a finite width. This width can be obtained from the Bloch equation above in the following way:

(a) When $\omega = \omega_0$, in the centre of the resonance peak, the term $(\omega - \omega_0)$ disappears, leaving $g(\nu)_{max} = 2T_2$.

(b) The half-height of the peak, where $g(\nu) = ½g(\nu)_{max}$, must occur when the bottom line of equation (2.1) is equal to 2, i.e. when $T_2^2(\omega_0 - \omega)^2 = 1$. In this case, $T_2 = 1/\omega_0 - \omega$ so that $1/T_2 = \omega_0 - \omega$. In other words, half the width of the resonance line, measured at half its height, is equal to $1/T_2$, and thus the linewidth is a direct measure of T_2. More efficient relaxation, resulting in smaller values of T_2, gives broader lines. This result is of great importance in biological NMR.

The magnetic noise at any given nucleus may be divided into two classes: that from all nuclei in the same equivalent set, and that from all other sources. We shall consider the former, simpler case first.

It is evident that each nucleus precessing with a given Larmor frequency is the source of a magnetic field varying with that frequency. This varying field is able to induce transitions in another nucleus having the same Larmor frequency but the opposite orientation. The effect is a two-way one; each nucleus is induced by the other to change states, and the result is termed a spin exchange. Since the state of affairs both before and after the exchange is one spin in each orientation, there is no net effect on M_z. However, during the transition the relative phase of the two spins changes. If there was no phase coherence between them before the transition, i.e. on average a zero contribution to M_{xy}, there will again be no observable effect. If, on the other hand, the spins were rotating in phase before the spin exchange, the result will be a dephasing and a consequent reduction in the contribution to M_{xy}. The rate of reduction of M_{xy} (which is exponential and characterized by the transverse relaxation time T_2) is therefore a function of the rate at which spin exchanges take place. For this reason, T_2 is often termed the spin–spin relaxation time.

Transverse relaxation

The rate at which spin exchanges occur, and hence the relaxation time T_2, depend on the extent to which nuclei will be exposed to each other's varying fields. In a rigid structure or one in which the relative motion of the nuclei is slow, the process is quite efficient and T_2 correspondingly short. As molecular motion speeds up, with smaller molecular weights, higher temperatures, or more flexible molecules, the efficiency drops away until in a very mobile liquid T_2, may reach as high as 10–100 seconds, corresponding to theoretical linewidths of less than 10^{-1} Hz. (Because of other limitations, particularly inhomogeneity in the magnetic field of the spectrometer, the smallest linewidth normally observable for protons is about 0.05 Hz.) It is convenient to be able to give quantitative expression to rates of motion of molecules relative to each other; this is done by means of a 'correlation time' τ_c which may crudely be defined as the time taken by a molecule to turn through one radian or move through one molecular distance.

As just mentioned, line broadening may be caused by inhomogeneities in the applied field H_0. If H_0 is not precisely the same over the whole sample, the spins in one part of the sample will precess at a slightly different rate from those in another part, and will therefore lose phase coherence with them at a rate determined by the inhomogeneity of the field. The resultant line broadening is generally undesirable, and explains why the attainment of very homogeneous fields is of prime importance in practical NMR.

Longitudinal relaxation

As well as the periodically varying magnetic fields of nuclei in the same equivalent set, a nucleus is subjected to magnetic noise from all other magnetic moments in the sample (these moments are collectively termed 'the lattice'). The frequency covered by this noise, or in other words, the range of frequencies at which components will be found in it, will depend on the correlation times, i.e. the relative rates of motion of the various groups involved. These will clearly be functions of molecular size and rigidity, of temperature and of solution viscosity. Some typical frequency spectra are shown schematically in Figure 2.23. The fields which interest us are those which vary at the Larmor frequency of our nuclei, since these are the fields which are able to induce transitions. Since such transitions will not be spin exchanges, they will have a net effect on M_z and hence will cause longitudinal relaxation. It can be seen from Figure 2.23 that the maximum quantity of magnetic noise, and hence the most efficient relaxation, occurs neither for very fast nor for very slow molecular motions, but for an intermediate value of the correlation time τ_c. Consequently, the longitudinal relaxation time T_1 passes through a minimum at some intermediate value of τ_c. The relationship between T_1 and τ_c is shown in Figure 2.24, where the minimum value of T_1 is clearly marked. It will also be seen that for values of τ_c less than about 10^{9} s, which is the condition obtaining in liquid solutions of small molecules, T_1 and T_2 become equal. Most of the terms used in the calculation of T_1 and T_2 are identical, and for small values of T_2 those terms which differ between the two calculations become negligible.

The net conclusion of these considerations of relaxation times is that the

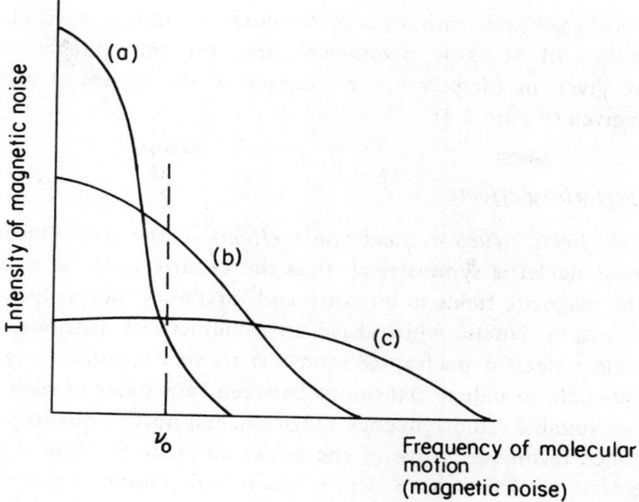

Figure 2.23 Frequency spectra of magnetic noise due to inter-molecular effects (spin–lattice effects). Note that the greatest intensity (most efficient T_1 relaxation) takes place at intermediate motion (b) and is lower for slower (a) and faster (c) motion

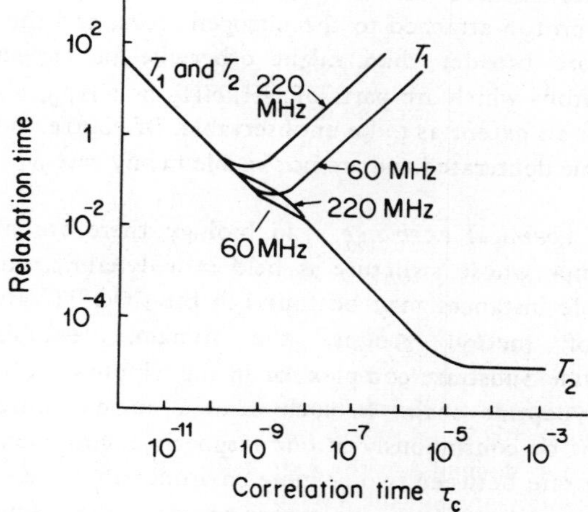

Figure 2.24 Relation between molecular correlation times and relaxation times for spectrometer frequencies of 60 MHz and 220 MHz

relaxation times of a given group of nuclei, as indicated by the linewidth of its resonance or by direct T_1 and T_2 measurements (see Chapter 5) may be used to indicate its rate of motion in solution. Biologically, this is very important, as the rate of motion of a given group of nuclei may be radically altered if the molecule or part of a molecule containing it either (a) changes from a flexible to a rigid form or vice versa, (b) aggregates with other molecules or (c) interacts with larger or more rigid molecules. All of these phenomena are very important in biology, and examples are given in Chapter 4. An example of the effects of aggregation has already been given (Figure 2.4).

Relaxation perturbing effects

(a) Electric fields. Nuclear quadrupole effects. The distribution of electric charge in most nuclei is symmetrical; thus the electric fields in a sample, which must rival the magnetic fields in intensity and variability, normally have no effect on their relaxation. Nuclei which have an asymmetrical distribution of electric charge (a nuclear electric quadrupole moment) are very sensitive to varying electric fields. It is possible to induce transitions between spin states of such nuclei by the application of suitable radiofrequency radiation, and nuclear quadrupole resonance is an established technique. None of the nuclei normally considered for biological nuclear magnetic resonance have electric quadrupole moments themselves; effects may nevertheless be seen in the NMR spectra of nuclei whose neighbouring nuclei have quadrupole moments. The prime example of this in proton spectroscopy is that of ^{14}N, the common isotope of nitrogen. This has a quadrupole moment and is therefore caused by the varying electric fields in a tumbling molecule to change its spin state (it has 3 allowed orientations) very rapidly. This enhances the relaxation of any proton attached to the nitrogen atom, and the resonance of the proton is therefore broader than might otherwise be expected. Indeed, the resonances of protons which are parts of NH, NH_2 or NH_4^+ groups are sometimes broadened to such an extent as to be unobservable. Of course, in solutions in D_2O, NH_2 groups become deuterated and are not visible in any case.

(b) Effects of chemical exchange. In biology there are many instances of molecules or groups whose structure is held in a dynamic, rather than a static equilibrium. Simple instances may be found in the COO^-H^+ and OH^- groups, in the rotation of methyl groups, the dynamic equilibrium Enzyme + Substrate ⇌ Enzyme/Substrate complex, or in the 'rippling' of helical segments up and down a polypeptide chain. In such cases a nucleus which gives an NMR spectrum may not be continuously in one magnetic environment, but rather may exchange at some rate between two or more environments. The effect that this will have on the spectrum depends on the extent to which the magnetic environments of the two forms differ and on the exchange rate. When the exchange rate is very slow, compared with the chemical shift difference of the two environments expressed in Hz, the nucleus precesses many times in one environment before moving to the other. In this case a separate signal will be observed for each environment, the relative sizes of the signals being a measure of the relative numbers of groups in each environment at a given time (i.e. on the equilibrium distribution of nuclei between the two states). On the other hand, if the exchange is very fast, nuclei do not stay long enough in either environment to adjust their frequencies and so effectively precess at an average frequency, the result in the

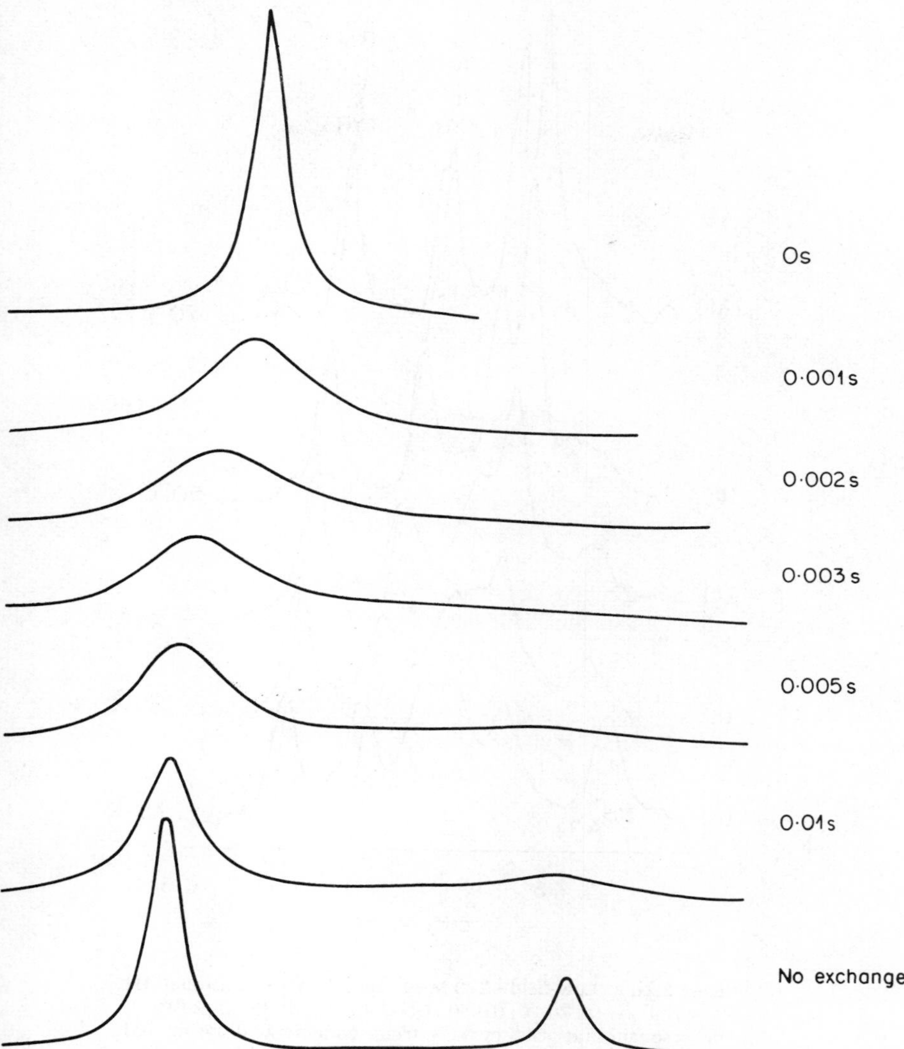

Figure 2.25 The effects of chemical exchange between two environments. The bottom spectrum represents two chemical environments respectively occupied by 75% and 25% of the molecules. Their signals are 10 Hz wide and separated by 100 Hz, and the number by each spectrum represents the lifetimes in seconds

spectrum being a single peak whose position is a measure of the relative time spent in each environment. For intermediate exchange rates, the spectrum to be expected in the simple case of two states which have relative populations of 75:25, is shown in Figure 2.25. If the exchange rates are in the intermediate range, they may be determined quite accurately by NMR, and even if they are outside the range, at

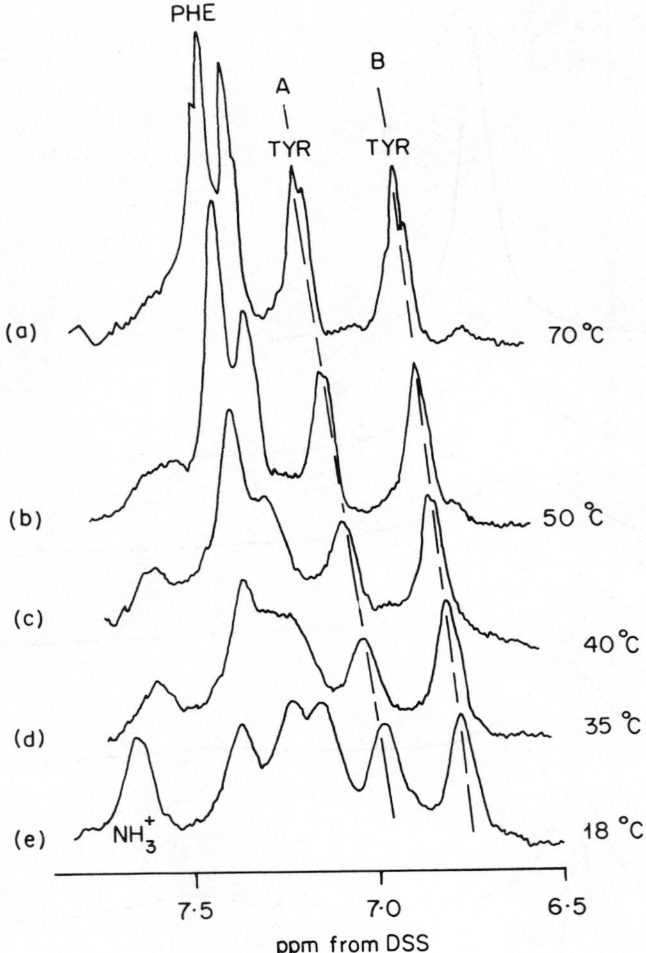

Figure 2.26 Low-field 270 MHz spectrum of histone H1, 40 mg/ml, at: (a) 70 °C; (b) 50 °C; (c) 40 °C; (d) 35 °C; (e) 18 °C. The resonance at +7.7 ppm is from undeuterated lysine NH_3^+ groups. Peaks A and B take up intermediate positions between their initial and final chemical shifts because they are in a fast exchange situation

least an upper or lower bound may be placed on them. Figures 2.26 and 2.27 give an example of the same histone molecule which is in the slow exchange state at room temperatures but in the fast exchange region at higher temperatures.

(c) Local paramagnetic relaxation probes. Paramagnetic ions may be divided into classes according to whether they have short electronic relaxation times, causing shifts without significant broadening, or long relaxation times, causing

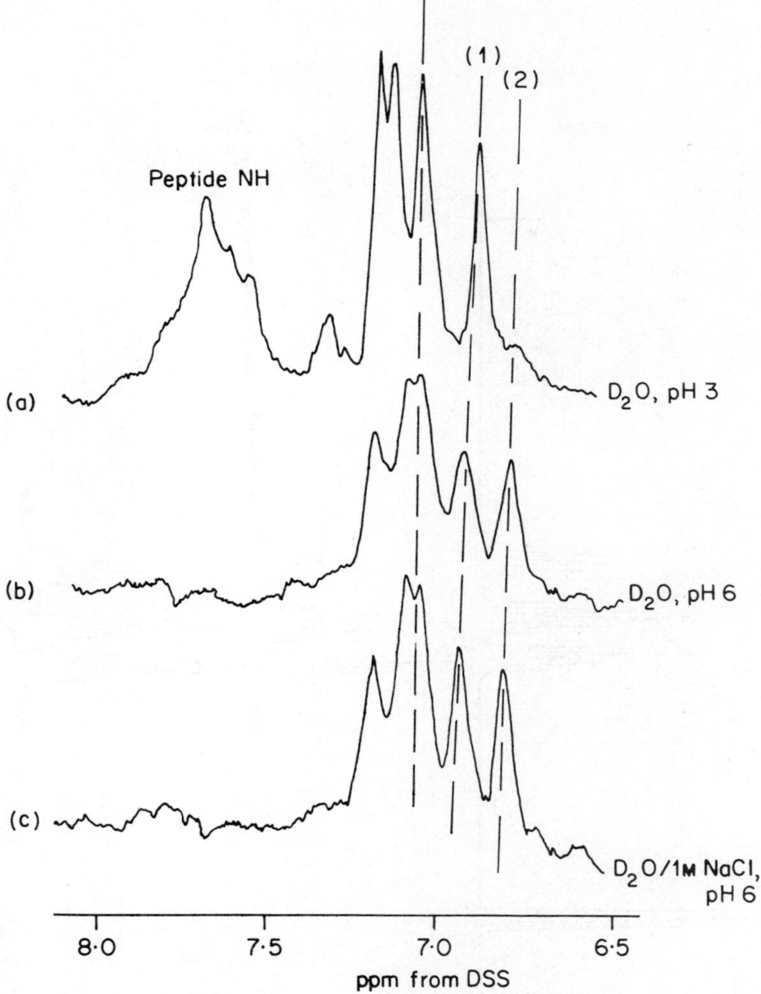

Figure 2.27 270 MHz downfield spectrum of histone H1, 50 mg/ml, in: (a) D_2O, pH 3; (b) D_2O, pH 6; (c) D_2O/1 M NaCl, pH 6. This is a slow exchange situation; the initial and final state resonances are present simultaneously and there is never a resonance at positions intermediate between positions (1) and (2). (Compare with Figure 2.26)

broadening without significant shifts. The latter are obviously the ones to use as relaxation probes; they include Mn^{++}, Gd^{+++}, Eu^{++}, Cu^{++}, and V^{++}. Relaxation may be caused by such ions either by direct dipole–dipole interactions or by scalar or hyperfine coupling transmitted through a chemical bond. The Solomon–Bloembergen equations which govern the effect of a paramagnetic ion on the relaxation times of nuclei bound nearby are complex but the main features of the

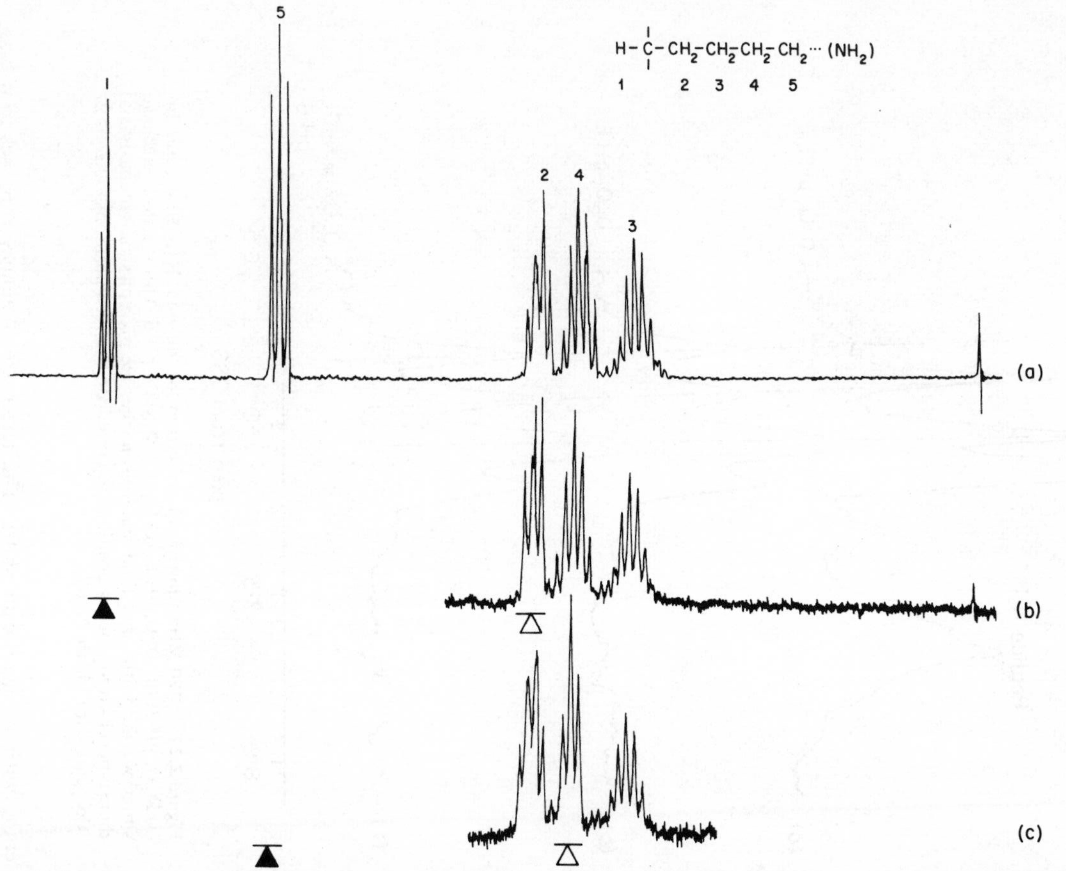

Figure 2.28 Spin decoupling of lysine. Spectrum (a) shows the undecoupled spectrum, while (b) and (c) show the effect produced (at △) by irradiation at ▲, and thus identify the groups which are coupled to those of peak

equations are a dependence on r^{-6}, where r is the electron–nucleus distance, and on two correlation times, τ_c, which refers to dipole–dipole interactions and τ_e which refers to scalar interactions. (A detailed analysis of the effects to be expected may be found in Dwek, 1973.)

In general we may note that difference spectroscopy may be used to identify the resonances of nuclei bound near a paramagnetic centre, since these will be almost completely broadened out, whereas the r^{-6} dependence ensures that nuclei at more than a few Å distant from the binding site of a paramagnetic ion are unaffected by its presence. The method is particularly applicable to the analysis of enzymes containing metals in which the metals may be replaced by paramagnetic analogues: this is particularly useful where, as in most enzymes, the metal ion is at or very near the active site. Further details of the method may be found in Chapter 5.

Spin Decoupling

In simple spectra where spin multiplets are visible, it is possible to infer which groups lie next to each other, and are therefore coupled, by measuring the value of J for the different multiplets; those with identical coupling constants must be coupled to each other. It is often the case, however, that several multiplets within one spectrum have J values which are the same, or at least the same within the available accuracy of measurement. In such cases, the technique of spin decoupling can be very useful. The principle is very simple: as has already been indicated, a proton which is subjected to a rapidly varying field will resonate at a frequency corresponding to the average value of the field. All that is necessary, then, to eliminate the effect of spin coupling between two nuclei is to cause one of them to undergo rapid and continuous transitions between its available energy states. The other nucleus then sees only the average value of the orientations, and the multiplet collapses. In order to make one of the nuclei undergo these rapid transitions, it is necessary to irradiate it steadily with radiofrequency radiation at its Larmor frequency while the signal of the other nucleus is being scanned. By irradiating the groups of a complex spectrum one by one and noting which other peaks are affected, it is possible to build up a complete picture of which groups are adjacent to each other. This might be done, for example, with the spectrum of lysine as illustrated in Figure 2.28. Irradiation at the frequencies marked on the spectrum by ▲̄ causes collapse of the multiplets marked by △̄, thus indicating that the groups are adjacent and allowing complete assignment of the groups along the lysine side chain.

2.5 Pulse and Fourier-Transform methods in NMR

Introduction

One of the major obstacles to the application of the continuous wave (CW) NMR method so described is its lack of sensitivity. The fundamental cause of this is the narrow gap relative to the thermal energies of the nuclei between the upper and lower energy levels of our nuclei, which means that upper and lower energy states are almost equally populated. There is little that can be done about this for biological samples; lowering the temperature would help except for the fact that our solutions would then freeze, and the energy gap itself is fixed by the nucleus being investigated and the magnetic field available. Higher-field spectrometers cause a larger population difference and would thus be expected to have a higher sensitivity than lower-frequency machines. Some improvement is found when running proton-decoupled ^{13}C spectra and will be covered in the section on ^{13}C spectroscopy. Apart from these, the only effective means of increasing our signal-to-noise ratio is by accumulating a number of spectra serially and adding them in a signal averaging device usually known as a CAT. In this way, the steady spectral signal accumulates and the randomly varying noise tends to cancel out. Such methods are virtually essential when studying biological molecules of molecular weight over a few hundred daltons. At once the researcher is faced with a dramatic increase in the time taken to obtain a spectrum: the improvement in signal-to-noise ratio is proportional to the square root of the number of scans, so that at two minutes per scan a tenfold improvement of signal-to-noise ratio requires over three hours accumulation, and a hundredfold would require nearly two weeks! – always assuming the spectrometer to be stable (and available) for so long. In practice, the sensible limit to CAT accumulation is 10–12 hours, which might be expected to yield signal-to-noise enhancements of the order of twentyfold. An example of what signal averaging can achieve is given in Figure 2.29.

One of the chief reasons for the slow rate of collection of data using a CW spectrometer is the serial way it is accumulated; only one resonance is being measured at one time, so that, for example, a resonance 2 Hz wide in a spectral width of 1000 Hz is only being sampled 0.2% of the time. Pulse-Fourier-transform methods overcome this difficulty by allowing simultaneous collection of all the data for one spectrum, typically in less than a second. The resultant increase in data-collection rate is sufficient to extend the usefulness of NMR to samples orders of magnitude more dilute than was possible previously.

To understand the Fourier-transform method it is necessary to understand, or at least accept, the following:

(1) Any waveform, however complicated, can be analysed into a number of simple harmonic (sine or cosine) waves of different frequencies; this process is known as Fourier analysis. The expression which relates any function of time to the sum of an infinite series of sine and cosine waves is

$$\star \quad f(t) = \sum_{n=0}^{\infty} A_n \cos\left(\frac{n\pi}{T}\right)t + \sum_{n=1}^{\infty} B_n \sin\left(\frac{n\pi}{T}\right)t \qquad (2.2)$$

(2) Since the original waveform usually describes the variation of some quantity with time, it is known as the time domain function. The *spectrum* of the frequencies into which the waveform is analysed is known as the frequency domain function.

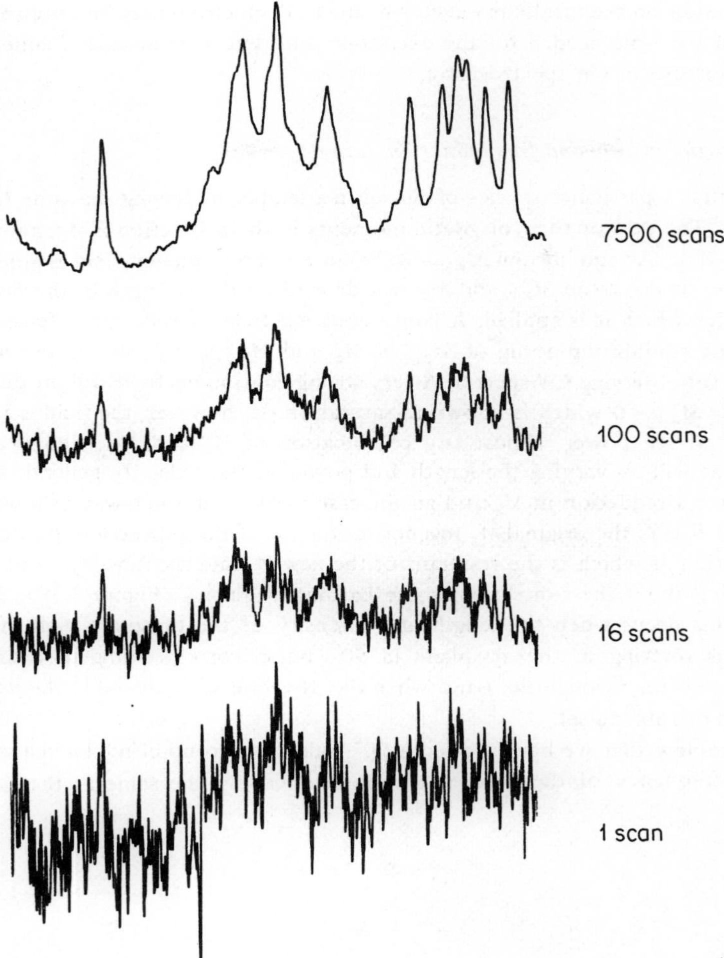

Figure 2.29 Signal-to-noise improvement obtained by adding and averaging a number of spectra

(3) Given one of these functions, it is possible to produce the other mathematically; the process is known as Fourier transformation, and the two functions are Fourier transforms of each other.

A 'normal' NMR spectrum, being a plot of the frequencies of absorbance of the various nuclei in the sample, is a frequency domain function. If all these frequencies are excited together, the resultant complex waveform which is the sum of all the resonant frequencies of the spectrum beating or interfering together, is a time domain function which is the Fourier transform of the normal spectrum. Thus by causing all the nuclei to resonate at the same time and performing a Fourier transformation on the resultant waveform, an NMR spectrum may be produced in a fraction of the time needed for the excitation and detection of each frequency in the serial manner of CW spectroscopy.

Nuclear magnetization and free induction decay

Consider first a particular species of nuclei in a sample, all having the same Larmor frequency. The sum of their magnetic moments in the z-direction is M_z, and in the xy plane, M_{xy}. At equilibrium $M_{xy} = 0$. When a radiofrequency field is applied to the sample, its effect on M_{xy} and M_z will depend on the strength of the field and the time for which it is applied. A continuous RF field of very low intensity will produce an equilibrium value of $M_{z_{eq}} < M_z$ and $M_{xy_{eq}} > 0$; this is the normal condition for observing CW spectra. A very strong continuous field will produce the effect $M_z = M_{xy} = 0$ which is known as saturation. If, however, the field is applied as a *pulse* of RF power, almost any combination of M_z and M_{xy} values can be produced at will by varying the length and power of the pulse. In general, a pulse will produce a reduction in M_z and an increase in M_{xy}; another way of looking at this is that it tilts the original M_z magnetization out of the z-direction, producing a magnetization M which is the resultant of the new M_z and the new M_{xy} and which is precessing about the z-direction at the Larmor frequency (Figure 2.30). Special cases of this occur when the length and intensity of the pulse are such that the M-vector is rotating in the xy plane (a 90° pulse, corresponding to tilting the original M_z vector through 90°) and when the M-vector is produced in the *negative* z-direction (a 180° pulse).

Suppose now that we have applied a 90° pulse to a group of nuclei in a sample. The radiofrequency of the pulse need not be precisely the same as the Larmor

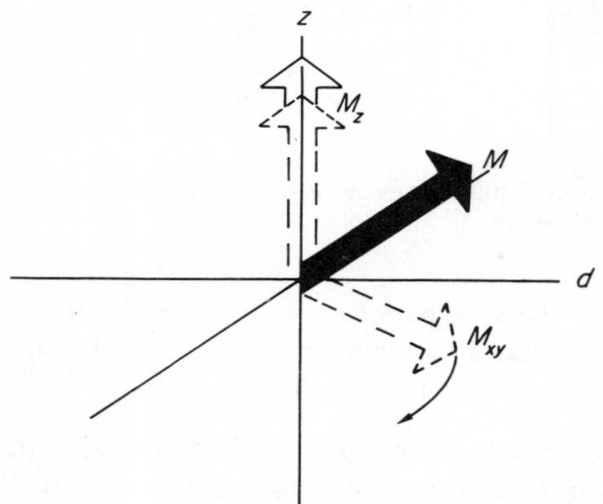

Figure 2.30 Reduction in M_z and production of M_{xy} by applied radiofrequency, represented as a tipping of magnetization M out of the z-direction

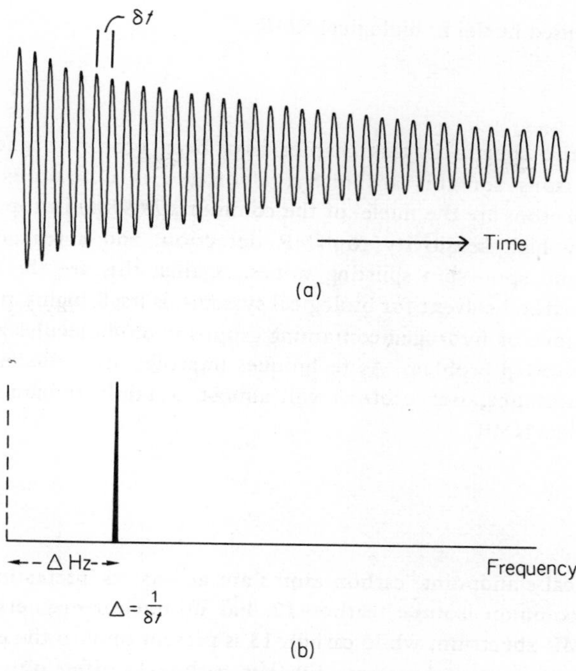

Figure 2.31 (a) Free induction decay of a spectrum containing a single resonance. (b) The resultant spectrum after transformation

frequency of the nuclei, since a short pulse of any frequency will also contain other frequencies in the same region. (In fact a short pulse can be built up by adding together a number of nearby frequencies.) A detector coil placed on the *x*- or *y*-axis will, after the end of the pulse, pick up the radiation due to the rotation of M about the *z*-axis. If a single group of nuclei is involved, the signal produced, which is known as the free induction decay or FID, will be a sine wave which has a frequency equal to the difference $\Delta\nu$ between the main RF frequency of the pulse (which is used in the detector circuit) and the Larmor frequency of the nuclei. It will also decay at a rate determined by the T_2 of that particular group of nuclei. If more than one group of nuclei is involved, then the resultant pattern will be the sum of the FIDs of all the groups. This overall FID is the time-domain function which is then transformed by the computer into the normal NMR spectrum. Typically it takes between 0.1 s and 10 s to record the FID for a single spectrum; many FIDs may be collected and summed in a short time to improve the signal-to-noise ratio of the resultant spectrum. The increase in data collection rate of about 100 times over that attainable with a conventional spectrometer is the seat of the greatly increased power of the FT machine. A simple FID and the resultant transformed 'spectrum' are shown in Figure 2.31. Further details of Fourier-transform spectrometers will be found in Chapter 3.

2.6 Commonly used nuclei in biological NMR

Protons

All the illustrative spectra in this chapter have been proton magnetic resonance spectra; the reasons for this are many. Hydrogen is ubiquitous in biological molecules and protons are the nuclei of the common (99.98%) isotope of hydrogen. They offer very high sensitivity to NMR detection, and a reasonable range of chemical shift and spin–spin splitting values. Against this are the considerations that water, the natural solvent for biological systems, is itself highly protic, and that the very abundance of hydrogen-containing groups in biomolecules is the source of the great peak-overlap problem. As techniques improve, other nuclei will doubtless increase in importance, but protons will almost certainly remain the most-used nuclei in biological NMR.

Carbon-13

From a biological standpoint, carbon atoms are at least as interesting as hydrogen. However, the common isotope, carbon-12, has no nuclear magnetic moment and thus has no NMR spectrum, while carbon-13 is present only to the extent of about 1.1% of all carbon in natural systems. Further, carbon-13 offers only about 1.6% of the sensitivity to NMR detection of protons, so that a natural-abundance ^{13}C spectrum has a several thousandfold disadvantage in signal-to-noise compared to a proton spectrum of the same sample. It is only since the advent of Fourier-transform spectrometers that ^{13}C spectroscopy has become a practical proposition. Now that the nucleus is available for use, the fact that its chemical shifts are far greater than those of protons (covering a range of 200 ppm or more) make ^{13}C increasingly attractive, especially when specific ^{13}C labelling is undertaken. More details of how ^{13}C techniques differ from proton techniques are given in Chapter 3.

Fluorine

Fluorine is not normally found in biological systems, but its nucleus is attractive from the NMR point of view in that it offers sensitivity almost as high as that of protons and because most proton spectrometers, particularly CW spectrometers, are readily converted to ^{19}F operation because of the closeness of the fluorine resonance frequency to that of protons at any given field. These factors have led to considerable use of ^{19}F as a label or heteronuclear probe; a small molecule such as an enzyme substrate may be synthesized or modified to contain one or more fluorine atoms, and the spectrum of these observed to follow changes in the environment of the labelled molecule consequent on, say, enzyme binding, enzyme action or changes in enzyme structure with pH. Alternatively, the macromolecule under investigation may itself be fluorinated in one or more sites.

Phosphorus

Like fluorine, phosphorus may be used as a heteronuclear label for the observation of changes in molecular environment. Its sensitivity relative to that of protons at the same field is only about 6%, against 83% for ^{19}F, but this is still adequate with CAT or FT facilities. In addition to use as a probe in this way, phosphorus is of course found naturally in biological molecules, notably nucleic acids, phospholipids and vital nucleotide molecules such as ATP and cyclic AMP whose structure and interactions are of great interest.

2.7 Summary

An NMR spectrum results from the action of a radiofrequency radiation on atomic nuclei precessing in a magnetic field. The resultant spectrum is characterized by

(a) the position ('chemical shift') of the resonances, which is characteristic of the chemical group of which it is part,

(b) the area of the resonance, which is proportional to the number of nuclei giving rise to it,

(c) the multiplicity of the lines and the relative intensities of their components, which may be analysed in terms of their neighbouring nuclei,

(d) the linewidths of the resonances, which may give information about the mobility and rigidity of the molecule and binding of small molecules to macromolecules.

The original method of obtaining an NMR spectrum by slowly sweeping the frequency of the applied radiofrequency is being replaced by the pulsed Fourier-transform method which allows for a very much faster accumulation of data.

References

Bradbury, E. M., and Rattle, H. W. E. (1972). *Eur. J. Biochem.*, **27**, 270.
Brame, E. G. (1962). *Anal. Chem.*, **34**, 591.
Breitmaier, E., Jung, G., and Voelter, W. (1971). *Angew. Chemie*, **83**, 659.
Cohen, J. S., Schrager, R. I., McNeel, M., and Schechter, A. N. (1970). *Nature*, **228**, 642.
Dietrich, M. W. and Keller, R. E. (1964). *Anal. Chem.*, **36**, 258.
Dwek, R. A. (1973). *N.M.R. in Biochemistry: Applications to Enzyme Systems*, Clarendon Press, Oxford.
Johnson, C. E. and Bovey, F. A. (1958). *J. Chem. Phys.*, **29**, 1012.
Kopple, K. D., Wiley, C. R., and Tanski, R. (1973). *Biopolymers*, **12**, 627.
McDonald, C. C. and Phillips, W. D. (1967). *J. Amer. Chem. Soc.*, **89**, 6332.
Roberts, G. C. K. and Jardetzky, O. (1970). *Adv. Prot. Chem.*, **24**, 447.

Reading List

Bovey, F. A. (1969). *Nuclear Magnetic Resonance Spectroscopy*, Academic Press, New York.

Bovey, F. A. (1972). *High Resolution N.M.R. of Macromolecules*, Academic Press, New York and London.

Carrington, A. and McLachlan, A. D. (1967). *Introduction to magnetic resonance*, Harper International Edition, Harper and Row, New York and London.

Emsley, J. W., Feeney, J. and Sutcliffe, L. H. (1965). *High Resolution Nuclear Magnetic Resonance Spectroscopy*, Pergamon Press, Oxford.

Farrar, T. C. and Becker, E. D. (1971). *Pulse and Fourier Transform N.M.R.*, Academic Press, New York and London.

Jackman, L. M. and Sternhell, S. (1969). *Applications of Nuclear Magnetic Resonance Spectroscopy in Organic Chemistry*, Academic Press, New York.

Levy, G. C., and Nelson, G. L. (1972). *Carbon-13 NMR for Organic Chemists.* Wiley–Interscience, New York.

Pople, J. A., Schneider, W. G. and Bernstein, H. J. (1959). *High Resolution Nuclear Magnetic Resonance* McGraw-Hill Book Co., New York, Toronto and London.

Roberts, J. D. (1961). *An Introduction to the Analysis of Spin–Spin Splitting in High Resolution Nuclear Magnetic Resonance Spectra*, Benjamin, New York.

Chapter 3
Practical Biological NMR

3.1 Introduction

Nuclear magnetic resonance is a very flexible technique: it can be used to determine many different molecular parameters from the measurement of chemical shifts, intensities, linewidths and multiplicities, and from perturbations of all these resulting from changes of molecular environment. A consequence of this flexibility is that the way in which a spectrum is run must be matched to the parameters which it is desired to measure — the operator must have a very clear idea of what is required in the way of signal-to-noise, resolution, expansions of part of the spectrum and so forth. The aim of this chapter is to introduce the reader to the most important parameters which are under the control of the spectrometer operator, and also to describe the way in which practical spectrometers work in order to help in appreciating their potentialities and limitations. However, the first requirement of the potential user of NMR is to know the sample requirements for the technique, which are therefore outlined below.

3.2 Sample requirements

The standard 5 mm proton NMR sample tube holds about 0..4 ml of solution when filled to an appropriate level; this may be reduced to 0.2 ml by the use of a suitable filler plug. The concentration of sample required in this volume, assuming that it is not already limited by solubility problems, is dictated by the sensitivity of the spectrometer, including the availability of a signal-averaging device, and by the signal-to-noise ratio which is acceptable in the final spectrum. Clearly if the requirement is to observe the arginine peaks in a protamine sample (protamine is 80% arginine) a much lower concentration is acceptable than for the observation of, say, a single histidine C-2 proton in a large protein. As a rough general guide, an acceptable *single-scan* proton spectrum of a protein should be attainable using a concentration of 0.005 molar (5 millimolar). This is a very high concentration for molecules of high molecular weight and explains why effective protein NMR had to await the availability of CATs and latterly of Fourier-transform machines. Bearing in mind that signal-to-noise ratio may be improved by a factor of $\sqrt{N}$, where N is the number of scans accumulated, concentration may be reduced accordingly. A Fourier-transform facility may, for example, be used with 10,000 pulses to reduce the sample requirement by a factor of 100. In this case, a concentration of 0.05 millimolar would be acceptable – say 0.4 mg of a protein of molecular weight 20,000 dissolved in 0.4 ml of solvent. These figures may vary considerably from sample to sample and of course depend also on the amount of machine time available for running each spectrum (for example, the practical limit to the number of scans using a CAT is probably an overnight run of the order of 250–1000 accumulated spectra, giving similar results to those of the Fourier-transform spectrometer with 10,000 pulses in something like 1½ hours). They should be used only as a general first guide.

The requirements for ^{13}C samples are much more stringent; for natural-abundance ^{13}C spectroscopy the common tube sizes are 10–12 mm, and the 1.5 ml of sample contained therein should be at concentrations around 1 molar for a single-scan spectrum – acceptable for small molecules, but quite impossible for

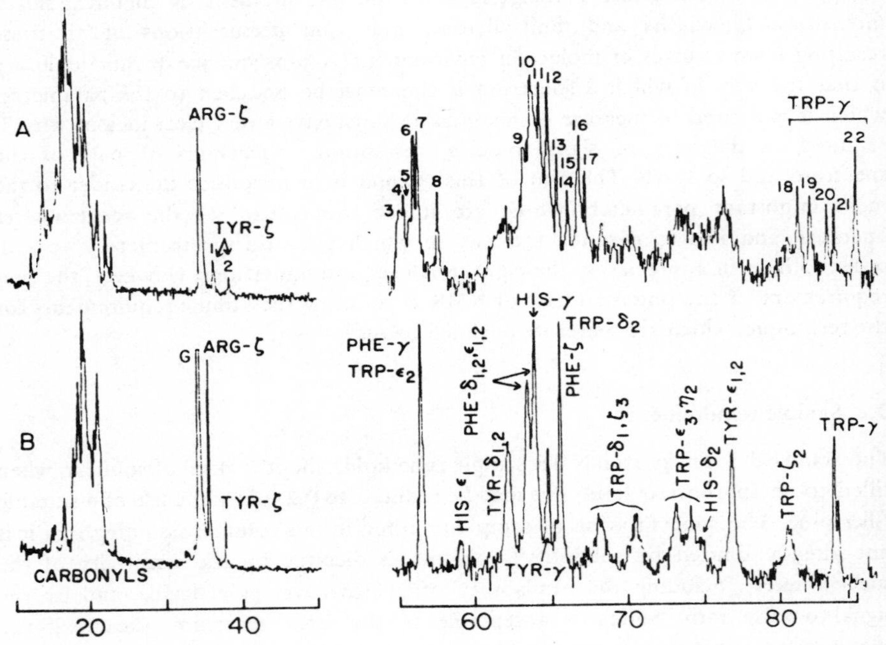

Figure 3.1 Unsaturated-carbon region in the proton-decoupled natural-abundance ^{13}C Fourier-transform NMR spectra of hen egg-white lysozyme (about 15 nM) at 15.18 MHz in a 20 mm sample tube, recorded with 1 Hz digital resolution, after 32,768 accumulations with a recycle time of 1.09 sec (9.9 hr total time). (A) Native lysozyme, in 0.1M NaCl, pH 4.0, 42 °C. Narrow aromatic carbon resonances, identified by noise-modulated off-resonance proton-decoupling (spectrum not shown), are numbered consecutively from left to right. (B) Guanidine denaturated lysozyme, in 0.1 M NaCl and 6.5 M guanidinium chloride, pH 3.9, 54 °C. Horizontal scale is in ppm upfield from CS_2. Assignments of non-protonated aromatic carbons are given with horizontal lettering. Assignments of aromatic methine carbons are shown vertically. Standard IUPAC–IUB designations for amino acid carbons are used. Peak G is the resonance of the guanidinium ion. (From Allerhand *et al.*, 1973. Reproduced by permission of the New York Academy of Sciences)

larger ones such as proteins. Using Fourier-transform techniques, 0.01 molar is an acceptable lower limit, a usable spectrum taking perhaps 12 hours to obtain. Even this is a considerable concentration – 100 mg/ml for a protein of 10,000 daltons molecular weight. Figure 3.1 shows parts of the spectrum obtained in 10 hours for lysozyme at 15 mM concentration in a 20 mm tube. Signal-to-noise is acceptable right down to single carbon atoms, but this spectrum obtained using a 'home- built' spectrometer probably represents the best obtainable anywhere at the time of writing.

In all cases it is possible, though inconvenient, to reduce the sample volume by a factor of about 10 by using microcells. Further details on sample preparation and referencing are in Section 3.4.

3.3 The NMR spectrometer

Figure 3.2 shows simplified block diagrams of continuous-wave and Fourier-transform spectrometers. Commercial realizations of these basic layouts are illustrated in Figure 3.3, which shows a continuous-wave spectrometer and its associated CAT, and in Figures 3.4 and 3.5, which show 270 MHz proton and 20 MHz ^{13}C spectrometers respectively. The following sections describe the subunits of the spectrometer separately.

The magnet

The primary requirements for a magnet for high-resolution NMR use are that it should provide a high field of good homogeneity and long-term stability. Homogeneity is the term used to denote the variation in magnetic field across the volume occupied by the sample, and is usually quoted as 'resolution', in terms of the best resolution obtainable on a sample, either in parts in 10^9 or directly as the width of a theoretically infinite sharp line produced by the spectrometer. A typical specification for resolution would be worded as '3 parts in 10^9 (0.3 Hz at 100 MHz)'. Magnets cannot be produced with an intrinsic field homogeneity of better than about 1 part in 10^7; the required improvement is brought about by the use of 'shim coils' (otherwise known as Golay coils) and of sample spinning. Shim coils are flat or printed circuit coils of various shapes attached to the pole faces of the magnet; the current through them is controlled by a set of multiturn potentiometers on the console of the spectrometer. By successive alteration of these controls and continuous observation of a reference signal, the resolution may be improved to the required value; usually most of the coils are set up only occasionally, leaving one or two which need to be adjusted for each sample. Even the use of shim coils leaves some inhomogeneities, which can at least partially be overcome by spinning the sample. Just as the rapid tumbling of molecules can average out the local magnetic inhomogeneities due to neighbouring molecules through regions of differing magnetic fields due to the inhomogeneities of the magnet, will average out the inhomogeneities. Figure 3.6 shows the proton spectrum of lysine obtained from a non-spinning sample and from spinning samples

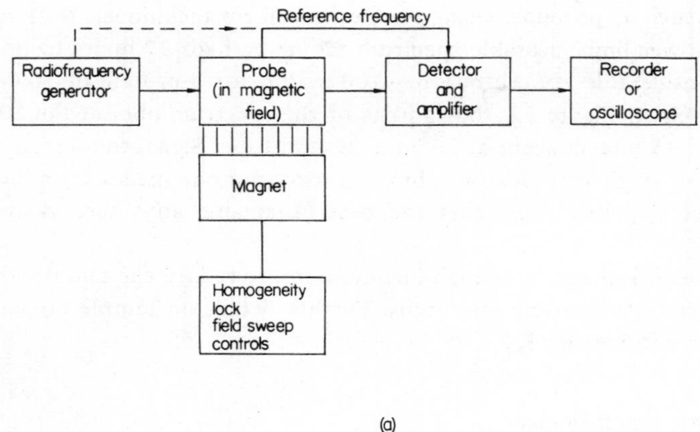

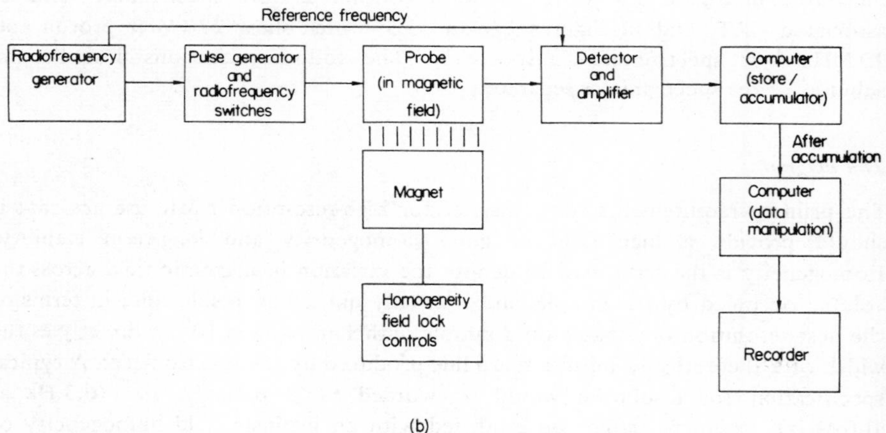

Figure 3.2(a) Block diagram of continuous-wave NMR spectrometer

Figure 3.2(b) Block diagram of pulse-Fourier transform NMR spectrometer

with various degrees of maladjustment of the shim coils. As with improvements to most things, sample spinning carried with it a penalty. In this case it is the production of 'spinning sidebands': small peaks distributed on each side of each peak of the spectrum and separated from it by the frequency of sample spinning. As Figure 3.6 shows, these sidebands may be reduced considerably by correct shimming, but it is rarely possible to eliminate them completely. Sidebands are not often a problem in biological NMR except when samples have to be run in a solvent which itself gives a large NMR peak; in this case the sidebands of the solvent peak may mean the loss of more spectrum than indicated simply by the width of the

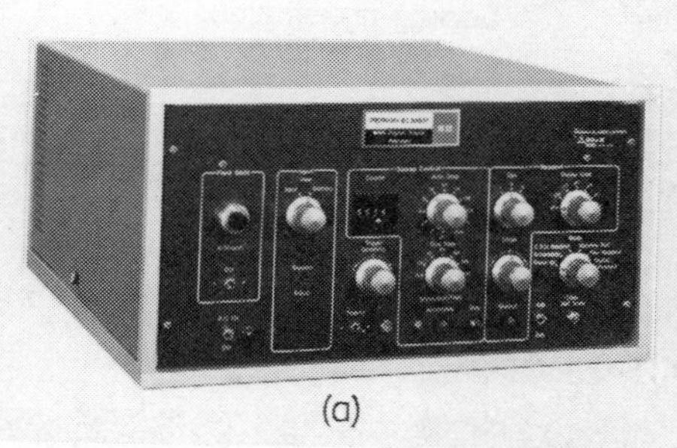

(a)

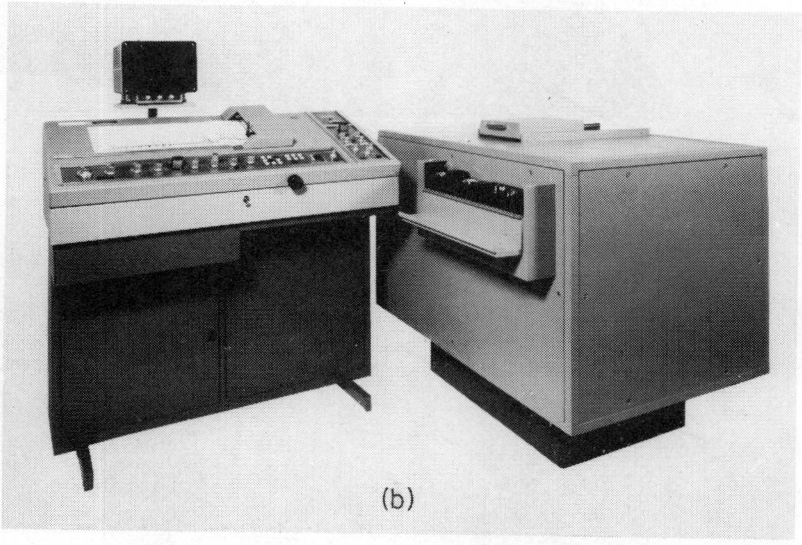

(b)

Figure 3.3(a) A Perkin–Elmer digital signal averager (CAT)

Figure 3.4(b) The Perkin–Elmer R32 90 MHz continuous-wave proton spectrometer

solvent peak itself. If it is suspected that a peak in a spectrum is a sideband, its nature may be determined (a) by checking whether there is an identical peak on the other side of the nearby 'real' peaks and (b) by seeing whether its position alters when the sample spinning rate is changed. Typical sample spinning speeds are in the region of 1000 rpm, and spinning is almost invariably brought about by a small turbine rotor slipped over the sample tube, which is then rotated by a jet of compressed air. The rate of flow of the air, and hence the spinning rate, is usually controlled by a valve on the spectrometer console.

Second only to resolution in importance is the stability over time of the field

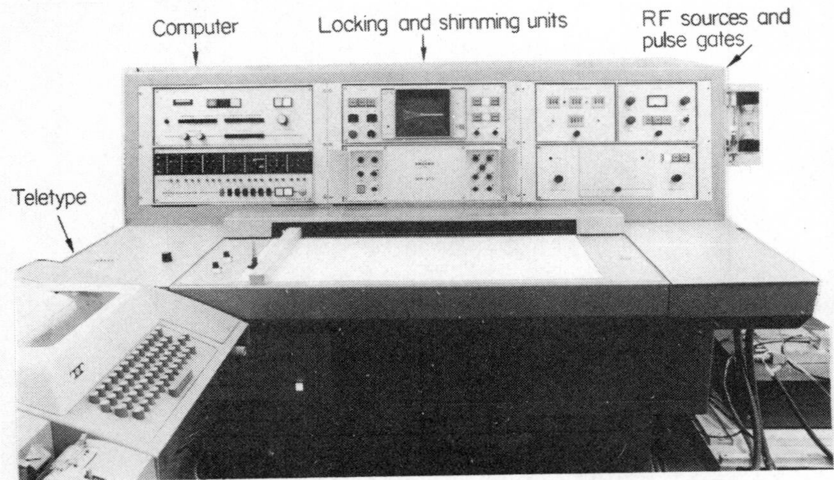

Figure 3.4 Bruker WH-270 270 MHz Fourier-transform spectrometer

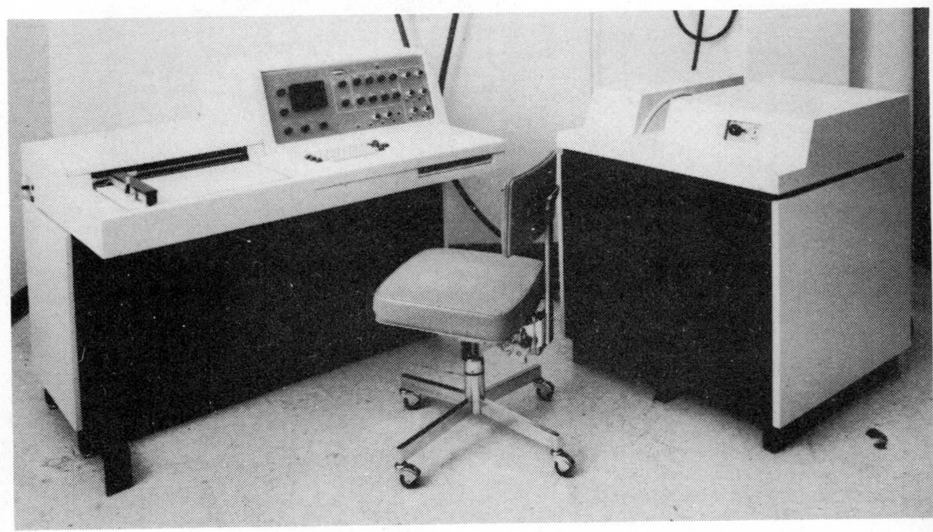

Figure 3.5 The Varian CFT-20 ^{13}C pulse spectrometer

produced by the magnet. This depends on the type of magnet under consideration, and may in general be divided into two parts: effects within the magnet system, such as variation in temperature or in the driving current of an electromagnet, and effects external to the magnet such as the movement of nearby masses of metal (it was at one time advised that the operator of a certain spectrometer removed keys from his pocket before using it!). These will be discussed further under the heading of individual magnetic types.

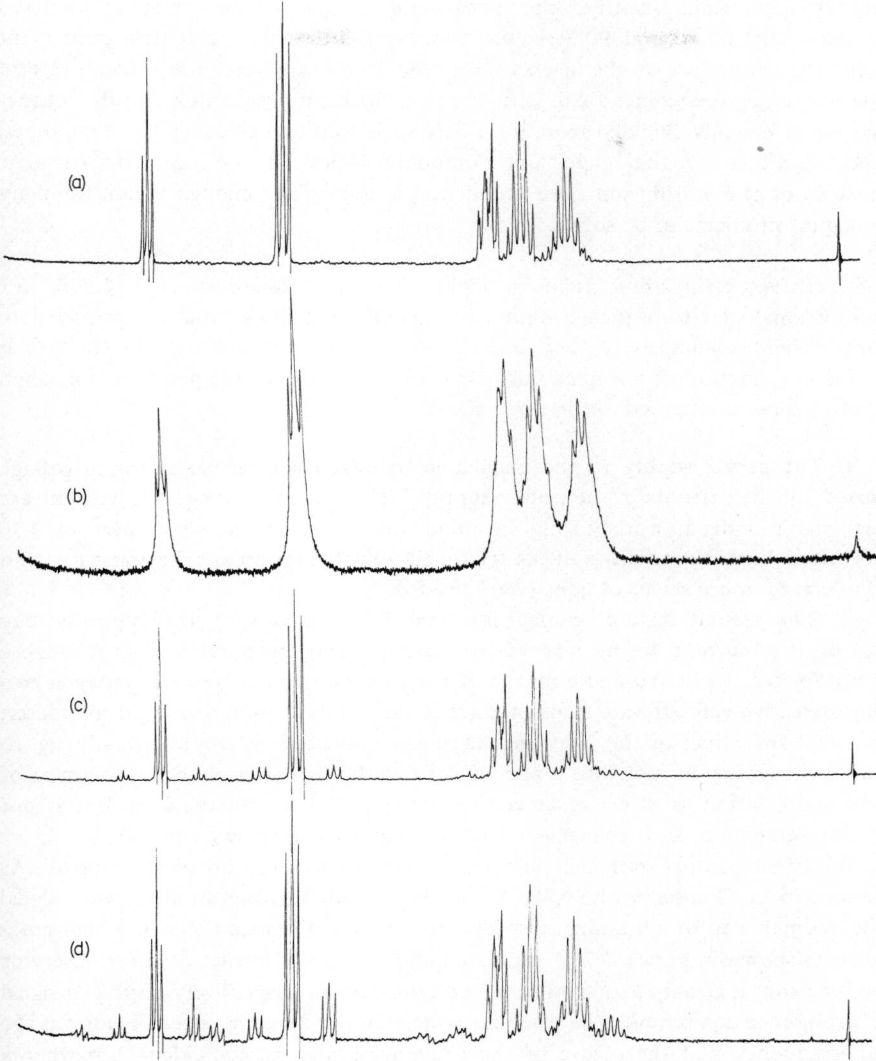

Figure 3.6 Spectra of lysine showing the effects of shimming. (a) Correct shimming, (b) non-spinning, (c) first-order transverse shim coils poorly adjusted, (d) first and second transverse shim coils poorly adjusted

Permanent magnets. The obvious advantage of a permanent magnet is that, being independent of an external power source, it is freed from bulky external equipment, large electricity bills and a major source of unwanted magnet field variation. Against this must be placed the fact that the useful field obtainable from a permanent magnet appears to be limited to about 2.3 tesla (corresponding to about 100 MHz for protons) and that even this is only obtainable over a restricted magnet gap. Consequently, the permanent magnet is at present restricted commercially to 60 and 90 MHz spectrometers, although a 100 MHz permanent magnet machine was on the market for a time. In this application it is ideal: careful thermostatting overcomes field drift due to temperature variations, and the magnet may be effectively shielded from local field variations by enclosing it in a mu-metal box. Machines of this type are commonly found in chemistry departments throughout the world, and their frequency is quite high enough to enable many biological problems to be solved.

Electromagnets. For field strengths in the region of 2.3–2.5 T, the conventional electromagnet is universally employed. Shim coils are provided to control field homogeneity, but control of the overall magnetic field strength is perforce a much more complex business than is the case for the permanent magnet. Control is usually carried out in three stages.

(i) The power supply to the magnet is stabilized against variations in voltage caused by fluctuations in the public supply. The resultant voltage and current are very stable indeed, but bearing in mind that fluctuations of 1 part in 10^9 (corresponding to a variation of 0.4 μV on a 400 volt supply) are the worst that can be tolerated, more stages of control are needed.

(ii) The second stage of control is a feedback mechanism which typically may measure the current at the magnet by passing a tiny proportion of it through a galvanometer. Light from the mirror of the galvanometer is beamed between two photosensitive cells. If variations in current cause a deflection of the galvanometer, the resultant effect of the light on one of the photocells is amplified and used to feed a correcting current into a pair of coils at the magnet pole face. This type of field stabilization is effective at coping with rapid field fluctuations, but is not sensitive enough to slow changes or drifts to enable them to be dealt with.

(iii) Final control over the field is effected by a 'lock' or 'NMR control'. As mentioned in Chapter 1, the NMR signal may be obtained as an absorption signal (the normal way of obtaining a spectrum) or as a dispersion signal, which has a shape as shown in Figure 3.7. A separate radio frequency to that used for observing the spectrum is arranged so as to be at the centre of the dispersively displayed signal of a reference compound. The resultant voltage in the detector is zero as long as the radiofrequency and the centre of the reference peaks are coincident, but when a change in the magnetic field causes a shift in the Larmor frequency of the reference material (dotted line in Figure 3.7) a voltage is produced which, amplified, may be used to return the signal to its central position by suitable alterations in the field strength. If the spectrum is being recorded in the frequency-swept mode, i.e. at constant field, the observing frequency may be constant, but if a field-swept mode is in use, then the reference observing RF must be altered in step with the main magnetic field so as to remain coincident with the reference signal.

The locking of a magnetic field may be either 'internal' or 'external'. In the former case, the reference compound is dissolved in the sample under observation, where it is usually required that it be the largest signal in the spectrum. Any

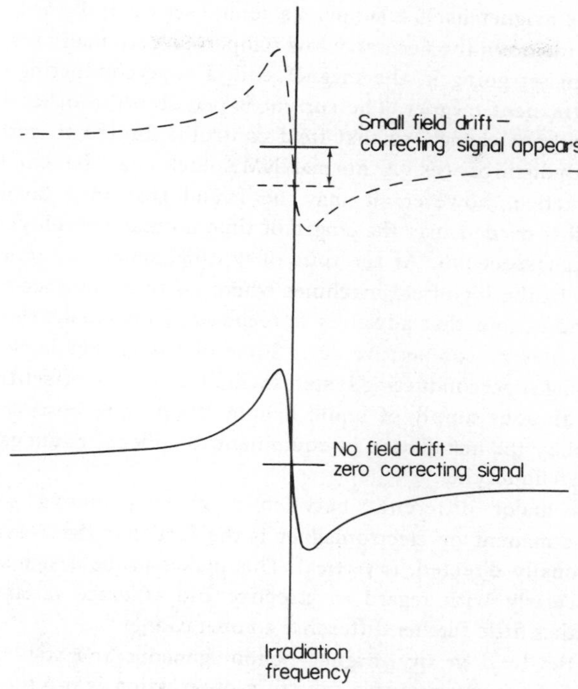

Figure 3.7 Field locking by use of dispersive mode signal

reference may be used, provided it has a single sharp peak, but the method has particular disadvantages when applied to biological samples. These usually lack any large sharp peak suitable for locking (concentrations are usually too low to allow of large signals at all) and the adulteration of the sample by reference compounds is usually undesirable. The problem may be overcome by the use of a concentric tube to hold the reference. More recently, the use of deuterium in the sample has become the method of choice for locking; most biological samples are dissolved in D_2O in any case.

External locking, as its name suggests, is field locking onto a reference which is not dissolved in the sample, but is contained in a separate tube, elsewhere in the magnet gap, with its own detector coil, bridge etc. This has the obvious advantage of being completely independent of the sample itself; to counter this is the fact that external locking is very slightly less effective at correcting varying fields at the sample.

An electromagnet stabilized and locked as described above should drift less than 0.2 Hz/hr.

Superconducting magnets. For the very high fields required for proton operating frequencies significantly above 100 MHz, only superconducting magnets are suitable. The magnet itself is simply a solenoid set vertically and surrounded by dewar flasks to maintain the necessary low temperature. In many respects, once the current has been set going in the magnet coil, a superconducting magnet is very similar to a permanent magnet. The current is persistent; in other words, it flows continuously without change, so that field control is limited to correcting for the effects of local disturbances. A normal NMR lock may be employed for this purpose; in practice, however, it may be found that in a favourable site no correction at all is needed over the length of time normally employed in running at least a single-scan spectrum. At the time of writing, superconducting magnets are limited by cost to the high-field machines where no other magnet can do the job, but there are indications that advances in technology may make them available for the lower fields at very competitive cost. Some of the savings in electricity supply obtained by using superconducting systems will of course be offset by the necessity to obtain a continuous supply of liquid helium; the running costs thereby incurred may be reduced by the installation of equipment to collect helium gas so that it can be returned for reliquefying.

An obvious major difference between a superconducting solenoid and a conventional permanent or electromagnet is the fact that the *Z*-axis, along which H_0 is conventionally directed, is vertical. This makes probe design somewhat more difficult, particularly with regard to effective and accurate variable temperature control, but makes little further difference to operation.

Given that the field in any magnet is homogeneous and stable, the necessary sweep of field for continuous-wave spectrum observation is produced by a pair of coils mounted on the pole-faces. The current through these coils is normally linked to the recorder pen or to the oscilloscope, so that the field is swept in precise step with the movement of the recording device, thus ensuring a repeatable spectrum. The amount by which the current in the sweep coils varies over the total pen travel is variable, so that the total width of the sweep may be chosen – a 'normal' sweep width for protons would be 10 ppm, corresponding to 1000 Hz at 100 MHz, while the range of sweeps selected for special purposes may vary from 0.5 ppm (50 Hz for the whole recorder span) to 200 ppm (20,000 Hz).

The probe

The probe is the part of the spectrometer which holds the sample tube and the radiofrequency coils. It also allows for spinning and temperature variation of the sample, and usually accommodates the first stages of signal detection, which are situated as close as possible to the sample coils in order to minimize the risk of picking up unwanted signals. The standard size of sample tube is 5 mm outside diameter, but 8 mm, 10 mm, 12 mm and even 15 mm probes are becoming available for use with dilute solution or samples where for other reasons very little signal is available, e.g. for natural abundance ^{13}C spectroscopy.

Single-coil probes. A single-coil probe is shown schematically in Figure 3.8. Such probes have the components of a detecting bridge incorporated, and two

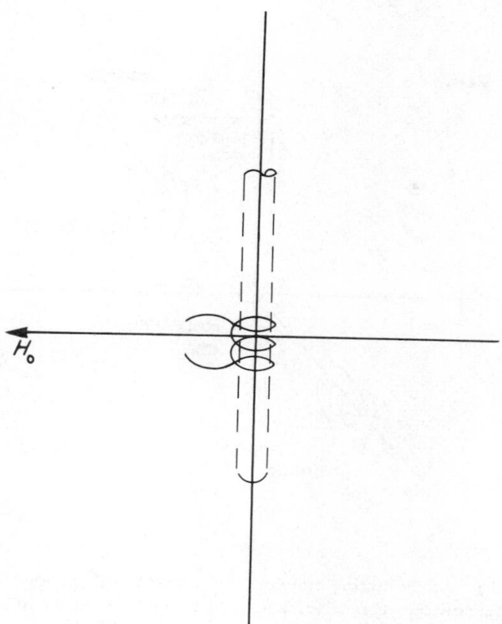

Figure 3.8 Positioning of transmitter/receiver coil in a single-coil probe. In superconducting magnets the field H_0 is in the vertical direction

controls for balancing the bridge are usually found on the probe; these are used in conjunction with a balance meter mounted on the console to ensure that the bridge is fully balanced each time a fresh sample is placed in the probe. This is necessary since the impedance of the single coil, which acts as the indicator of NMR absorption, is also sensitive to the precise magnetic nature of the sample – effects due to changing the sample must therefore be cancelled out by balancing the bridge before running the spectrum.

Crossed-coil probe. A schematic drawing of a crossed-coil probe is shown in Figure 3.9. The major apparent difference apart from the coils is that there is no bridge, the probe instead housing a preamplifier to amplify the extremely small signals from the receiver coil at the earliest possible stage. Normally no allowance need be made for the varying magnetic properties of different samples, although these do of course affect the coils. In exceptional cases, perhaps when high concentrations of metallic salts are present in the sample, the effects on the coil must be balanced out, a single control being provided for the purpose. A photograph of a crossed-coil probe is shown as Figure 3.10.

It is desirable, and indeed necessary, that some of the signal from the transmitter coil passes directly into the receiver coil in order to provide a reference for both the intensity and the phase of the received NMR signals. Such a 'leakage' is provided by

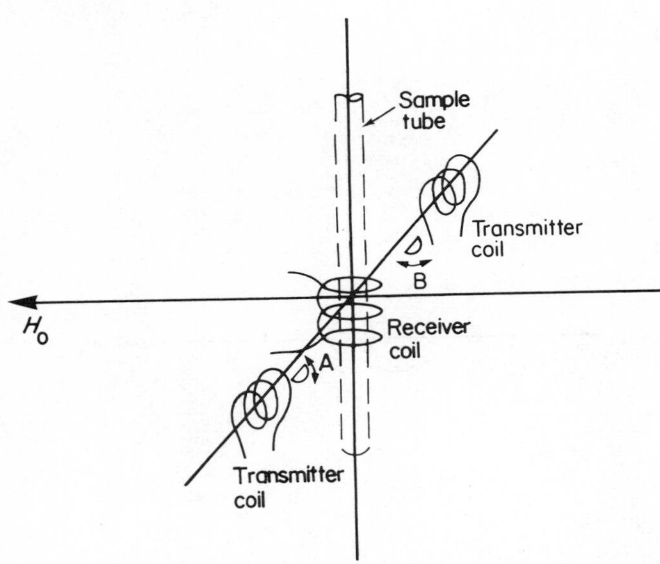

Figure 3.9 Schematic drawing of crossed-coil probe. Leakage from transmitter to receiver coils can be controlled by 'paddles' A and B

a suitable arrangement of the coils relative to each other, and controlled by fine manipulation of small metal 'paddles' which are used to deflect the course of the radiofrequency radiation until the correct amount of leakage flux is obtained.

The probe, whether single or crossed-coil, is mounted between the magnet poles. On some spectrometers, it is rigidly fixed in place; on others, the probe is withdrawn each time the sample tube is changed, and may be mounted on an adjustable holder which enables it to be placed in the most homogeneous part of the field. Other machines incorporate an automatic sample-loading device which places the sample into the probe in the correct, gentle manner each time; this eliminates the risk of breaking off a sample tube in the probe – very easy to do with careless handling of the thin-walled glass sample tubes, and usually entailing a complete stripdown of the probe to remove solvent, sample and pieces of broken glass from the probe.

All current spectrometers incorporate sample spinning by means of a small turbine rotor slipped onto the sample tube; most ensure even spinning by supporting the spinning tube on air-lubricated bearings. This enables a slightly unbalanced tube to rotate about its own centre of mass, thus minimizing mechanical vibration effects and spinning sidebands.

Radiofrequency generation and detection

Clearly the frequency of irradiation of the sample must be stabilized to the same extent as the magnetic field; this is usually achieved by basing the frequency on an

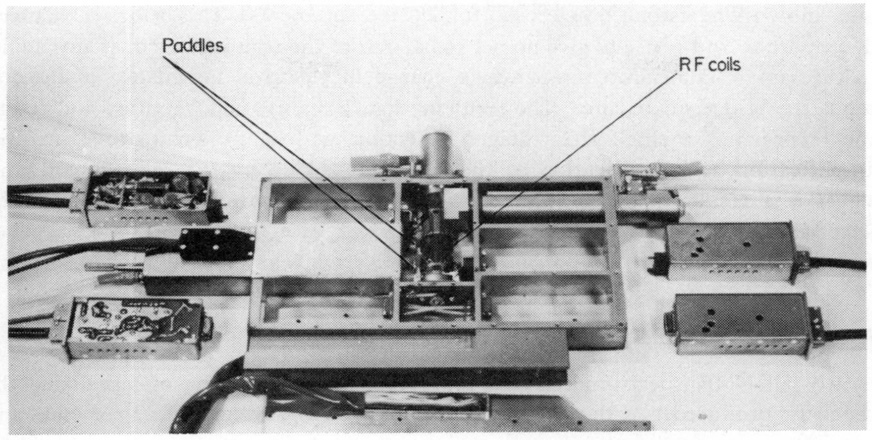

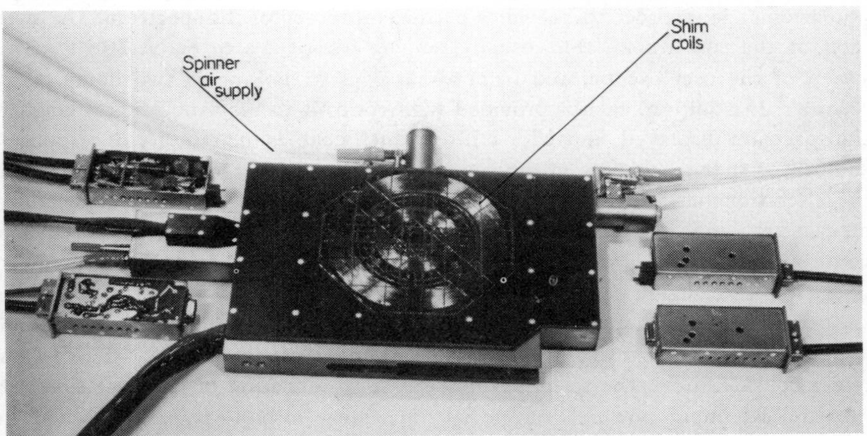

Figure 3.10 A JEOL Crossed-coil probe

oscillating crystal, which is a very stable source of radiofrequency alternating voltage provided that it is maintained at a constant temperature. Good crystal oscillators may be built at frequencies of a few MHz, so the higher frequencies needed for most NMR spectrometers are obtained by electronic multiplication of the crystal frequencies. After amplification, the radiofrequency is usually modulated for use in a CW spectrometer by the addition to it of a lower frequency of a few thousand Hz before passing it into the probe: this is done because in the later stages of amplification and detection of the signal, the main frequency may be subtracted from the combination, leaving the lower frequency upon which these operations may be performed with greater ease.

The detection of the signal caused by the sample in the probe coil differs slightly according to whether a single-coil or crossed-coil probe is used. For the single coils the coil itself is made into one arm of a radiofrequency bridge (analogous to the well-known Wheatstone bridge used for DC measurements). This bridge is balanced in amplitude and phase to give no net signal before the scan is started; as any nuclei in the sample come into resonance, a change in electrical impedance of the coil sends the bridge off balance. The resultant signal is amplified, rectified and fed to the recorder as a small DC voltage. Detection with a cross-coil probe involves amplification and rectification of the signal picked up by the receiver coil; this signal is a result of the motion of the M_{xy} magnetization in the sample. The necessary phase information is obtained in this case by allowing a leakage of radiofrequency direct from transmitter to receiver coil as already described.

Recorders (continuous-wave spectrometers)

Nearly all NMR spectrometers are provided with two means of visualizing the spectrum produced: a cathode-ray oscilloscope which provides a means of rapid and continuous sweeping over all or part of the spectrum for setting-up purposes, and a potentiometric recorder to provide a permanent record of the spectrum. The sweep rates of the two are variable, usually ranging from 0.5 s to about 20 s for a full sweep of the oscilloscope, and from about 30 s to as long as two hours for the recorder. In addition, each is provided with controls to vary the vertical height of the spectrum displayed, and with a filter which enables the rapidity of response to the pen or spot to changes in the spectrum to be varied. This latter is achieved by the alteration of the 'time constant' of a small additional circuit in the pen-drive mechanism, and is extremely useful in minimizing the effects of noise. Time constant is usually expressed in seconds or milliseconds, and response in the inverse unit, the Hz. Figure 3.11 shows the effects of different response times on a spectrum. All of the spectra were run at the same speed, and the response times used are (a) about right, (c) too long and (d) unnecessarily short for the spectrum under consideration. The selection of the best combination of response time, scan rate and RF input power is of special importance in biological NMR, where low signal strength is frequently a problem; it will be dealt with after the next section.

Fourier-transform spectrometers

The requirements for a FT spectrometer are, in general, very similar to those of a conventional one, with the addition of the necessary radiofrequency switches and pulse programmer to produce the pulse. It is of great importance that the radiofrequency amplifiers are powerful enough to give a 90° pulse of short duration; long pulses tend to produce some distortions in the spectrum because relaxation processes are well under way before the end of the pulse. It is also a great advantage for the magnetic field locking to be heteronuclear so that the radiofrequencies used for locking purposes are different from those used for spectra. Most current FT spectrometers have magnets locked on the resonance signal of deuterium. An additional radiofrequency channel will also be needed for decoupling experiments, either homonuclear or heteronuclear.

The central frequency of the pulse is normally placed at one end of the spectral

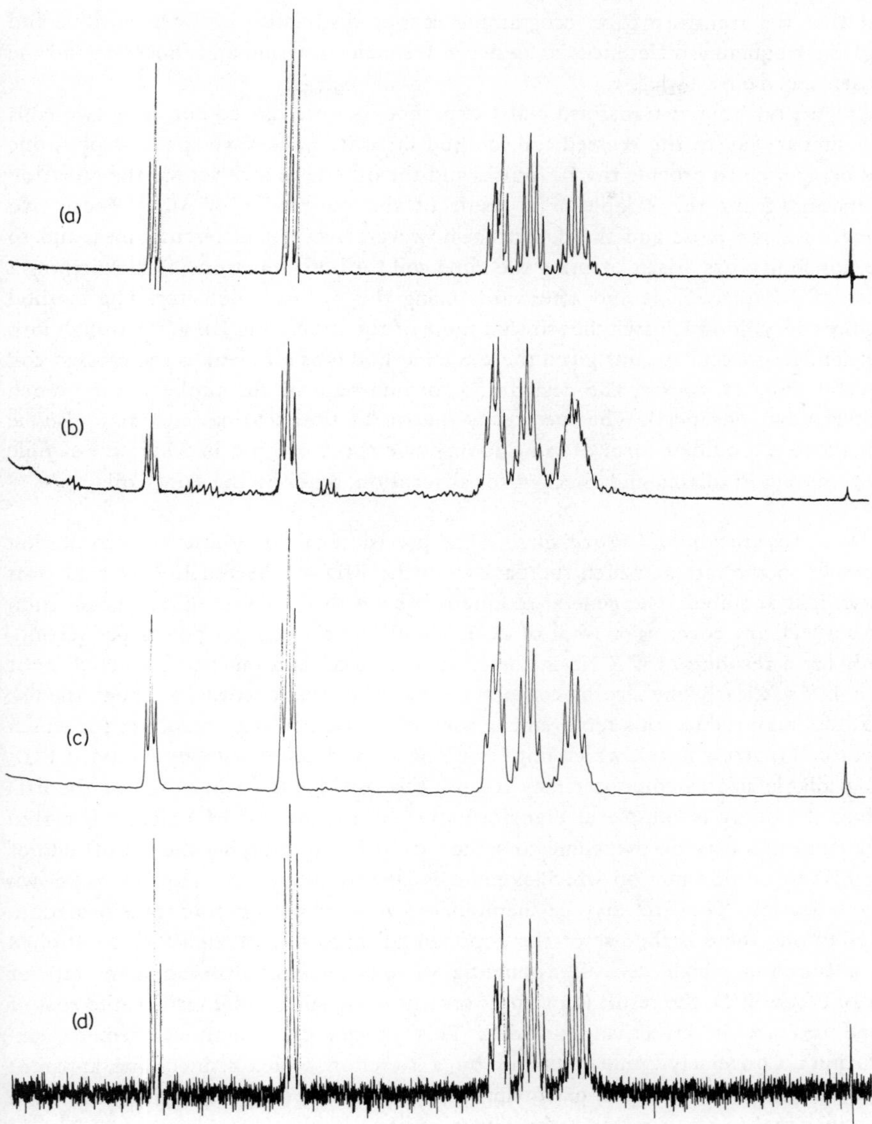

Figure 3.11 Spectrum of lysine, showing the effect of RF level and filters in a continuous-wave spectrometer. (a) Correct, (b) too much RF power, (c) too long time constant (filter frequency too low), (d) too short time constant (filter frequency too high)

range to be measured; this avoids difficulties due to 'folding back', a phenomenon which appears if the irradiation is within the spectral range and which is due to the fact that the transformation programme cannot distinguish between positive and negative frequency differences or between resonances within and those beyond the chosen spectrum width.

Originally, Fourier-transform NMR experiments were carried out using two coils in a similar way to the crossed-coil method in continuous-wave spectroscopy, one coil being used to provide the RF pulses and the other as a receiver for the radiation emanating from the sample as a result of the movement of M_{xy}. These two operations, the pulse and the detection, however, occur at different times, and so the possibility has arisen of using the same coil for both functions, first switching a pulse of RF through it and afterwards using the coil as a detector. The method requires very good RF switches so that none of the irradiating RF gets through into the detecting circuitry, but given these the method is as efficient as the crossed-coil method and, of course, the design and manufacture of the probe is very much simpler (and cheaper!). The method is known as time-sharing, and may also be applied to a modified form of continuous-wave spectroscopy, in which the sample is alternately irradiated and checked for absorption, again by the same coil.

Data Acquisition and Processing. The precision of the Fourier transformation depends on the rate at which the data from the FID is collected and the time over which it is acquired. The general requirements are that the rate of data acquisition for a spectrum covering a total of Δ Hz should be at least 2Δ points per second, while for a resolution of R Hz in the final spectrum, data must be collected for at least $1/R$ s. Clearly the size of computer required is $2\Delta/R$ words, although the use of filters may reduce this requirement somewhat. Particularly in spectra for which R is small (narrow lines), which implies a long T_2 and hence a slowly decaying FID, the available size of computer may require the cutting-off (truncating) of the FID before the decay is complete. Transformation of a truncated FID gives a distorted spectrum; this may be overcome to some extent by multiplying the cut-off end of the FID by some function which slopes more gently to zero. This process is known as apodization. The FID may be manipulated in other ways before transformation; chief among these is the use of the exponential multiplier. If the FID is multiplied by a function which decays exponentially, thus increasing the apparent rate of decay of the FID, the result is an improvement in signal-to-noise ratio at the cost of some increase in effective linewidth. This process is sometimes termed 'convolution'. Conversely, multiplication by a function which reduces the apparent decay rate gives an artificial narrowing of the lines and increase in resolution, at a cost in signal-to-noise ratio. An example of the effect and its results are given in Figures 3.12 and 3.13.

After transformation, both the absorption and dispersion mode spectra are available. Usually these are mixed somewhat, a situation similar to that when a conventional spectrometer has its phase control badly adjusted, except that the phase error may vary linearly through the spectrum. Phase correction must then be applied to produce the pure absorption spectrum. The computers supplied with FT

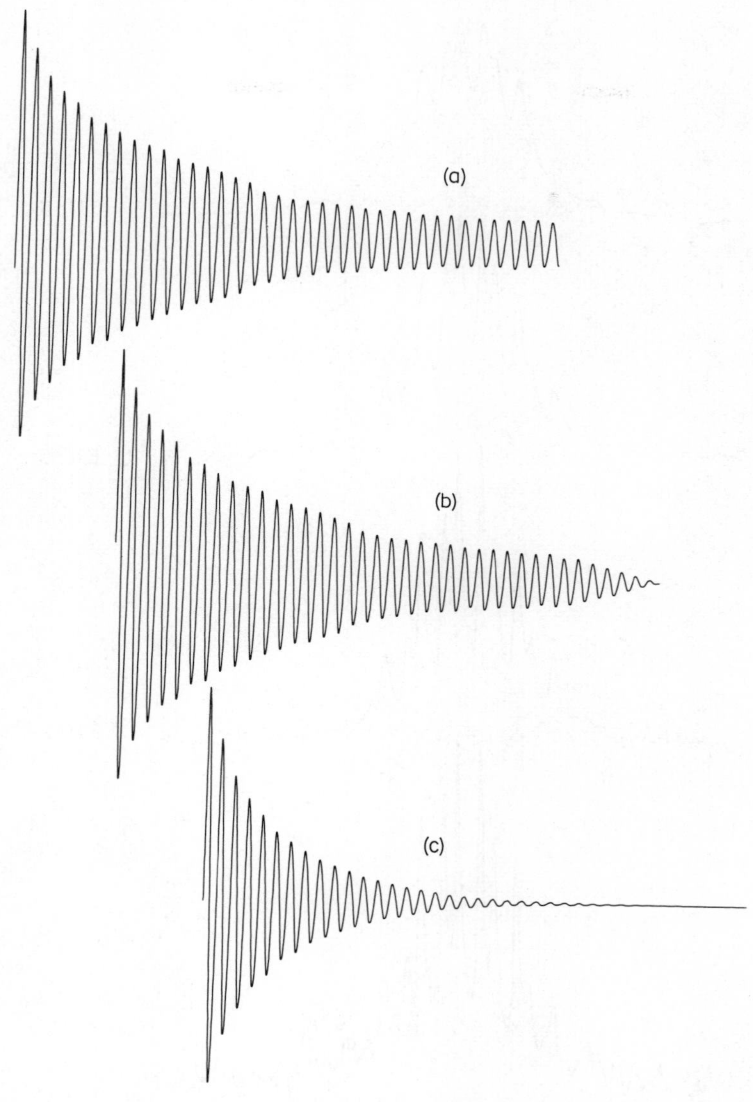

Figure 3.12 (a) A simple single-resonance FID as accumulated in truncated form, (b) after apodization, (c) after exponential multiplication by a negative exponential (convolution)

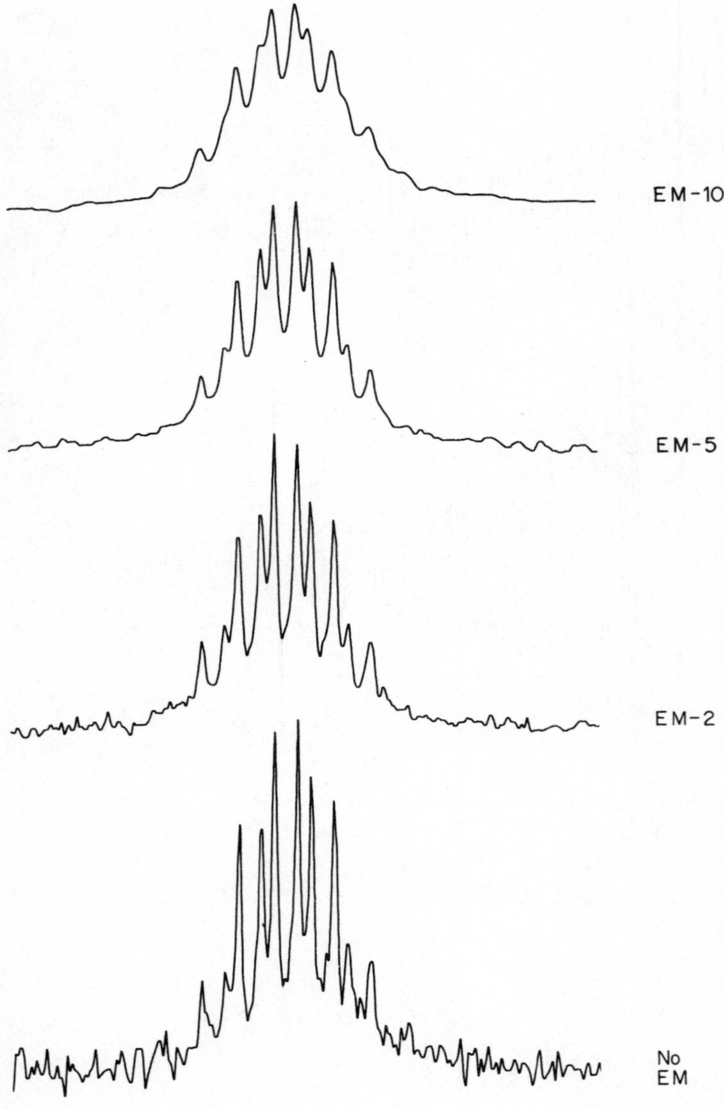

Figure 3.13 α-CH resonance of alanine, showing improvement in signal-to-noise ratio coupled with loss of resolution using different exponential multipliers

spectrometers usually require only single commands to perform such processes as exponential multiplication, apodization, Fourier transformation, phase correction, baseline correction, selection of data for recording, integration and so forth.

3.4 Practical spectrometer operation

The precise details of operation of any particular spectrometer, with details of the locations of the various controls, is of course the province of the instruction manual rather than this book, but there are some general observations which may be made on the choice of parameters which will be common to all machines and which may be helpful. This section is intended to help the molecular biologist to get the best from his samples, particularly when the machine is being operated by someone else.

Continuous-wave spectrometers

(1) If the whole spectral region is not to be run, select the appropriate scale expansion and the region to be scanned. If calibrated paper is being used ensure that any reference peak is appropriately placed. Ensure that any magnetic field lock is operating.

(2) If not already checked, set up the resolution (magnetic field homogeneity). With a spinning sample, this usually involves the successive operation of two shim-coil controls.

(3) Select the appropriate combination of RF power, scan speed and response (time constant). Experience plays a large part here, but one or two pointers may help. Scan speed may be selected first; this will vary with the sharpness of the lines in the spectrum, but typically may be five minutes for a single scan spectrum with broad lines, up to 20 minutes for sharp lines. Rather faster scan speeds may be used if CAT accumulation is required; scan times of about a minute are permissible for proton spectra with broad lines. Next the RF level may be selected: this may be optimized by increasing RF power until signs of saturation appear in the spectrum (i.e. an increase in RF produces no corresponding increase or even a decrease in the height of the sharpest signals in the spectrum; or running the spectrum at a slower speed causes a slight reduction in the height of the sharpest peak), and then reducing the RF one or two steps from this value. The effects of too high a value of RF are shown in Figure 3.11; note the loss of height in the signals and the degradation of resolution. Surprisingly high RF levels may be found to be acceptable for biological molecules with broad lines (short relaxation times), and time spent on careful selection of the appropriate maximum RF level is well repaid in maximum signal-to-noise ratio. Finally, response or time-constant is chosen by trial and error so that noise is minimized without visible distortion of the spectrum. Examples of various values of response or time constant are also given in Figure 3.11.

(4) Adjust phase control. The detector of a CW NMR spectrometer allows detection of signals in the absorptive or dispersive modes or a combination of both. It is very important to ensure that your spectrum is exactly absorptive, especially

when there is a large solvent peak in the spectrum. With a CW spectrometer, there is nothing that can be done about phase after the spectrum has been run, which is especially annoying in the case of long CAT runs.

(5) A single scan should then show whether all is well, and if a CAT is to be used, will enable a selection of the number of sweeps likely to be required to obtain the desired signal-to-noise ratio.

Fourier-transform Spectrometers

The parameters under the operator's control are rather different on a pulse spectrometer, and a rather different approach is needed since at least some of the processes are carried out after the accumulation of the data. After checking that lock and resolution are satisfactory, the main parameters to consider are:

(a) *Position of centre of pulse relative to spectrum frequency.* This should be arranged so that the pulse frequency spread adequately covers the whole spectrum width, while the central pulse frequency itself is clear of the spectrum to avoid any possibility of 'folding back'.

As already indicated, the main pulse frequency is the centre of a spread of frequencies wide enough to encompass all the spectrum resonance frequencies. After the pulse, all these frequencies are found in the FID, and the position of each in the spectrum is expressed relative to the main pulse frequency. The way in which this is done relies on the *difference* between the central pulse frequency and the resonance frequencies, but there is no way of telling whether this difference is positive or negative. The assumption is therefore made that they are all of the same sign, and the spectrum computed accordingly. However, if resonances are in fact on both sides of the central pulse frequency, this assumption means that a peak, say 1000 Hz downfield of the pulse frequency, while all the others are upfield, will be plotted as if it were 1000 Hz upfield – an effect analogous to folding the spectrum back about the pulse frequency. Thus the pulse frequency should always be selected to be one side of all the peaks in the spectrum. Further, if the spectrum width chosen is not adequate to cover all the resonances in the spectrum, those beyond the end of the chosen width will also be folded back into the main part of the spectrum.

(b) *RF pulse intensity and length* is of relatively little concern unless a specific pulse, i.e. a 90° or 180°, pulse is required. Most pulse spectrometers in normal use produce a 30°–60° pulse.

(c) *Dwell time.* The length of time taken to accumulate a single FID is governed by the number of memory channels used to store it and by the length of time spent in sampling the signal for each channel, which is known as the dwell time. The choice of these parameters is primarily governed by the requirements already stated, firstly that for a spectrum of width Δ Hz, data must be accumulated at 2Δ points per second or faster, which means that dwell time must be equal to or less than $1/2\Delta$ seconds, and secondly that for a resolution of R Hz, data must be collected for at least $1/R$ s. If after satisfying these requirements it is found that

$1/R$ s is shorter than four or five times the T_1 of the sample, so that application of the next pulse immediately after the end of accumulation would find the sample incompletely relaxed, a waiting time should be allowed before the next pulse. This point bears watching particularly if it is suspected that some lines in the spectrum may be sharper than the others – for example the histidine C-2 and C-4 resonances in some proteins. A pulse repetition rate which is acceptable for the rest of the spectrum may be too rapid for such resonances which will therefore appear reduced in area.

(d) *Delay time and phase problems in FT spectroscopy.* When the applied RF pulse is switched off at its end, a finite time elapses before all traces of it disappear from the probe circuits. Consequently a delay time must be left before data acquisition is started, otherwise some of the pulse would break through into the accumulated data with resulting spectrum distortions. This delay time, usually of the same order as the dwell time, leads to some problems. In particular, if all of the precessing groups of nuclei are in phase at the end of the pulse, by the time data acquisition starts they will all be out of phase with each other as well as with the irradiating RF which is used in continuous form in the detector circuitry. To take a simple example: suppose the delay time to be 100 μs. A sharp resonance which is 1000 Hz from the irradiating frequency, and which therefore appears in the FID as a 1000 Hz sine wave, will have advanced one-tenth of a cycle during the delay time, i.e. is 36° out of phase with the measuring frequency when data acquisition starts. This is readily corrected, of course, but a resonance 2000 Hz from the main RF will have advanced 2/10 of a cycle, or 72°, during the same time. Thus a phase correction will be required which is frequency dependent and varies from one end of the spectrum to the other. Note, too, that particularly if the spectrum width is large, so that peaks far from the main RF appear as high frequencies in the FID, phase corrections may vary by more than 360° from one end of the spectrum to the other. So we must apply two phase corrections to a Fourier-transformed spectrum: a frequency dependent correction which ensures that all the peaks have the same phase, and another to ensure that this phase corresponds to the absorption mode. Figure 3.14 shows spectra with both frequency dependent and frequency independent phase errors, and Figure 3.15 indicates a systematic method for correcting them.

(e) *Filtering.* In common with all other electronic signals, the FID resulting from the detection of our sample resonances contains a certain amount of noise which by definition covers a very wide frequency range. It is advantageous to remove as much as possible of this noise from the FID, since its Fourier transform will also be noise on the baseline of our spectrum. Clearly all frequencies within the spectrum must be unhindered; the range covered depends on the frequency of the applied RF relative to that of the spectrum resonances. But in fact the combination of many frequencies in the FID leads to an effective high-frequency range which should also be allowed to pass. Thus our filtering is restricted to the very highest frequencies only, and must be a compromise between noise and spectrum distortion. Trial and error is the best way of arriving at a suitable value, although most spectrometers will have 'normal' settings and these may often be used without

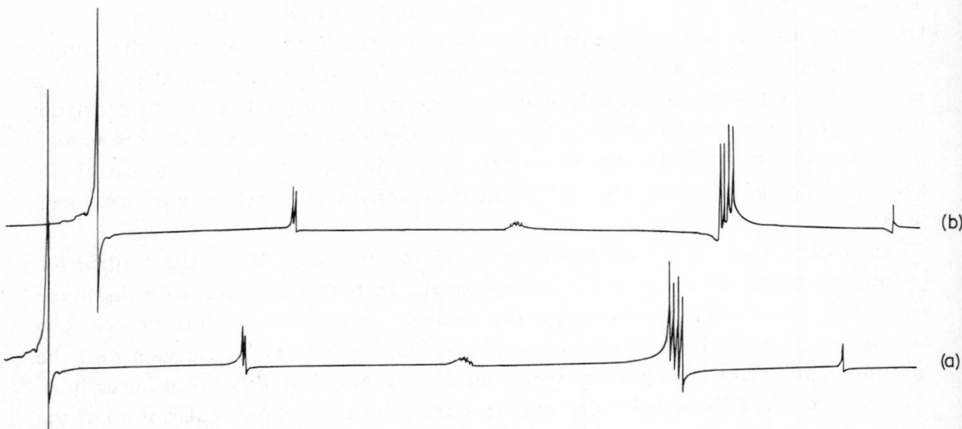

Figure 3.14 (a) Spectrum with frequency-independent phase error, (b) spectrum with frequency-dependent phase error

further trial, as filter selection is not so critical in FT as response time in CW spectroscopy.

(f) After setting up, accumulation and Fourier transformation are normally automatic. Phase correction may then be performed (Figure 3.15) and regions of the spectrum selected for writing out on the recorder. Some manipulation of the FID may be required before transformation; in this case it is wise to keep a copy of the original FID as a safeguard against accidental loss or other mismanagement of data. Several useful techniques for subsequent data manipulation are available and will be described in Chapter 5.

Special considerations for ^{13}C resonance

The resonance frequency of a carbon-13 nucleus in a given field is about one-quarter of that of protons in the same field. This is a consequence of its smaller magnetogyric ratio, which also leads to the unfortunate conclusion that the sensitivity of ^{13}C NMR detection can only be about 1.6% of that for protons. Since ^{13}C occurs naturally only to the extent of about 1.1% of all carbon, it is clear that an NMR experiment entailing observation of natural abundance ^{13}C resonance starts off with about 0.01% of the available signal strength of a proton spectrum of the same sample. Until the advent of Fourier-transform spectroscopy, experiments involving such low sensitivities were clearly not a matter of routine; even now, quite high concentrations of sample and large-bore sample tubes are required.

Against these difficulties may be placed the vast potential of ^{13}C spectroscopy. The chemical shift range for ^{13}C is much greater than that for protons (about 350 ppm) and the shift values are very sensitive to the electronic environment. Coupling constants with protons directly bound to the carbons are in a range ~120–250 Hz. Spin coupling between ^{13}C atoms does not appear in natural

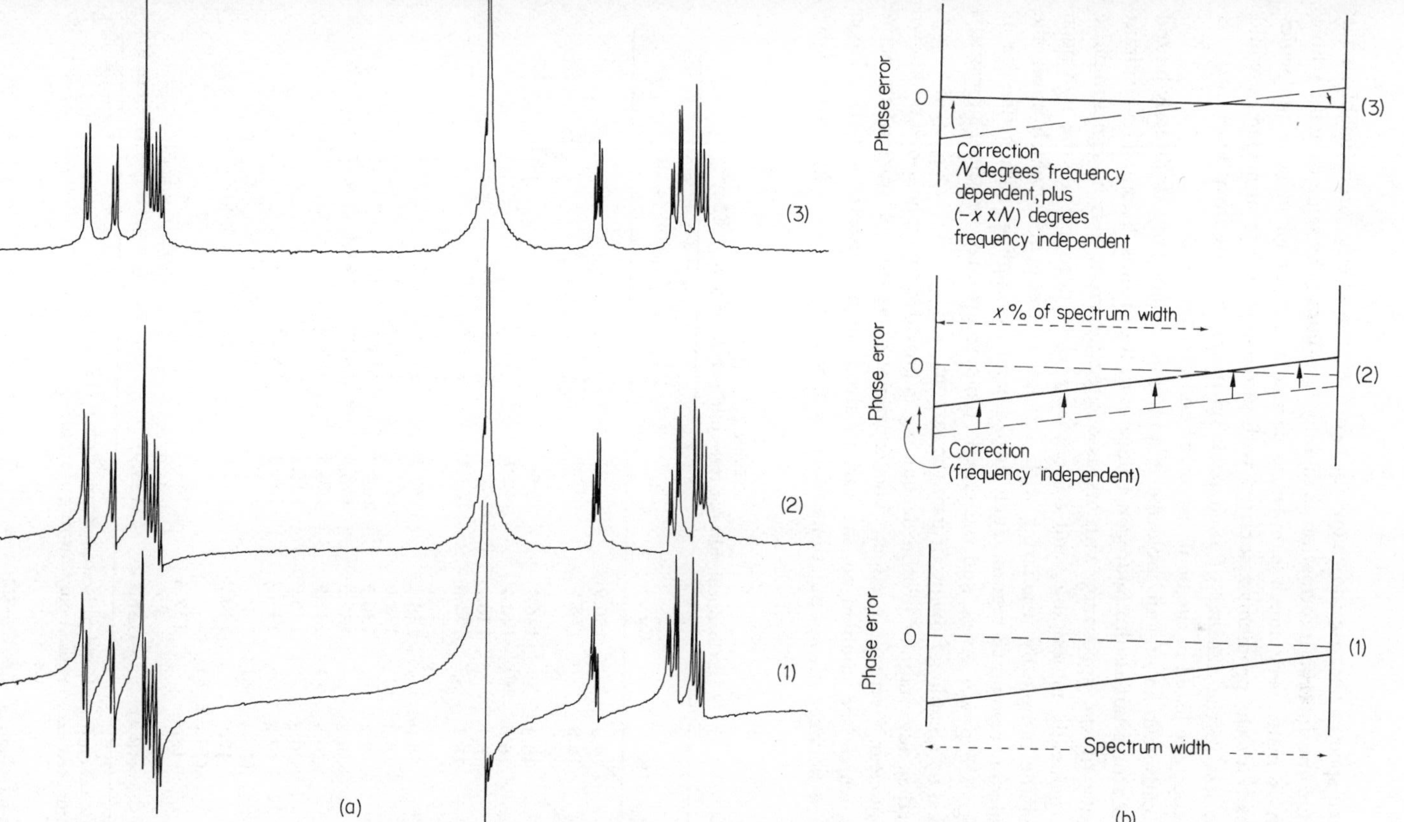

Figure 3.15 (a) Spectrum of tryptophan in D_2O in successive stages of phase correction. (b) Phase error diagrams in successive stages of phase correction: (1) Diagram for uncorrected spectrum showing both frequency-dependent and frequency independent phase errors. (2) Application of frequency independent correction. This brings prominent peak to correct phase as shown in spectrum (2). (3) Application of N degrees of frequency-dependent phase correction, coupled with $-x \times N$ degrees of frequency independent correction to maintain prominent peak at correct phase

abundance spectra because the chance of two ^{13}C atoms being direct neighbours is only about one in 10^4; information is thereby lost, but at the same time the whole spectrum is made very much simpler, a particular advantage in large molecules where many of the problems associated with peak overlap in proton spectra would be much less in the absence of such peak splittings. Introductory texts for ^{13}C spectroscopy are listed in the book list at the end of Chapter 2.

Each carbon in an organic molecule is spin coupled not only to directly bound hydrogen atoms but also to hydrogen atoms up to four bands distant. The resultant complexity of the spectrum, with its associated apparent loss in signal-to-noise ratio, is generally undesirable, and so it is normal to decouple all the hydrogen nuclei in the sample by irradiating with a range of frequencies which cover the whole proton resonance region. Such 'broad-band decoupling' entails the use of quite high RF power levels, and the sample temperature may be raised unless it is controlled by a cooling flow of air past the sample.

A further advantage of proton decoupling is provided by a phenomenon known as the nuclear Overhauser effect. The continual excitation of transitions in the protons which are coupled to the carbon atoms being observed causes a larger difference between the populations of the upper and lower energy states of the

Table 3.1
^{13}C Chemical shifts of free amino acids relative to CS_2 [a]

	C_0	Cα	Cβ C2[b]	Cγ C3[b]	Cδ C4[b]	Cε C5[b]	C6[b]
Gly	19.9	150.9					
Leu	16.8	138.7	152.4	168.0	170.2 171.2		
Phe	18.3	136.1	155.9	56.7	62.6	62.6	64.3
Ala	16.6	142.1	176.1				
Met	18.1	138.3	162.4	163.3	178.2		
Val	18.1	131.8	163.1	174.2 175.8			
Lys	18.0	138.1	162.7	171.0	166.2	153.4	
Pro	18.8	131.8	163.7	169.0	146.9		
Arg	18.2	138.3	164.9	168.5	151.9	35.9	
Ilu	18.2	132.5	156.3	167.7	181.1	177.5[c]	
Thr	19.4	131.9	126.3	172.9			
Ser	20.3	136.0	132.1				
Glu	17.8 (11.1 C_0δ)	137.7	165.3	158.9			
Asp	17.9 (14.6 C_0δ)	140.2	155.8				
His	18.5	137.6	164.2 56.2		75.2	N.O.	
Tyr	(18.4)[d]	(136.1)[d]	(155.9)[d]		(62.9)[d]	(75.9)[d]	(36.9)[d]

[a]Data taken from Horsley, Sternlicht and Cohen (1970).
[b]Numbered carbons used only for ring protons.

[c]Ilu sidechain is —Cβ(—Cε)—Cγ—Cδ.
[d]Figures in brackets are calculated.

carbon atoms than in an undisturbed system; the result is that more carbon transitions are observable. The full value of the nuclear Overhauser enhancement is just under 3; in other words the integrated area of proton-decoupled ^{13}C peaks is about 3 times that of undecoupled peaks. Further uses of proton decoupling in ^{13}C spectroscopy are discussed in Chapter 5.

Two factors make the measurement of peak areas in ^{13}C spectra difficult; the first is the fact that for small molecules in particular, the nuclear Overhauser enhancement may not reach its full value for all carbons. The second effect, which is perhaps of more importance for the larger molecules of concern here, is due to the long longitudinal relaxation time (T_1) often found for ^{13}C nuclei. It takes $\sim 5T_1$, for 99% of the original M_z to be restored; FT experiments with pulse repetition rates faster than this will find some at least of the nuclei still not fully relaxed. The problem may sometimes be overcome to some extent by 'doping' the sample with paramagnetic ions; further details will be found in Chapter 5, but normally it is necessary to have a long waiting time between pulses, which of course destroys much of the advantage of the FT method. For the above reasons, integrated peak areas are often not used in routine ^{13}C spectroscopy.

Chemical Shifts for biopolymers. Tables 3.1 and 3.2 give the ^{13}C chemical shift values for amino acids together with the ranges of chemical shift changes to be expected from incorporation of these amino acids and N and C terminal residues. Non-terminal amino acids in proteins at neutral pH would be expected to have much the same shifts as the free amino acids.

Table 3.2

^{13}C Chemical shift changes (ppm) of amino acids on incorporation in peptides. These shift values should be added to the chemical shifts of free neutral amino acids to arrive at the value for the residue when incorporated in a peptide. Shifts may vary with pH for residues with titrable groups. Data taken from Christl and Roberts (1972)

	C_o	$C\alpha$	$C\beta$	$C\gamma$
Peptide shift (N-terminal)	5.4 ± 1	1.3 ± 0.4 (Gly 0.7 ± 0.2)	−0.2 ± 0.5	0.4 ± 0.5
Peptide shift (C-terminal)	−3.5 ± 1	−1.0 ± 0.5 (Gly 2.0 ± 0.2)	−1.2 ± 0.6	−0.4 ± 0.3
Peptide shift (Non-terminal)	1.0 ± 1	0.6 ± 0.4 (Gly −1.1 ± 0.1)	0.0 ± 0.5	0.0 ± 0.1

3.5 Sample Preparation and referencing

Sample requirements

The signal-to-noise ratio available from a given sample is determined by how much of the sample is actually within the probe coils. Various arrangements may be used for containing the sample in order to obtain maximum value from the sample available.

(i) Normal samples, where a reasonable quantity of sample is available and the concentration of its solution is not limited by solubility or other considerations, may be run in the standard NMR tube, which is of 5 mm outside diameter. Probe design is usually such that about 3 cm depth of liquid is required in the tube, so that a total sample volume of about 0.4 ml is usually the minimum required. This may be reduced to about 0.25 ml by the introduction of a close-fitting plug of nylon, PTFE, glass or other material and about 1 cm long into the bottom of the tube to take up what is effectively 'dead volume'. It is difficult to give any rule concerning the required concentration of the sample, because features such as the sharpness of the peaks affect the available signal-to-noise ratio considerably, but in general a reasonable *single-scan* spectrum can, with care, be obtained from a solution made up to about 5 millimolar. Peaks due to single protons should be at least visible on such a spectrum, provided that they are not too broad. 5 mM corresponds to about 100 mg/ml for a protein of molecular weight 20,000; a concentration of 100 mg/ml is frequently referred to as '10% w/v' (weight/volume) or simply 10%.

(ii) In the investigation of biological molecules, a concentration of 100 mg/ml is usually much too high. Solubility is rarely a problem, but biological macromolecules often have a strong tendency to aggregate at high concentrations, and the experimenter may well be forced to work at concentrations of 1 mg/ml or even less. The availability of CAT or Fourier-transform facilities is a key factor here, but a considerable saving in time can be obtained by using a larger-diameter sample tube, which, by placing a larger volume of solution within the probe coils, increases the available signal. A 10 mm tube will put about 4 times, and a 15 mm tube about 10 times, as much sample in the coils, and these represent a theoretical reduction in the required number of accumulated sweeps of between 16 and 100 times – obviously an improvement well worth having, even if the factors are somewhat less in practice.

(iii) Some samples are limited in the quantity available rather than in the solubility or permitted concentration; in such cases the best use of the sample is made by putting as much of it as possible into the coils. This is commonly done by using a spherical microcell, which may consist either of a pair of plugs with hemispherical cavities in their ends or of a separate glass cell (Figure 3.16). In either case the volume in a 5 mm outer tube is about 30 μl, so that the concentration of 10 mg/ml can be achieved with only 0.3 mg of sample, all of which is within the sample coil. As is normal in a fallen world, the full advantage which might be expected is not available, partly because of the thickness of the microcell walls, and partly because a spherical cell does not 'fill' the coil as effectively as does a cylindrical sample. Nevertheless, microcells are on occasion extremely valuable.

Sample requirements for ^{13}C spectroscopy are even more difficult; for a spectrometer employing 10–12 m tubes, sample concentrations of the order of 0.5–1 Molar are required for a normal spectrum at natural abundance; about 1.5 ml of solution would be required, although the use of a microcell can reduce this to about 0.3 ml. If, however, a 5 mm ^{13}C probe is available, putting your 0.3 ml of sample into a 5 mm tube is a better proposition because the sample will fill the coil

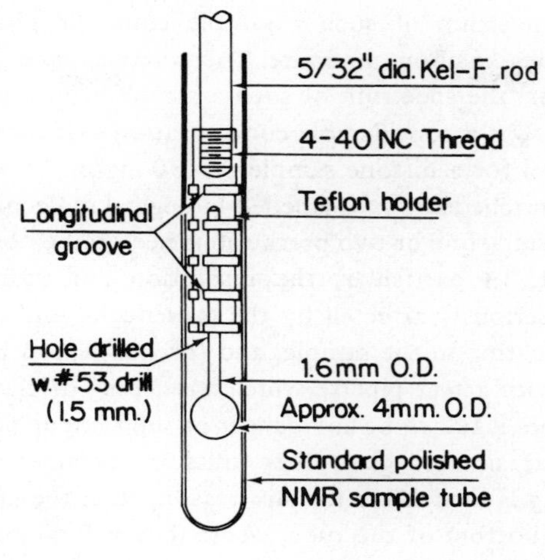

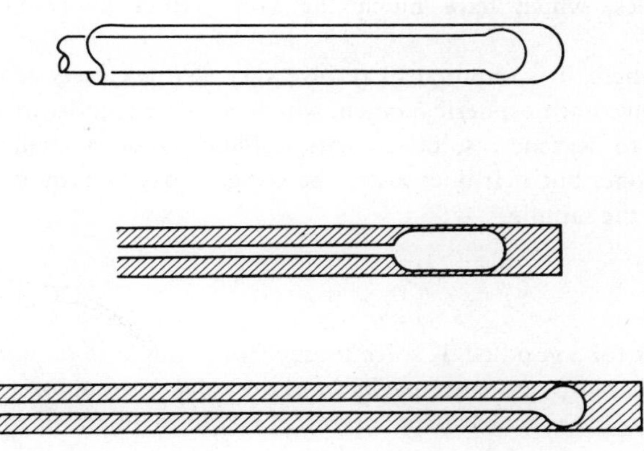

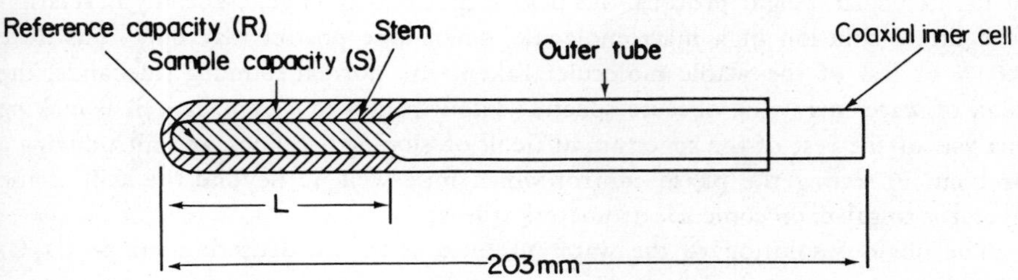

Figure 3.16 Microcells and reference capillary. (Reproduced by permission of Wilmad Glass Co., Inc.)

better. A useful spectrum of such a sample could be obtained, using Fourier-transform techniques, in about a minute. The practical lower limit of concentration is about 0.01 Molar; the spectrum of such a sample would take about 12 hours to obtain. Even 0.01 M is a considerable concentration – it corresponds, for example, to about 100 mg/ml for a histone sample or 130 mg/ml for cytochrome-*c*! Clearly the field for ^{13}C enriched and ^{13}C-labelled biological molecules is very inviting.

For the best results, one or two precautions need to be observed when preparing samples for NMR. In particular, the resolution and spinning sidebands of a spectrum may be seriously affected by the presence of undissolved sample, dust or other impurities floating in the sample, and for this reason it is a good idea to fill the sample tube with a teat pipette which has a plug of glass wool or other filter medium in it if there is felt to be any danger of solid impurities being in the sample. Small purpose-made sintered glass filter units are commercially available for this purpose. If filtering is inadvisible for any reason, then the impurities may often be spun down to the bottom of the tube, where they will do no harm, by the use of a small hand-operated bench centrifuge. This tool can be an essential part of sample preparation when the samples are viscous or gel-like; it offers the easiest means of getting the sample to the bottom of the tube, and is also a convenient way of getting rid of air bubbles, which have much the same effect on resolution as solid impurities.

For spectra where it is required to resolve very sharp, closely spaced lines, the presence of dissolved atmospheric oxygen, which is paramagnetic, may broaden the lines sufficiently to degrade resolution. This problem is more a small-molecule than a large-molecule one, but if it does arise, the oxygen may be removed by bubbling nitrogen through the sample.

Solvents

The requirements for a good NMR solvent vary from sample to sample, but perhaps the main one is that any resonance peaks from the solvent should not interfere with the part of the spectrum which is of interest. It is unfortunate in this respect that water, the most generally useful of biological solvents, has a peak at about 4.7 ppm, more or less in the centre of the 'normal' proton spectrum, and that with over 5% of its molecular weight protons, this peak is particularly large, especially in relation to a dilute solution of a macromolecule, where one proton may only constitute 0.01% or less of the whole molecule. Taken with normal spinning sidebands, the peak of water may well obscure spectral detail from 4 to 6 ppm, as well as making analysis of the rest of the spectrum difficult on sloping baselines, and introducing a problem in setting the phase control which may well be beyond the skill of the operator to solve, on some spectrometers at least.

The obvious solution to the water problem is to use deuterium oxide (D_2O) which has no protons in it but otherwise is effectively the same as ordinary water. In practice, D_2O which is 100% pure is very expensive, and it is usual to employ D_2O containing from 0.1% to 0.2% of protons; the resultant proton peak is not large enough to cover much of the spectrum (though it may obscure the backbone α–CH proton signals of proteins). The use of D_2O is complicated by the following disadvantages:

(a) D_2O exchanges protons quite readily with atmospheric water, and precautions must thus be taken to exclude air, especially in long experiments.

(b) Any exchangeable protons in the sample will be replaced by deuterium, which may remove useful peaks from the observable spectrum (this may be an advantage if their removal reveals other, more useful, peaks). In particular, –NH and –OH protons are not visible in spectra taken in D_2O.

(c) The use of a pH meter on solutions in D_2O yields a false result. This may be corrected by adding 0.4 pH units to the reading of the meter.

(d) The position of the residual proton peak of D_2O varies with temperature, with pH and with ionic strength. This makes it unsuitable for locking and reference purposes.

(e) D_2O is relatively expensive, especially for experiments which involve dialysis of D_2O into 'wet' samples.

Despite these drawbacks, D_2O is the most commonly used solvent in biological NMR. Methods for reducing the size of a water or residual water peak will be found in Chapter 5.

For purposes other than the direct simulation of biological conditions, of course, any solvent in which the sample is sufficiently soluble may be employed. Prominent among these have been trifluoroacetic and dichloroacetic acids, which are good polypeptide solvents (some polypeptides are notoriously difficult to dissolve) and give an acid-proton signal at about 11 ppm, well clear of the normal proton spectrum, and dimethyl sulphoxide, dimethyl formamide, pyridine, methanol and many others. Most of these are available, at a price, in deuterated form. Table 3.3 gives a short list of those parts of the NMR spectrum which may be expected to be affected by a selection of solvents in protonated and deuterated form. A table of solvents for proton NMR, with an indication of the region of the spectrum they affect in undeuterated form, has been published by Henty and Vary (1967).

Reference compounds

The general requirements for a reference compound are that it should have a single sharp resonance which is affected as little as possible by changes in temperature, pH or other solution conditions, and which does not intereact with the sample. Table 3.3 gives some of the more common solvents and reference compounds with comments on their suitability for various applications. If for any reason it is undesirable to mix the reference with the sample, then the most usual method for referencing is to use a coaxial inner cell (Figure 3.16) in which a solution of the reference compound is placed. This raises problems since the magnetic field inside the coaxial cell may not be quite the same as that in the outer tube due to difference in the magnetic properties of sample and reference solutions so that the reference peak may not be in the expected position. A straightforward way of overcoming this is to run a duplicate spectrum in which conditions are as close as

Table 3.3
Some common solvents and references

Compound	Chemical shift (ppm from TMS)	Remarks
(a) For proton NMR		
TMS (tetramethyl silane)	0	Common reference. Immiscible with water.
DSS (2,2-dimethyl silapentane 5-sulphonic acid)	0	Water-soluble variant of TMS. Interacts readily with basic residues in proteins.
D_2O (deuterium oxide)	~4.7	Common protein solvent. Shift varies with temperature and pH
Dimethyl sulphoxide	2.7	
Dimethyl sulphoxide (deuterated)	2.6	
Methanol	3.4, N5 (CH_3) (OH)	
Dimethyl formamide	8.1, 2.9	
Dioxane	3.6	
Acetone	2.2	Useful approximate reference
Trifluoroacetic acid	11.5	Good polypeptide solvent.
Chloroform	7.3	Good polypeptide solvent.
(b) For ^{13}C NMR		
Acetone	30.4	
Acetic acid	178.3	
Chloroform	77.2	
Carbon tetrachloride	96.0	

possible to those in the real spectrum except that there is a reference compound in the outer as well as the inner tube. If the effect is significant, two reference peaks will then appear and the difference between them may be used as a correction factor.

3.6 Summary

(1) Useful spectra can be obtained from quantities of the order of 0.02–0.5 μ moles of material for FT or CAT accumulated proton spectra. Perhaps a hundred times this amount or more is required to obtain any spectrum using natural abundance ^{13}C. The majority of biological NMR spectra are of samples dissolved in D_2O and referenced to DSS.

(2) The NMR spectrometer has as its main components a magnet, a device for generating radiofrequency radiation, a probe, amplifiers and detectors and a recording system.

(3) For a continuous-wave spectrometer, the main parameters under the operator's control are radiofrequency level, scan speed, time constant (filtering), region of the spectrum to be scanned and the number of CAT scans.

(4) On a Fourier-transform machine, the parameters are spectrum width, delay time, dwell time, number of pulses and the use of exponential multiplication.

References

Allerhand, A., Childers, R. F. and Oldfield, E. (1973). *Ann. N.Y. Acad. Sci.*, **222**, 764.

Christl, M., and Roberts, J. D. (1972). *J. Amer. Chem. Soc.*, **94**, 4565.

Henty, D. N., and Vary, S. (1967). *Chemistry and Industry*, p. 1783.

Horsley, W., Sternlicht, H., and Cohen, J. S. (1970). *J. Amer. Chem. Soc.*, **92**, 680.

Chapter 4
NMR Applied to Biomolecules

4.1 Introduction

The attack on a biological problem by NMR methods may be usefully divided into three phases: (1) Resolve the resonances; (2) Assign them to individual chemical groups or types of group within the molecule; and (3) Interpret the data, usually by explaining changes in assigned resonances from one spectrum or sample to the next. The amount of resolvable data is primarily a function of spectrometer frequency and the type of molecule under investigation, although resolution enhancement by convolution difference and the sensible use of other forms of difference spectroscopy (all described in Chapter 5) will increase the quantity of available information. General assignments may then be made from chemical shift and multiplicity of the resolved resonances, with spin decoupling as a powerful aid. How much further the assignment can go depends largely on the molecule in question, on how much is known about it from other sources and on the amount of work the investigator is prepared to put into the study. For example, some assignments may be made using proteins with only slightly differing sequences from the one being analysed, or specific chemical modifications may be introduced; the molecule may be fragmented and the pieces investigated separately, or (as in the case of oxytocin mentioned later) a synthetic version of the molecule built up, residue by residue, with assignments made step by step. Assignment at this level is undoubtedly the hardest part of biological NMR. Once the required assignments have been made, stage 3, the interpretation of the data, may be started. A surprising amount of the 'biological NMR' literature is taken up with studies which never get past stage 1 (resolution) and only a few can honestly be stated to be genuinely in the third stage of development. The casual reader of the literature may be readily guided: papers which begin or end with a statement to the effect that 'NMR is a promising technique for the investigation of biological molecules' are probably still in stage 1 or early stage 2, since promise speaks of hope rather than fulfilment.

In the sections that follow some studies which the authors consider important in illustrating these points and the ways through them are outlined. This chapter is in no sense a review, but is intended to discuss in a straightforward way, not overburdened with detail, some of the more successful attempts of recent years to apply NMR to biomolecules. A short list of review articles is given at the end of the chapter, and these will open the doors to the literature rather wider.

4.2 Oxytocin

Oxytocin is a nonapeptide with a hexapeptide cyclic portion closed by a disulphide bond and a linear tripeptide segment terminated by a carboxamide group

H—Cys—Tyr—Ile—Gln—Asn—Cys—Pro—Leu—Gly—(NH_2)

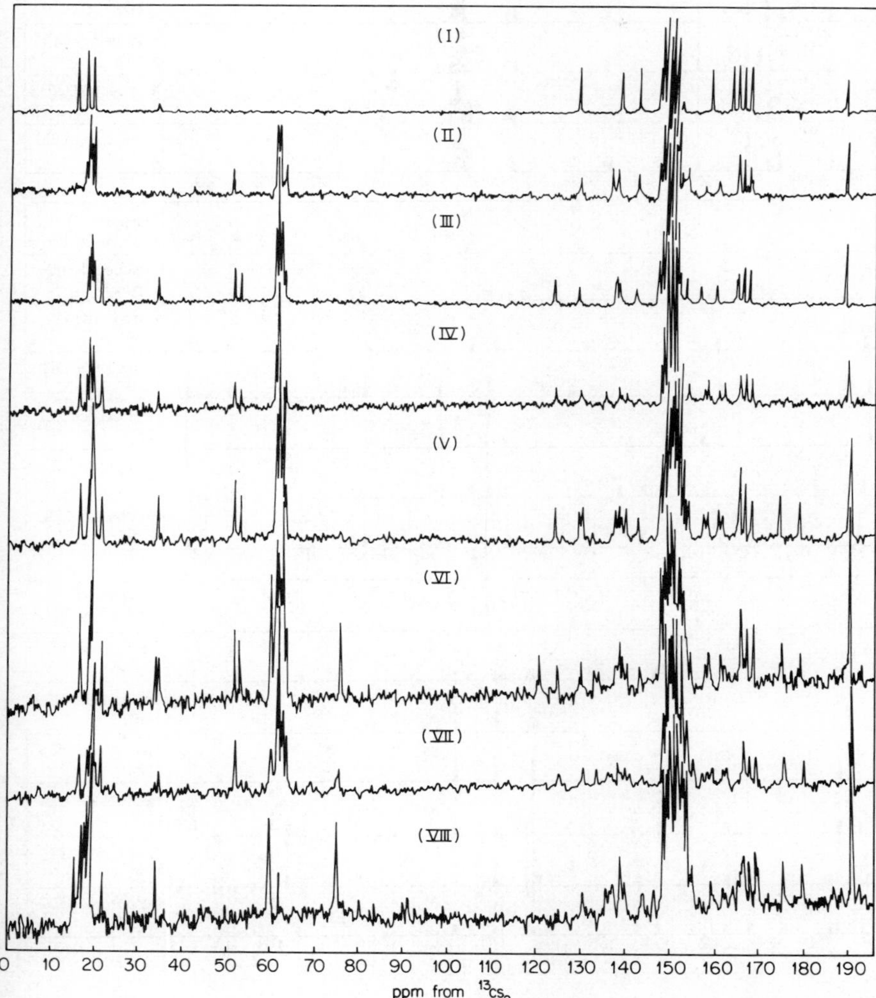

Figure 4.1 Spectra of seven precursors of oxytocin and of oxytocin: (I) Pro-Leu-Gly-NH_2, (II) (*S*-Bzl(Cys-Pro-Leu—Gly-NH_2, (III) Z-Asn-(*S*-Bzl)Cys-Pro-Leu-Gly-NH_2, (IV) Z-Gln-Asn-(*S*-Bzl)Cys-Pro-Leu-Gly-NH_2, (V) Z-Ile-Gln-Asn-(*S*-Bzl)Cys-Pro-Leu-Gly-NH_2, (VI) Z-(*O*-Bzl)Tyr-Ile-Gln-Asn-(*S*-Bzl)Cys-Pro-Leu-Gly-NH_2, (VII) Z-(*S*-Bzl)Cys-Tyr-Ile-Gln-Asn-(*S*-Bzl)Cys-Pro-Leu-Gly-NH_2, (VIII) oxytocin. Me_2SO-d_6 appears as the large multiplet between 151 ppm and 156 ppm. (Reprinted with permission from Brewster, A. I. R., Hruby, V. J., Spatola, A. F., and Bovey, F. A. (1973). *Biochemistry,* **12**, 1643. Copyright by the American Chemical Society)

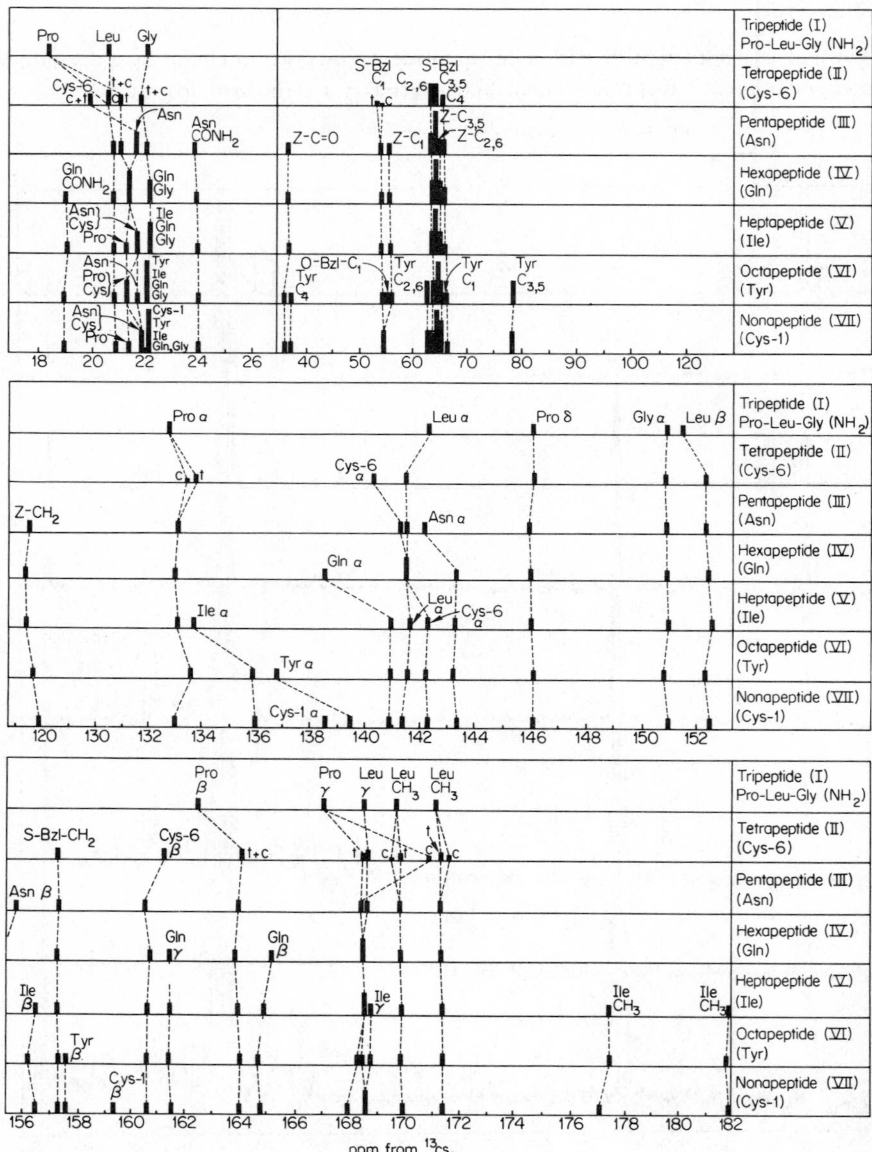

Figure 4.2 Assignment of resonances in seven precursors of oxytocin: (I) Pro-Leu-Gly-NH$_2$, (II) (*S*-Bzl)Cys-Pro-Leu-Gly-NH$_2$, (III) Z-Asn-(*S*-Bzl)Cys-Pro-Leu-Gly-NH$_2$, (IV) Z-Gln-Asn-(*S*-Bzl)Cys-Pro-Leu-Gly-NH$_2$, (V) Z-Ile-Gln-Asn-(*S*-Bzl)Cys-Cys-Pro-Leu-Gly-Nh$_2$, (VI) Z-(*O*-Bzl)Tyr-Ile-Gln-Asn-(*S*-Bzl)Cys-Pro-Leu-Gly-NH$_2$, (VII) Z-(*s*-Bzl)Cys-Tyr-Ile-Gln-Asn-(*S*-Bzl)Cys-Pro-Leu-Gly-NH$_2$. Internal Me$_4$Si appears at 192.8 ppm from the CS$_2$ resonance. (Reprinted with permission from Brewster, A. I. R., Hruby, V. J., Spatola, A. F., and Bovey, F. A. (1973). *Biochemistry*, **12**, 1643. Copyright by the American Chemical Society)

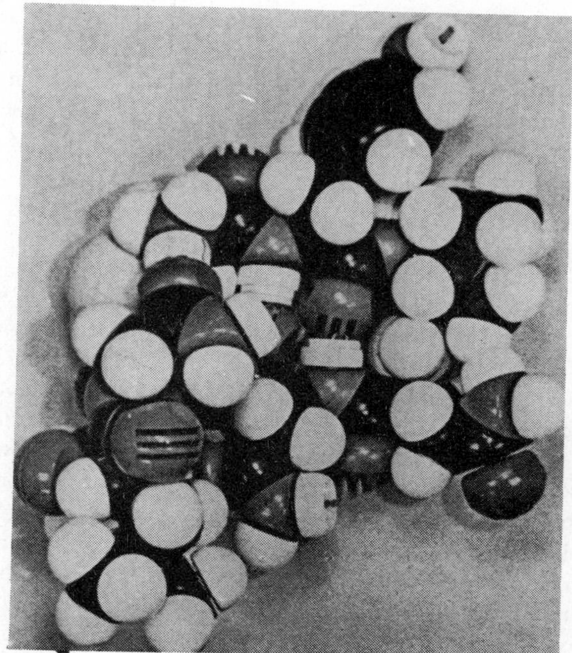

Figure 4.3 Proposed conformation of oxytocin in solution. (Reprinted with permission from Brewster, A. I. R., Hruby, V. J., Spatola, A. F., and Bovey, F. A. (1973). *Biochemistry*, 12, 1643. Copyright by the American Chemical Society)

Its ^{13}C spectrum is quite complex, containing 43 carbon resonances, and complete assignment is clearly difficult. Assignments have been made using the straightforward, but by no means easy, method of building up the molecule synthetically, residue by residue, and assigning the spectra of the partial molecules step by step (Brewster *et al.*, 1973, Deslauriers *et al.*, 1972). Figure 4.1 shows the spectra of seven precursors of oxytocin and of the whole molecule, while Figure 4.2 shows the assignments of the resonances for the seven precursors; an idea of the difference between the chemical shifts of carbons, particularly the α- and β-carbons, in the terminal and non-terminal positions in the peptide may also be gained from this diagram (see Table 3.2). Difficult assignments were assisted by selective deuteration and the selection of appropriate analogues of oxytocin, modified in one position only from the normal molecule, with appropriate analysis of the resulting spectral changes. One of the most interesting features was the observation of conformation-dependent shifts which should enable the solution structure of the molecule to be completely determined by NMR, particularly when the ^{13}C data is combined with the considerable volume already available from proton NMR studies. Smith *et al.* (1973) from ^{13}C work report that the proline residues in oxytocin are in the *trans* form, and that in cyclization of the linear nonapeptide precursor substantial shifts of the α-CH resonances of the cyclic moiety occur. These may be compared with these found on α-helix formation in polypeptides, and lead to a model for the structure as shown in Figure 4.3. This structure had already been proposed on the basis of proton resonance, studies from which dihedral angles had been found.

4.3 The unfolding of staphylococcal nuclease

As we have just seen, spectral assignments even for a nonapeptide involve a great deal of labour; the difficulty increases rapidly with increasing molecular weight. One method of simplying a proton spectrum before assignment is available in selective deuteration, a technique which has so far been used only by a few workers because of the considerable expenditure of effort and money entailed. Basically a supply of fully deuterated amino acids is obtained, usually by growth of algae in D_2O, and these are then used in the growth medium of the organism which produces the protein of interest. The growth medium is modified by the addition of wholly or partially protonated amino acids, so that there are only a few proton sites in the resultant sample. An example of the application of this method to staphylococcal nuclease may be found in Jardetzky *et al.* (1971) and references therein. The protein was grown as described in a medium in which one site only on

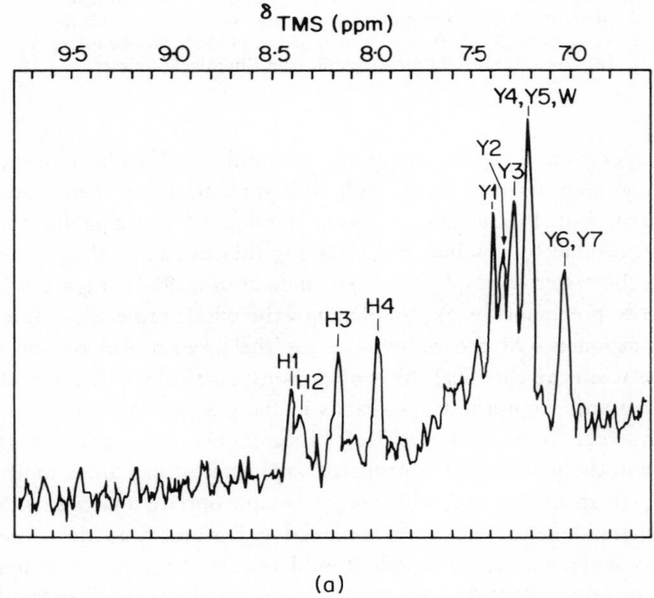

Figure 4.4(a) 220 MHz NMR spectrum of the aromatic region of selectively deuterated staphylococcal nuclease, showing resolution of individual amino acid peaks. H = histidine, Y = tyrosine, W = tryptophan

each histidine, tryptophan and phenylalanine in the molecule was protonated – a total of 15 protons in each molecule. As Figure 4.4(a) shows, the resultant low-field spectrum of the molecule in its native state shows nine separated resonances for the twelve protons of histidine (4), tyrosine (7) and tryptophan (1). As the pH of the solution is raised from 8 to 11 and the protein unfolds, these peaks shift until only three are visible, one for the histidine protons, one for the tyrosine and one for the tryptophan. However, the resonances shift at different pH values, implying that the unfolding is a sequential process and providing a way of determining the order in which the unfolding takes place. Since the denaturation is reversible, the order of refolding may also be observed, and this is of great importance to an understanding of the mechanisms of protein folding in general.

Assuming that the structure of the native protein is known from X-ray studies (a prerequisite for these experiments) and that each of the peaks now made visible in the NMR spectrum may be assigned to a specific amino acid residue in the chain, a clear idea of the order of unfolding may be obtained. Methods of assignment are given by Jardetzky and Wade-Jardetzky (1971), and the resultant order of unfolding is shown in Figure 4.4(b).

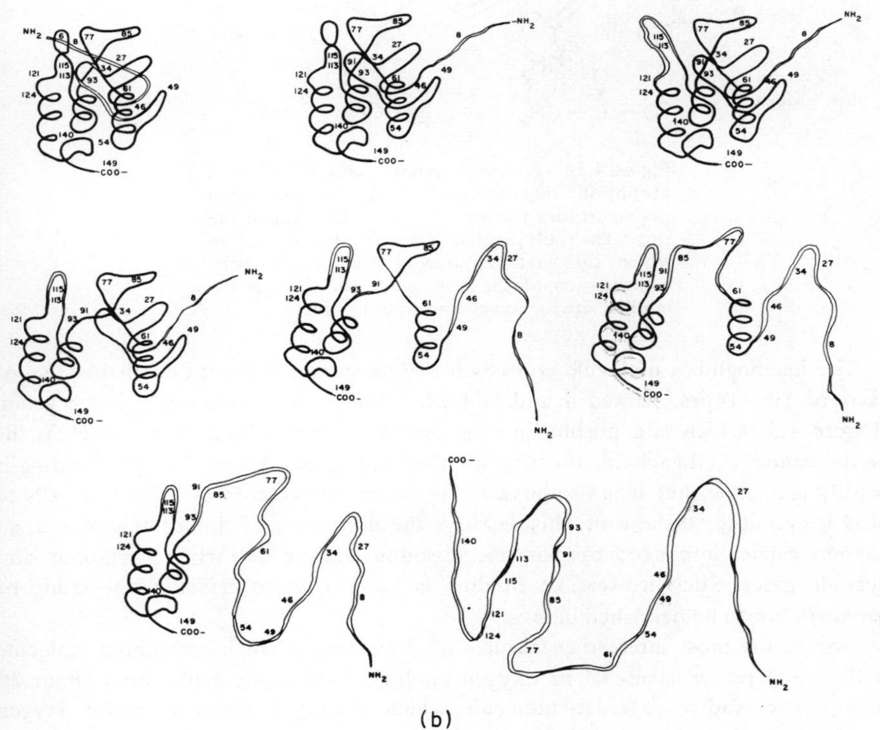

Figure 4.4(b) Sequence of folding and refolding of staphylococcal nuclease proposed from changes in NMR spectra. (Jardetzky, *et al.*, 1971)

4.4 Haemoglobin (Ogawa *et al.*, 1972)

The haemoglobin molecule is another system which lends itself to investigation b NMR; although it is a very large molecule, containing same 3500 protons, man resonances are shifted outside the normal 0–10 ppm region by interactions wit the haem iron atoms. Most of the useful information in the spectrum lies in th regions 10–25 ppm downfield and 2–6 ppm upfield of the DSS reference signal.

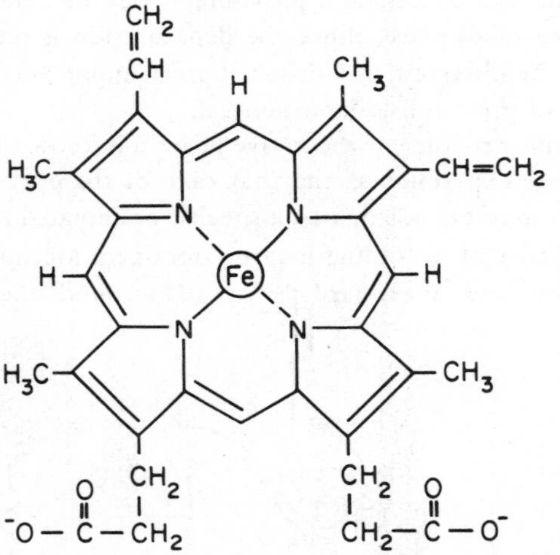

$$
\begin{array}{c}
\text{[Haem structure: porphyrin ring with central Fe bound to four N; substituents } CH=CH_2,\ CH_3,\ H_3C,\ CH=CH_2,\ H,\ CH_3,\ H_3C,\ CH_2CH_2COO^-\ (\times 2)]
\end{array}
$$

Figure 4.5 A haem group, consisting of a porphyrin ring structure with an iron atom bound to four nitrogen atoms in the plane of the ring. The polypeptide chain of the protein in which the haem is situated provides the fifth coordination of the iron, while the sixth is the binding site for oxygen or other ligands

The haemoglobin molecule consists of four separate polypeptide chains, two of each of two types, named α and β. Each subunit chain contains a haem group (Figure 4.5) which is a porphyrin ring complexed to an iron atom which is the active centre of the chain, the site for the binding of oxygen. Oxygen binding is readily reversible, but it is also possible for other groups, notably –CO and –CN to bind irreversibly to the iron; this destroys the usefulness of the haemoglobin as an oxygen carrier and accounts for the poisonous nature of carbon monoxide and cyanide gases. Such irreversible binding is used to good effect in the study of haemoglobin to be described below.

One of the most interesting features of the action of the haemoglobin molecule is the cooperative nature of its oxygen binding. Oxygen molecules bind about 20 times more readily to a Hb molecule which already has one or more oxygen molecules bound than to one which has none. Clearly the binding of an oxygen molecule to one subunit of the tetramer modifies the binding energy of the others in some way so as to increase their oxygen affinity, but the mechanism of this change has been the subject of much discussion for some time. In a series of papers by Ogawa *et al.*, different models were considered; the first, originally proposed by Monod *et al.*, is an allosteric model in which the quaternary structures of the tetramer (i.e. the precise interrelation between the four subunit chains) can exist in two different forms, one of intrinsically low oxygen affinity and the other of intrinsically high affinity. Binding of an oxygen molecule to one subunit causes a shift towards the high-affinity structure. Evidence for this model came from the X-ray observations of Perutz that the quaternary structures of fully oxygenated and fully deoxygenated forms were different. However, there were barriers to accepting the model in that no evidence existed either for an equilibrium mixture of the two forms or for a dependence of oxygen affinity on the quaternary structure.

An alternative model, originated by Koshland *et al.*, proposed that the binding of a ligand to one subunit altered the tertiary structure (the chain folding and arrangement) within that subunit, and that the effect of this change on the other subunits was to alter their tertiary structure and degree of oxygen affinity. There is X-ray evidence for ligand-induced tertiary structure changes as well as the quaternary changes already noted. It can be seen that the two models are not diametrically opposed, but that their emphasis is quite different. (Another model, the so-called 'Tension model' has recently been proposed on the basis of ESR data (Asakura (1973)).

A solution to the question as to whether it is the quaternary structure of the Hb molecule, or the tertiary structures of its subunits, that is responsible for the cooperative binding of oxygen has been indicated using NMR in a series of papers by Ogawa, Shulman and others. Firstly, they closely examined the shifted peaks in the spectra of the individual α- and β-chains in their ferricyanide form (the ferric iron in this form is paramagnetic and gives shifted peaks, while iron in the ferrous form, as is found in the oxygenated form of Hb, is diamagnetic and gives no shifted resonances) and then observed the changes in the spectrum (corresponding to structural changes in the region of the shift-producing haem group) consequent on association of the α- and β-subunits to form the tetramer. To do this they prepared 'valency hybrid' tetramers, such as $(\alpha^{III}CN\beta^{II}O_2)_2$, where the β-chains, with their haem in the ferrous oxygenated state, gave no shifted resonances, so that the $\alpha^{III}CN$ spectrum in the tetramer could be compared directly with that of the free $\alpha^{III}CN$ chain. The resultant spectra can be seen in Figure 4.6; the overall pattern of the spectra is the same whether or not the subunit is incorporated into a tetramer, but there are a number of small but definite changes. Another difference was that many of the lines in the spectrum of the tetramer showed pH dependence, while most did not in the isolated chain.

The last step in the series of NMR experiments was to prepare Hb in the half-ligated state, e.g. $(\alpha^{III}CN\beta^{II})_2$, where the α-chain were in the ferric form while the β-chains were deoxygenated, being still in the diamagnetic ferrous form. The effect of oxygenating the β-chains, or of other changes such as the addition of phosphate, could then be monitored as changes in the spectrum of the α-chains, reflecting changes in the haem environment. Similar observations could be made on the $(\alpha^{II}\beta^{III}CN)_2$ tetramer. The results and conclusions of these observations may

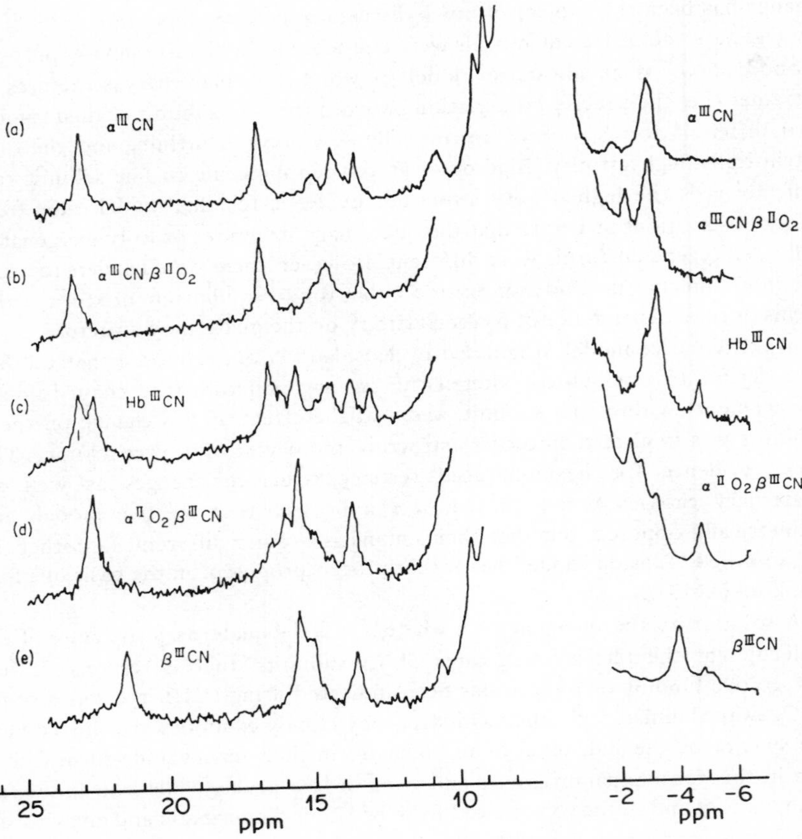

Figure 4.6 NMR spectra of fully ligated haemoglobins at pH 6.6 in 0.1 M phosphate buffer in D_2O at 20°C. (Ogawa *et al.*, 1972)

be summarized as follows:

(1) In the deoxygenated $(\alpha^{III}CN\beta^{II})_2$ hybrid, two different NMR spectra of the α^{III}CN subunits could be observed (Figure 4.7a and c). One spectrum (a) was very similar to the fully ligated hybrid's spectrum (b), and is referred to as the unchanged spectrum. It was obtained when the solution was phosphate-free and at pH values above 7. The similarity of spectra (a) and (b) implies that deoxygenation of the β-chains has little effect upon the haem environment of the α-chains under these conditions. On the other hand, the changed spectrum (c) was quite different in all peak positions. This changed spectrum was observed in the presence of phosphates or at pH below 6.7.

(2) In the case of the $(\alpha^{II}\beta^{III}CN)_2$ hybrid, a changed spectrum was not produced by the very mild changes in solution outlined above, but was produced in the presence of inosine hexaphosphate (IHP).

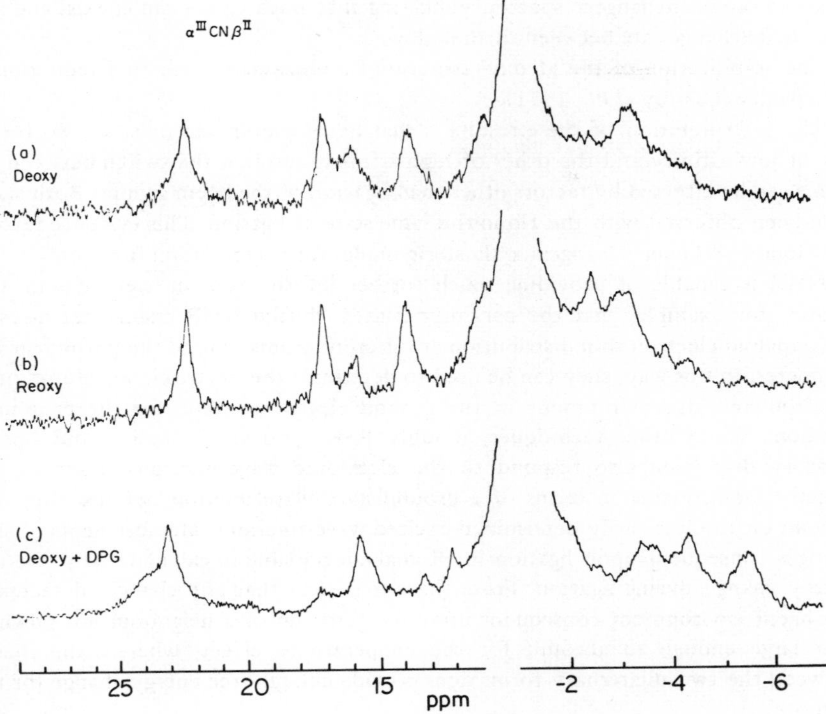

Figure 4.7 NMR spectra of the $(\alpha^{III}CN\beta^{II})_2$ hybrid (a) Deoxy $(\alpha^{III}CN\beta^{II})_2$ in Bis Tris, pH 7.4, (b) reoxygenated sample from (a). Haem concentration was approximately 8×10^{-3} M. Signal accumulation time for the downfield spectrum was 1 hr and for upfield 0.5 hr. Vertical gain is twice as small for the upfield region. (c) The deoxygenated $(\alpha^{III}CN\beta^{II})_2$ with one diphosphoglycerate per tetramer in Bis Tris buffer, pH 7.0 at 15 °C. The haem concentration was 7×10^{-3} M. (Ogawa *et al.*, 1972)

The explanation proposed for these changed spectra is that they correspond to changes of the quaternary structure of the tetramers. In cases where the spectra of the cyano subunits of the deoxygenated hybrids are extremely similar to those of the fully ligated hybrids, Ogawa and Shulman postulate that the whole tetramer is in the 'fully ligated' or 'oxy' tetramer structure. The changed spectra which can be obtained for both deoxygenated hybrids indicate that the molecule is in the 'deoxy' quaternary structure. In this view, the 'oxy' quaternary structure is much more favoured in $(\alpha^{II}\beta^{III}CN)_2$ because of the need for strong allosteric effectors like IHP to produce the 'deoxy' form, in contrast to the ease with which the $(\alpha^{III}CN\beta^{II})_2$ hybrid can be switched, indicating that in the latter case the two structures are closer in energy.

An important aspect of this two-state model is seen in cases where IHP was present in ratios of less than one per tetramer of the deoxygenated $(\alpha^{III}CN\beta^{II})_2$ hybrid. In this case, a spectrum is obtained which is clearly a superposition of both 'changed' and 'unchanged' spectra, indicating that both forms can coexist and also that the exchange rate between them is slow.

The stabilization of the 'deoxy' structure by phosphate leads to a reduction in CO affinity (Cassoly *et al.*, 1971).

The interpretation of these results is that haemoglobin can exist in two forms, one of low affinity and the other of high affinity, and that the switch between the forms can be effected by factors other than ligation of the haem groups. Both states have been observed with the Hb in the same state of ligation. This evidence favours the Monod–Wyman–Changeaux allosteric model for haemoglobin function.

NMR is capable of providing much further information on haemoglobin. It is known, for example, that the paramagnetically shifted NMR resonances measure the unpaired electron spin distribution at different atoms around the porphyrin ring perimeter. In this way, they can be used to determine the electronic wavefunction of the iron and its environment in the ground electronic state, for the protein in solution. While other techniques, notably ESR, optical absorption and optical rotatory dispersion also respond to the electronic wavefunctions, they are not directly interpretable in terms of a ground-state wavefunction because they also depend on the less easily determined excited wavefunctions. Measurements of shift changes consequent upon ligation in Hb make it possible to calculate ΔF_1, the free energy change during ligation. From these it is clear that any changes detected in the haem environment consequent upon oxygenation of a neighbour are nowhere near large enough to account for the cooperativity effect, whereas the change between the two quaternary forms does provide enough free energy change for this purpose.

4.5 Cytochrome-c_3

The cytochrome-c_3 of *Desulphovibrio vulgaris* is a small (14,000 daltons) multi-haem protein which is part of the complex sulphate reduction mechanism of the organism. Its sequence is known, as are the sequences of several related cytochrome-c_3s, and it has been the subject of two recent studies by proton NMR which reveal much about its structure and properties. (Dobson *et al.*, 1974; McDonald *et al.*, 1974). The methods and results may be summarized as follows:

(a) Measurement of the magnetic susceptibility of the oxidized form of *D. vulgaris* cytochrome-c_3 by an NMR method reveals a susceptibility per haem group appropriate to iron atoms in the low–spin ($s = ½$) state, on the assumption that there are four haem groups in each molecule. This latter assumption is born out by ESR and absorption spectroscopy measurements, and also by the fact that almost the only amino acid residues which are invariant between several different cytochrome-c_3s are for groupings of the type Cys(x)$_2$CysHis or Cys(x)$_4$CysHis, which are obvious sites for haem binding via thioether linkages. Other invariant histidine and lysine groups may also be associated with haem binding.

(b) Oxidation and reduction of the protein may be followed by observing the changes in the paramagnetically shifted peaks in the low-field regions of the

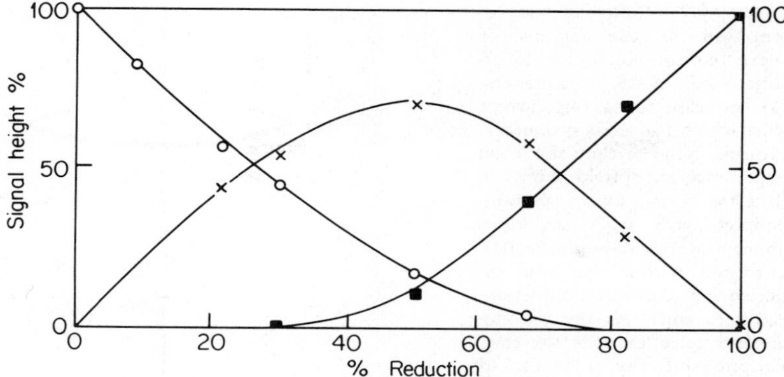

Figure 4.8 Appearance and disappearance of NMR lines associated with the three different redox states of cytochrome-c_3. ○, Concentration of the fully oxidized state which has been followed by measuring the area of several contact shifted methyl resonances at very low field; x concentration of the intermediate form, followed by the appearance and disappearance of the new contact-shifted methyl resonances on addition of reducing agent, sodium dithionite; ■, the appearance of the diamagnetic form, followed by the appearance of the single proton resonances at very low field attributed to two histidines. (From Dobson *et al.*, 1974. Reproduced by permission of Macmillan (Journals) Ltd)

spectrum. As reduction proceeds, some resonances gradually disappear, others slowly appear, while still others appear and then disappear again (Figure 4.8). The titration appears to pass from four oxidized haem groups (12–16 low-field shifted methyl resonances) to two (7–8 low-field methyls) and then to the fully reduced state (no methyls). McDonald and Phillips also observe a second intermediate state with only one haem oxidized.

(c) The low-spin state of the iron requires that at all times the iron is bound by at least one other strong ligand as well as the histidine of the binding Cys(x)$_n$CysHis sequence. This group might be methionine, histidine or lysine; the *g*-values revealed by ESR measurements seem to rule out methionine but the NMR spectra show that although there are five histidine residues not in the specific 'binding' sequences, only one has a resonance in a normal position in the spectrum, the others being highly perturbed. Since the lysine resonances show no such perturbation, it is concluded that these histidines are bound to the iron.

(d) The use of resolution enhancement techniques and changes of temperature to distinguish between normal and ring-current shifted (non-temperature-dependent) and pseudocontact and contact-shifted (temperature-dependent) resonances reveals some high-field temperature-dependent peaks which either must be in the plane of the haem or must be contact-shifted (i.e. bonded to the iron). Obvious candidates for such shifts are methene and propionionic acid groups of the haem porphyrin, and methyls of the thioether links (see Figure 4.9). In cytochrome-*c* spectra the highest shifted methyl is one of the latter, at 2.2 ppm. In contrast, in cytochrome-c_3 at least six methyl groups appear between 2 and 5 ppm, and other resonances at still higher fields, including two single

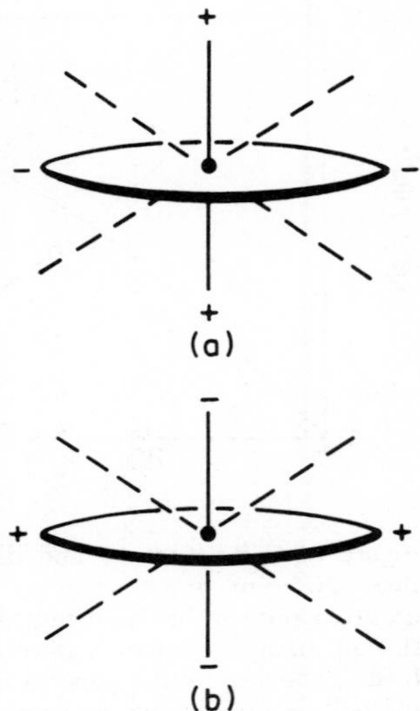

Figure 4.9 Schematic representation of the regions of space (cones) which give rise to shifts of NMR resonances. (a) The case for a ring-current shift which has axial symmetry. Protons lying within the cone experience an upfield shift (+). (b) Case for axial pseudocontact shift with the signs appropriate for low-spin Fe(III), a proton within the cone experiencing a downfield pseudocontact shift. As the pseudocontact term exceeds the ring-current shift by a factor of three, shifts in Fe(III) porphyrin complexes are in the opposed sense to those in diamagnetic FeII porphyrin complexes. (From Dobson *et al.*, 1974. Reproduced by permission of Macmillan (Journals) Ltd)

protons at ~−15 ppm. Such large shifts could be produced by two haem groups edge-to-edge, so that protons situated between them were shifted cooperatively by the two paramagnetic irons.

(e) In addition to the histidines, the whole of the aromatic region of the spectrum and the whole of the methyl region are very highly perturbed, indicating that nearly all aromatic and apolar residues are interacting with haem groups.

(f) In the half-oxidized state, half the low-field shifted methyls remain, indicating that two of the haem groups are still fully oxidized; however, only two methyl resonances remain above −1 ppm – the cooperativity required to produce very large upfield shifts has disappeared. (N.B. the ring-current effects of the porphyrin conjugated systems will act in opposition to the pseudocontact effects of the iron atoms, as shown in Figure 4.9.)

In the reduced state, the only perturbed shifts are due to ring-current or contact effects, since the iron is now diamagnetic. A number of such resonances, attributable particularly to histidine residues bound to iron or to sidechain groups of the porphyrin ring, are still visible.

A notable difference between the observations of McDonald *et al.* and Dobson *et al.* is that the latter report a large number of very slow-to-exchange N–H groups (still undeuterated even at high temperatures and after complete oxidation–reduction cycles) while the former specifically note the absence of any such groups.

On combining all the conclusions outlined above, Dobson *et al.* (1974) propose the structural model shown in Figure 4.10 for the cytochrome-c_3 of *Desulphovibrio vulgaris*. No X-ray data on this protein is yet available; it will be interesting to compare such data with the predictions of NMR when it does appear.

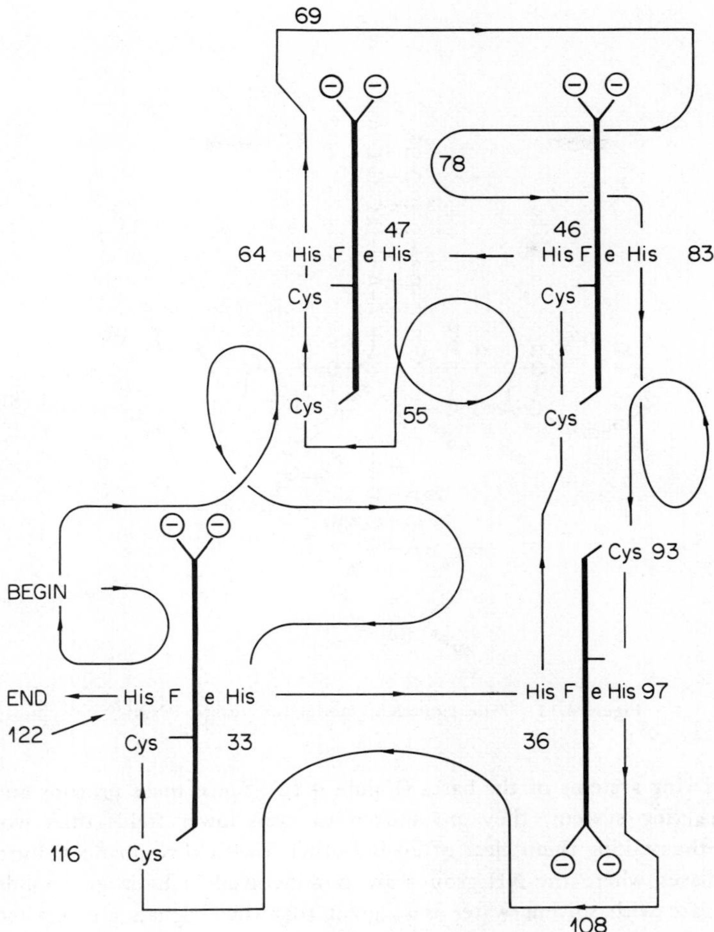

Figure 4.10 Proposed outline structure of cytochrome c_3 from *Desulphovibrio vulgaris*. (From Dobson *et al.*, 1974. Reproduced by permission of Macmillan (Journals) Ltd)

4.6 Transfer RNA

The relatively small (~80 nucleotides) and compact t-RNA molecules which are an essential part of protein synthesis have proved to be a very fruitful field for proton NMR as is shown in elegant studies by Kearns *et al.* (1973). Their sequences have been known for some time, and careful matching of base sequences to give double-helical segments led to the 'clover-leaf' model in which four short lengths of double helical RNA radiate from a common centre (Figure 4.11). Particularly interesting from an NMR spectroscopist's point of view are the NH protons of the

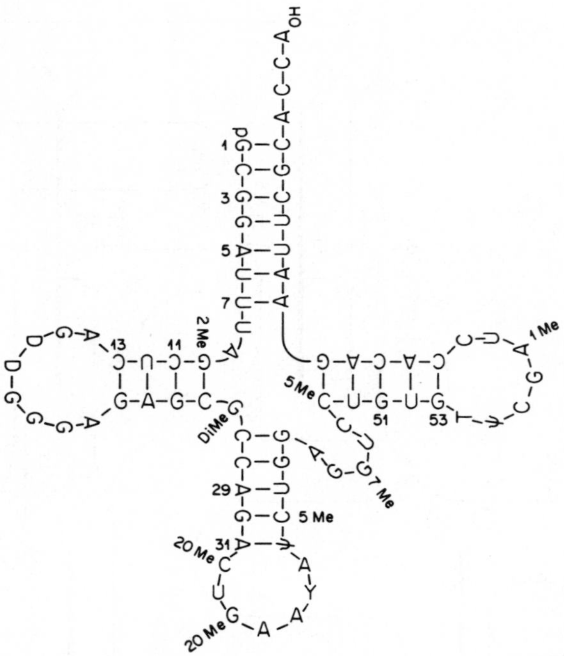

Figure 4.11 The cloverleaf model for yeast t-RNA^{Phe}

conjugated ring systems of the bases (Figure 4.12). Since these protons are in the plane of a ring system, they are shifted to even lower fields than would be expected, thus taking them clear of all the other low-field resonances. Further, in unpaired bases where the NH groups are not involved in hydrogen bonds, their exchange rate with solvent water is so great that their signals are lost from the low-field region completely. However, when the bases are paired, it is found (a) that the exchange rate is slowed down to a rate which is too low to perturb the resonances and (b) that these protons, being now in a double helical RNA structure, are subject to upfield ring-current shifts from the base pairs between which their own base pair is stacked. The magnitude of these shifts depends on the base pairs concerned, and may be calculated. Thus in a region clear of the rest of the spectrum we find one proton resonance per base pair, the chemical shift of which depends in a predictable way on its neighbours in the RNA sequence. One drawback is that of course NH protons are exchangeable with the deuterium in D_2O, so that all spectra have to be run in water; fortunately the resonances are a long way from the H_2O resonance, but even so this is probably a case where continuous-wave spectrometers with CAT are essential – the dynamic range of Fourier-transform analog-to-digital converters is really insufficient to cope with the tiny single-proton resonances as well as taking in the whole of the water resonance (protons in water are at a concentration ~ 110 molar).

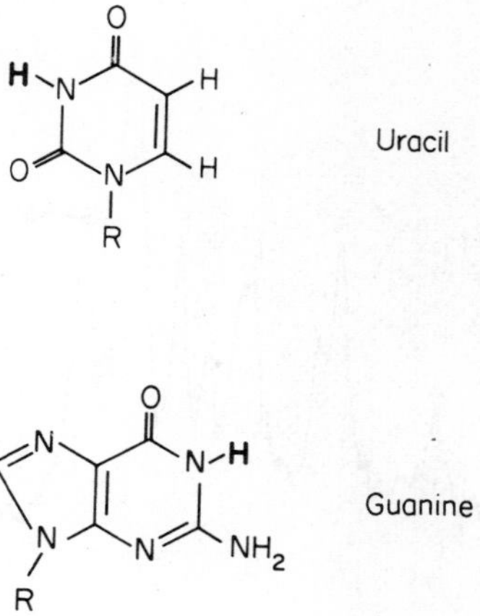

Uracil

Guanine

Figure 4.12 Ring NH protons whose signals are used in the study of t-RNA by proton magnetic resonance

Table 4.1
A summary of the assignments of the low-field resonances in t-RNA^{Phe} yeast

Base pair		Calculated position (ppm)	Peak	Observed resonances: relative intensity	Observed resonances: position (ppm)
AU	6	−14.4	A	1	−14.4
AU	12	−13.8	B		−13.8
AU	52	−13.9		3	
AU	7	−13.5	C		−13.7
AU	50	−13.5			
AU	29	−13.5	D	3	−13.2
Aψ	31	−13.2			
GC	11	−13.3	E	1	−12.9
GC	10	−12.7[a]			
GC	2	−12.6			
GC	51	−12.4			
GC	53	−12.4			
GC	3	−12.3	F		−12.8
GC	30	−12.3	G	10	−12.5
GC	49	−12.3[a]	H		−12.2
GC	1	−12.2[a]			
GC	27	−12.2[a]			
GC	28	−11.9			
GC	13	−11.5[a]	I	1	−11.6

[a]Resonances associated with base pairs at the termini of helices which are susceptible to large ring-current effects from adjacent bases in single-stranded regions.

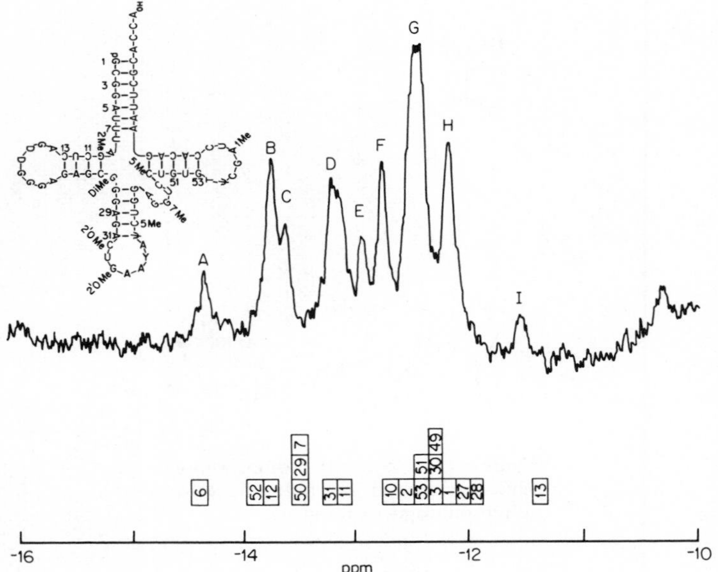

Figure 4.13 High-resolution 300 MHz NMR spectrum of t-RNA^{Phe}. The predicted locations of resonances associated with all base pairs in the molecule are shown by the numbered boxes. (From Kearns *et al.*, 1973. Reproduced by permission of the New York Academy of Sciences)

From a study of model compounds, Kearns *et al.* (1973) assigned 'unperturbed' chemical shifts of 14.5 ppm to AU base pairs, 13.5 ppm for GC and 13.5 ppm for Aψ. Initial measurements of integrated area of the signals revealed between 19 and 23 base pairs for various t-RNA molecules, in close agreement with the cloverleaf model predicted from base sequences. The next step, and a most difficult one, was to assign the individual resonances. This was done for t-RNA$^{phe}_{yeast}$ by cleaving the molecule into parts: the 5′ half, a fragment of about half the molecule centred on the anticodon, the 3′ half, and the 3′ three-quarters of the molecule. In each case only a few of the resonances were visible, and careful analysis of temperature dependence and other features enabled the peaks to be assigned (Figure 4.13) and their shifts compared with those calculated on the basis of the ring-current effects of nearest neighbours (Table 4.1). The results very strongly supported the cloverleaf model, which has since been confirmed by X-ray diffraction results (Suddath *et al.* (1974)).

The results obtained for t-RNA$^{phe}_{yeast}$ have been applied (Kearns *et al.*, 1974) to the unusual t-RNA$^{Leu}_{3}$ of yeast which has been found to have *two* stable conformers – a native (N) form and a denatured (D) form which is inactive with respect to aminoacylation and is hence a possible source of information on synthetase recognition. Little is known about the secondary or tertiary structure of the D-conformer, particularly in solution. The 300 MHz resonance spectrum of the D-form was obtained and assigned as above (Figure 4.14). It contained ~18 base

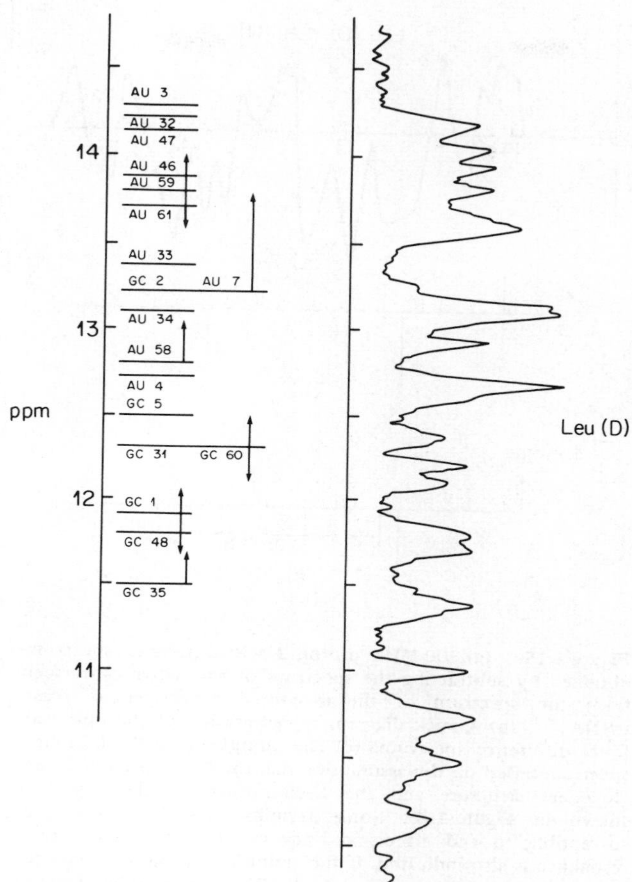

Figure 4.14 The 300 MHz proton NMR spectrum of the denatured conformer of yeast t-RNA$_3^{Leu}$ at 45 °C in a solution containing 0.1 M NaCl and 10 mM cacodylate buffer at pH 7. The t-RNA concentration was 60 mg/ml. A stick diagram representation of the NMR spectrum computed for the model shown in Figure 4.16 is also presented, together with assignments. The length of one of the smaller horizontal bars represents one resonance. (From Kearns *et al.*, 1974. Reproduced by permission of Macmillan (Journals) Ltd)

pairs, about 4 fewer than the N-form. A difference spectrum between N- and D-forms was then obtained (Figure 4.15), and this suggested that at least 5 base pairs were lost and two gained on going from the N- to the D-form (see Figure 4.15b). Following this, the expected spectra and difference spectra were computed for a number of possible base-pairing arrangements of the D-conformer. Only one of these satisfactorily accounted for the observed spectra; it is shown in Figure 4.16. The model is consistent with other data on the D-form, and is thus a valuable contribution to our precise knowledge of the mechanisms of protein synthesis.

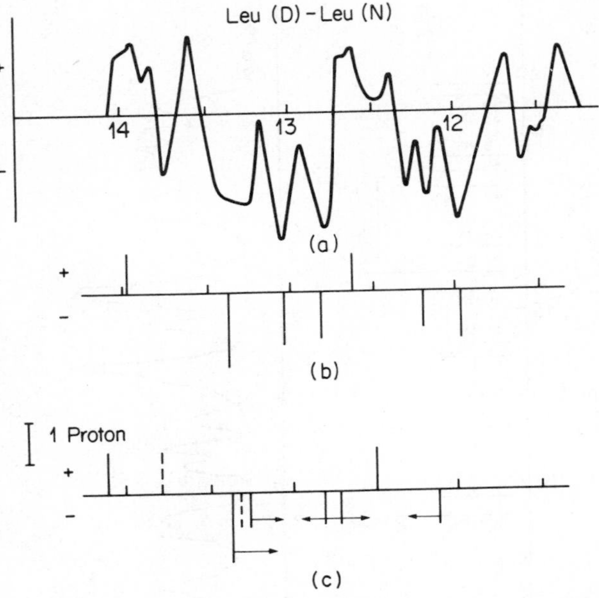

Figure 4.15 (a) 300 MHz proton NMR difference spectrum obtained by subtracting the spectrum of the native conformer from the spectrum of the denatured conformer of yeast t-RNA$_3^{Leu}$. (b) A stick diagram representation of the observed D–N difference spectrum. (c) The computed D–N difference spectrum based on the assumption that the N-conformer has the cloverleaf structure and the D-conformer has the structure shown in Figure 4.16. Some terminal base pairs may be susceptible to end effects and the expected range for these resonance is also indicated. If the amino acid acceptor stem and the TψC stem are not stacked in the D-conformer, there will be additional changes (indicated by dashed lines). (From Kearns *et al.*, 1974. Reproduced by permission of Macmillan (Journals) Ltd)

4.7 Histone fraction H1

The histones are a small group of basic proteins found in association with DNA in the chromosome. Their precise purpose is still being investigated, but they are at least partially responsible for maintaining the three-dimensional structure of the chromosome and also for altering it at various stages of the cell cycle. Control of chromosome conformation is intimately related to cell growth and division. Histones may also be involved in the repression of genetic activity, although present knowledge suggests that they do this in a blanket way rather than being themselves responsible for the very precise control of repression exhibited in living organisms.

Nuclear magnetic resonance has played a major role in the progress so far made

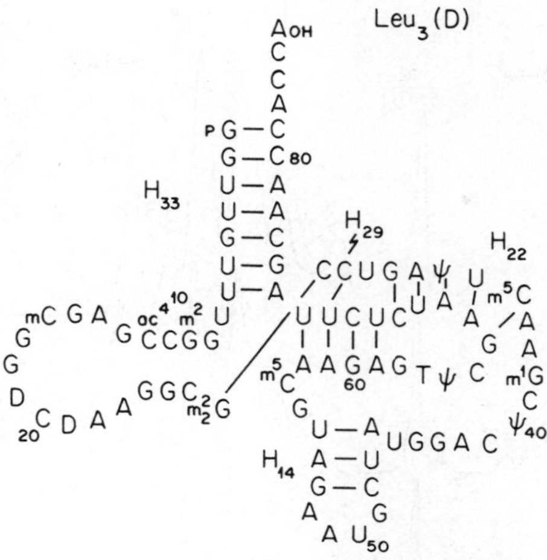

Figure 4.16 Proposed model for the secondary structure of the denatured conformer of yeast t-RNA$_3^{Leu}$. (From Kearns *et al.*, 1974. Reproduced by permission of Macmillan (Journals) Ltd)

in evaluating the role of histones; as an example we may take the role and mode of operation of one histone fraction, H1. Calf thymus H1 is an extremely lysine-, alanine- and proline-rich protein, containing only three arginine residues out of its total of 216.

NMR Studies of isolated H1 (Bradbury *et al.*, 1975a)

Figure 4.17 shows 270 MHz spectra of calf thymus total H1. Sequence data show that in fact this material is a mixture of several subfractions with slightly differing sequences; this does not alter the conclusions which may be drawn about the general behaviour of the molecule in differing solution conditions. The spectrum is dominated by a few readily identifiable resonances, notably those of lysine and alanine and of the terminal methyl groups of leucine, valine and isoleucine sidechains. Raising either the ionic strength or the pH of the solution causes a marked fall in the height of the terminal-methyl peak at ~0.9 ppm relative to the others, and at 270 MHz with convolution difference spectra it is possible to see that the area lost from the main peak is reappearing in the form of ring-current shifted resonances between 0.8 ppm and −0.1 ppm (see also Figure 5.2 which shows the high-field region of an H1 spectrum after resolution enhancement). This observation is important in that it implies that at least part of the molecule is taking part in a very rigid, stable structure, a feature previously not associated with histone molecules, and also that this structure must closely involve the single tyrosine and phenylalanine residues found in the molecule as well as the apolar residues. A simple analysis of the loss in area of the apolar resonance implies that the region

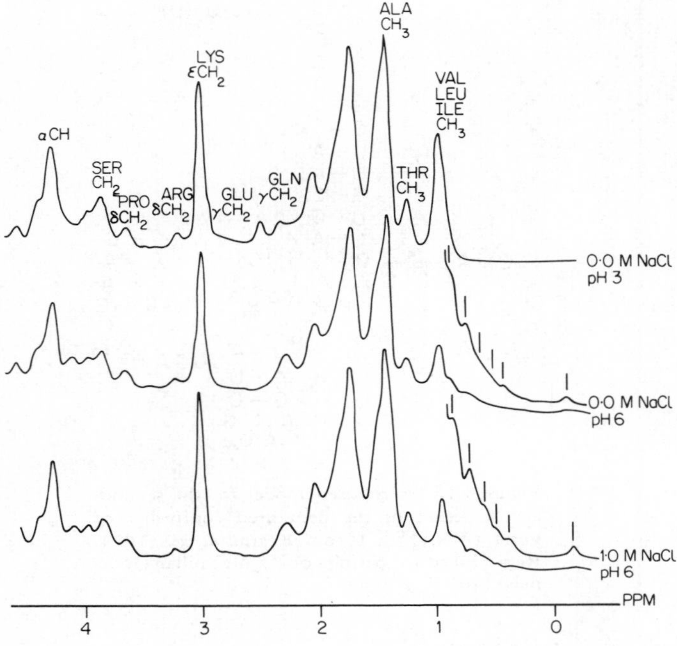

Figure 4.17 270 MHz upfield spectrum of histone H1, 50 mg//ml, in: (a) D_2O at pH 3; (b) D_2O at pH 6; (c) D_2O/1 M NaCl at pH 6. Note ring-current shifted resonances between −0.2 and 1 ppm. (From Bradbury *et al.*, 1973. Reproduced by permission of the New York Academy of Sciences)

involved in the structure formation must contain well over half the total apolar residues in the molecule, and examination of the sequence reveals that the only region answering to this condition is the part of the molecule from residue 40 to about residue 95 – the involvement of the phenylalanine residue extends this region to at least 104. An earlier study, in which peaks in a simulated spectrum were broadened on the assumption that residues involved in structure would be restricted in motion, provided the prediction that residues 47–106 would be taking part in structure formation (Figure 4.18).

The interactions of H1 in chromatin (Bradbury *et al.*, 1975b)

Chromatin in water is a diffuse fibrous gel. Increasing the salt molarity to 0.1 M NaCl causes a contraction of the gel to about one-tenth of its original volume. As the molarity is increased above 0.3 M NaCl the gel disperses and by 0.6 M NaCl the Hl molecules are fully dissociated. NMR spectra recorded over this range of molarities are shown in Figure 4.19. Figure 4.19(a) is the control and shows the signals from Hl-depleted chromatin in 0.6 M NaCl. Only weak broadened

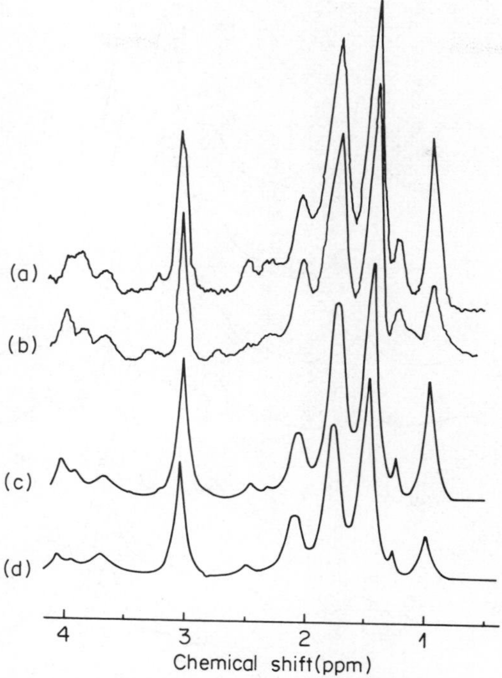

Figure 4.18 Observed 220 MHz upfield spectra of histone H1 in (a) D_2O and (b) 1 M NaCl/D_2O; simulated spectra (c) of the random-coil form of H1 and (d) of that obtained by broadening resonances from residues in segment 47 to 106. (From Bradbury and Rattle, 1972. Reproduced by permission of the Federation of European Biochemical Societies)

resonances are observed and it is assumed therefore that in the range of salt molarities 0 to 0.6 M the observable NMR signals from the gel will come only from the Hl molecules. The almost complete absence of signal in Figure 4.19(b) indicates that in the non-condensed gel in D_2O, virtually all the histones including Hl are bound firmly to the complex. The addition of 0.1 M NaCl (Figure 4.19c) which is accompanied by gel condensation causes a large change in the spectrum; peaks appear which correspond mostly to alanine, proline and a few lysine residues, with little other observable change. Increase of NaCl to 0.25 M (Figure 4.19d) made little difference either to the spectrum or to the state of condensation, but further increase to 0.5 M (Figure 4.19e) which corresponds to both complete reexpansion of the gel and to complete removal of the Hl, yields a spectrum which is identical to that of Hl alone in 0.5 M NaCl, with the sole difference that all the linewidths are greater by a factor of approximately 1.8.

The most remarkable change in the spectrum between 0.25 and 0.5 M NaCl is the sudden appearance of the lysine ϵ CH_2 peaks at an ionic strength which corresponds

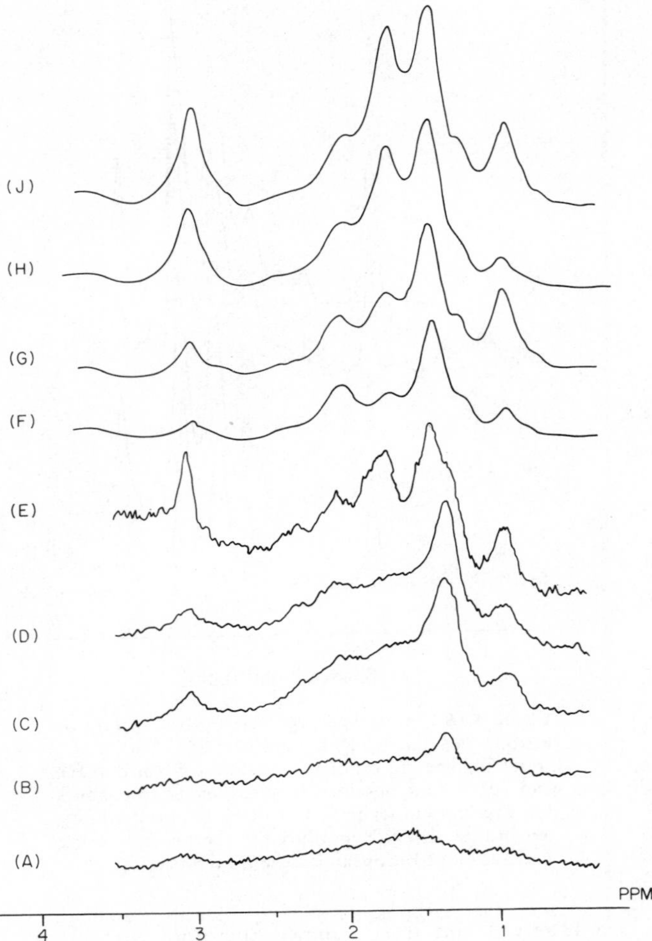

Figure 4.19 High-field parts of (A): 100 MHz NMR spectrum of H1-depleted chromatin; and 220 MHz spectra of total chromatin in (B) D_2O, (C) 0.1 M NaCl, (D) 0.25 M NaCl and (E) 0.5 M NaCl; simulated 220 MHz spectra of histone fraction H1, (J) in random-coil form, (H) with signals from residues 47–106 broadened, (F), and (G) as (H) and (J) but with resonances of 40 lysine residues removed. (From Bradbury *et al.*, 1973. Reproduced by permission of the New York Academy of Sciences)

to the release of H1 from the complex. The spectrum at 0.25 M NaCl may be closely simulated by a model which assumes that 40 of the 60 lysine residues of each molecule are rigidly held to the complex. The best simulations are made on the additional assumption that the apolar region from 47–106 is fully in its interacted state. We may thus draw the following conclusions from the NMR spectra of chromatin:

(1) Under the solution conditions used, no spectrum appears which is not directly attributable to the molecule of H1 in the complex. Removal of H1 also removes almost the whole of the observable spectrum. The implication of this is that all the remaining components of the system (other histones, non-histone proteins and DNA) are too rigid to give a high-resolution NMR spectrum. A corollary to this observation is that the resonance of any part of the H1 which becomes bound to the rest of the complex must also be broadened to the point of invisibility.

(2) Under conditions of low ionic strength, where there is no condensation of the gel, all the H1 is firmly bound to the complex.

(3) Under conditions corresponding to gel condensation, most of the H1 lysine residues remain bound to the complex, and the rest of the molecule, while free from the complex, exhibits its own structure formation in residues 47–106.

(4) Complete removal of the H1 occurs concurrently with the freeing of the bound lysine residues.

We may conclude that histone H1 is essential to, and is almost certainly the agent of, the contraction of chromatin gel induced by changes in ionic strength *in vitro*. H1 is implicated by biological methods in the contraction of chromosomes before mitosis *in vivo*; it is hoped that further investigation will establish a close relation between the two phenomena.

4.8 NMR of phospholipid membranes

Flexibility gradients

Aqueous dispersions of pure phospholipids spontaneously form multilamellar structures which can be disrupted into single bilayer vesicles by sonication (Figure 4.20). The sonicated material is very suitable for NMR studies; ^{1}H and ^{13}C NMR spectra of dipalmitoyl lecithin (DPL) are shown in Figure 4.2, (a) and (b). The assignments given are the results of selective proton decoupling studies. It can be seen that in the ^{13}C NMR spectrum at least some of the alkyl chain methylene groups are resolved. Fourier-transform methods allow measurement of several ^{13}C T_1s which are shown in Figure 4.22. The T_1s increase along the alkyl chains away from the glycerol backbone, which suggests that the centre of the bilayer is more mobile than the polar surface. However, it is a more difficult task to separate the contributions to T_1 from the various motions involved. These include tumbling of the whole vesicles, rotation of the alkyl chains as rigid units about their long axis and motion about individual carbon–carbon bonds in the alkyl chains. Calculations by Levine *et al.* (1972) suggest that the motion about carbon–carbon bonds dominates and, since this is cumulative down the chain, explains the increasing T_1 values. In other words, the terminal methyl group is affected not just by the motion about its own carbon–carbon bond but also by all the others up to the carbonyl of the backbone. However, this model is not completely satisfactory; a better fit to the data would be a model allowing similar rates of motion for methylenes close to the backbone but with a sharp increase towards the terminal methyl.

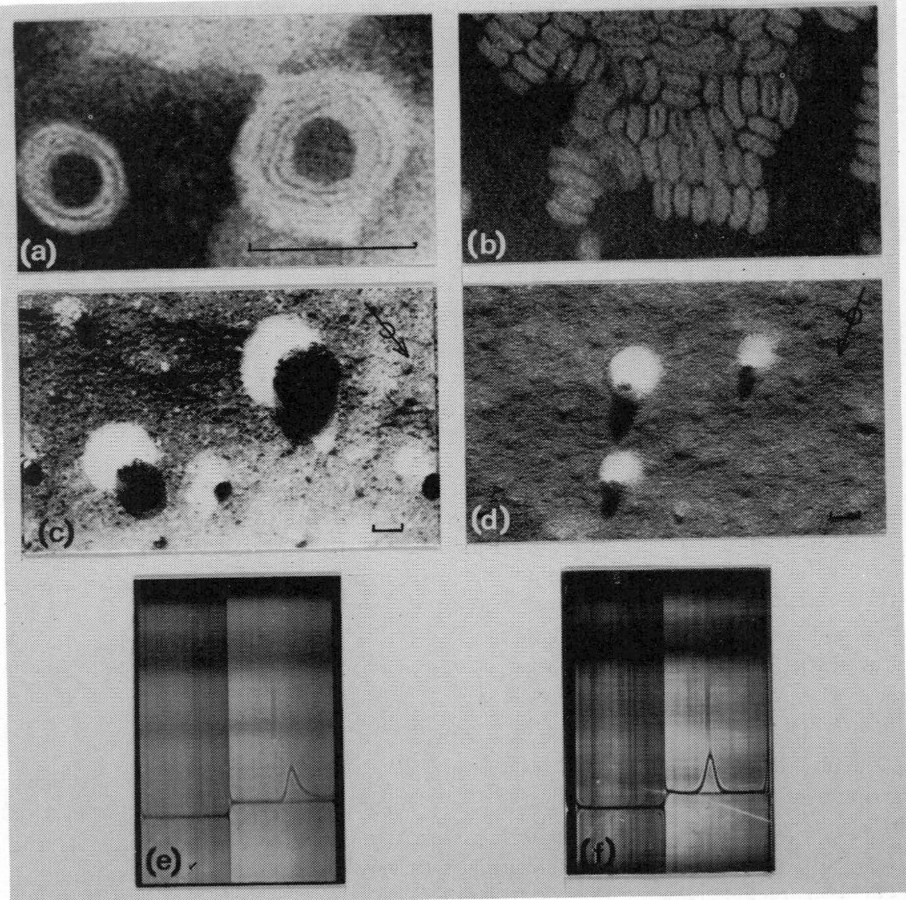

Figure 4.20 Electron microscopic and ultra centrifuge characterization of phospholipid vesicle fractions. Dimension markers represent 500 Å. (a) and (b) Show negative stained electron micrographs of phospholipid dispersions and single bilayer vesicles respectively (c) and (d) show freeze-etched electron micrographs of dispersions and single bilayer vesicles. (e) and (f) Show the sedimentation velocity ultracentrifuge schlieren peaks of the dispersions and single bilayer vesicles respectively. (From Marsh *et al.*, 1972. Reproduced by permission of Academic Press Inc.)

Lateral diffusion

Metcalfe and coworkers (Birdsall *et al.*, 1971; Lee *et al.*, 1972) noted an increase in proton T_1 for DPL preparations as increasing amounts of DPL deuterated in the alkyl chains were added. This shows that *inter* chain relaxation is important in the fully protonated bilayer. From a consideration of the various possible motions occurring in the membrane (see Section 8.4), it was concluded that lateral diffusion

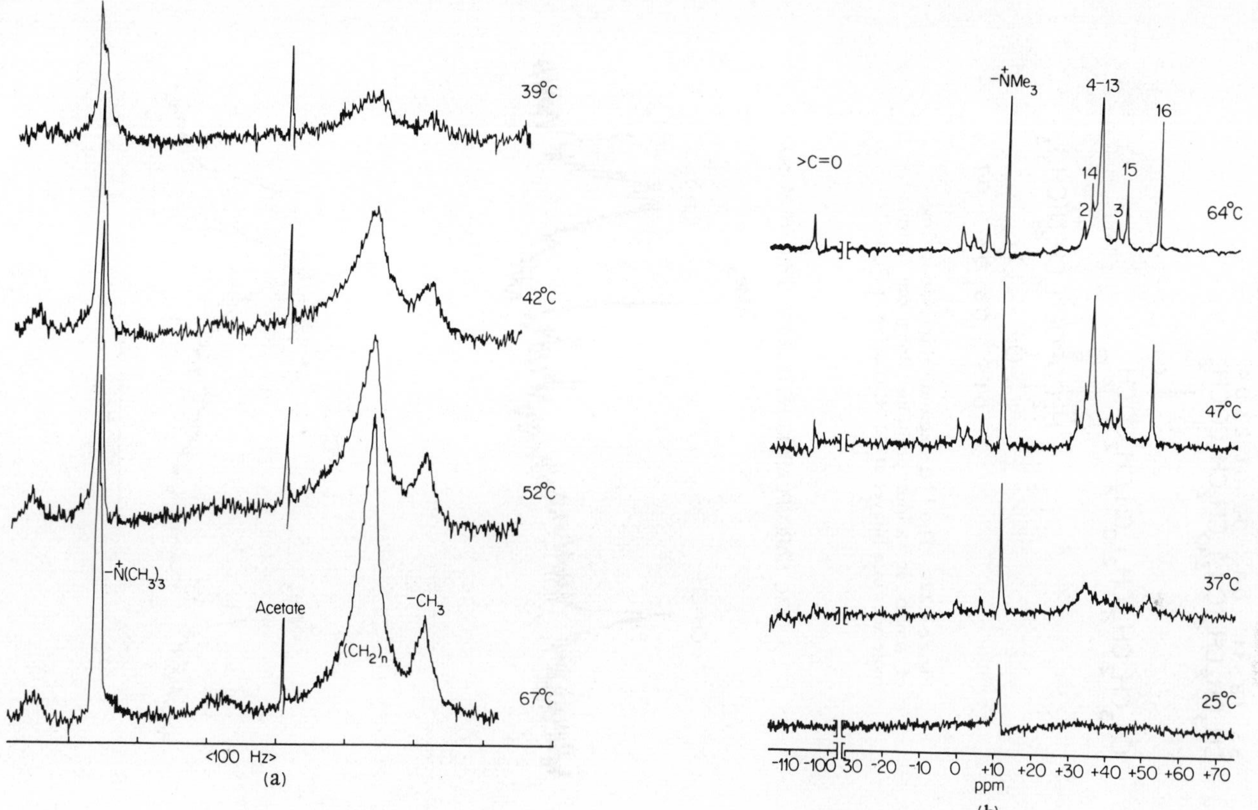

Figure 4.21 (a) Proton and (b) ^{13}C spectra of dipamitoyl lecithin. (Levine *et al.*, 1972)

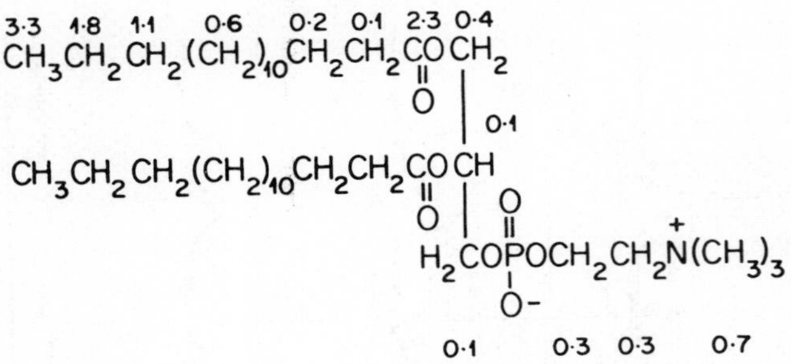

Figure 4.22 The ^{13}C longitudinal relaxation times of nuclei at various positions along the lecithin molecules in a bilayer at 52 °C (Levine *et al.*, 1972)

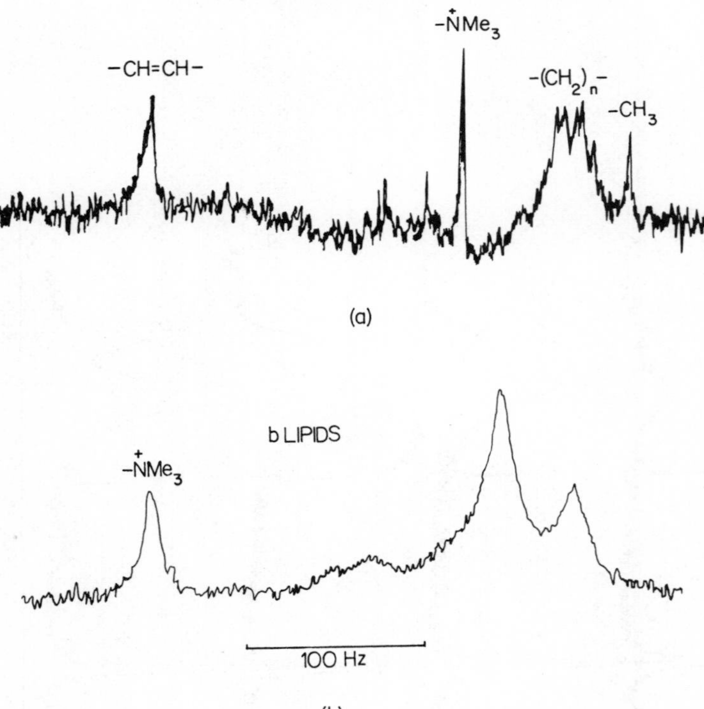

Figure 4.23 (a) The ^{13}C and (b) ^{1}H NMR spectra of vesicles prepared from sarcoplasmic reticulum. (Lee *et al.*, 1974)

of lipid molecules in the plane of the bilayer dominates the T_2 of the protons. The T_2 values determined from linewidths gave a lower limit for the lateral diffusion coefficient which agreed reasonably well with that obtained using the spin-labelling technique. (Traube and Sackmann 1972).

Biological membranes

The ^{13}C and $.^{1}H$ NMR spectra of vesicles prepared from sarcoplasmic reticulum are shown in Figure 4.23(a) and (b). As for the model membranes, the ^{13}C NMR spectra are better resolved; terminal methyl, methylene and quaternary amine methyl resonances can be distinguished. Comparison of the relative intensities in the ^{13}C spectra from the membranes and extracted lipids shows that three-quarters of the lipids contribute to the membrane spectrum. This correlates with the proportion of the membrane which is fluid. Proton T_1 studies on the fluid portion of the sarcoplasmic reticulum membrane suggest that the lateral diffusion coefficient is comparable to that in pure lipid bilayers (1×10^{-8} cm^2 s^{-1}) (Lee, Birdsall and Metcalfe, 1973). It is interesting to note that no $-NMe^{3+}$ resonances appear in the ^1H spectrum of the membrane which suggests that these groups are involved in interaction with proteins. Further information about both fluid and non-fluid regions of the biological membrane and protein–phospholipid interactions will require NMR studies using phospholipids selectively labelled with isotopes (e.g. ^{13}C or ^{19}F).

4.9 Collagen hydration

Although the collagen molecule, which is of such great importance in the structure of connective tissue, is a relatively simple one, the elucidation of its basic structure has occupied a great deal of time and effort. It is now known that each molecule consists of three polypeptide chains rich in glycine, proline and hydroxyproline, arranged as a triple helix. The resultant composite molecules are then packed hexagonally in solid collagen. It has been known for some time that collagen can take up water, and Berendsen (1962) performed an early experiment on the NMR spectrum of this water. The close association of the water molecules with the solid collagen naturally made the linewidths very large, but the investigation produced the extremely interesting result that in oriented samples of collagen, the water resonance was in the form of a symmetrical doublet resulting from a dipolar interaction between the protons of the water molecules. Berendsen proposed that the water in collagen was in the form of hydrogen-bonded chains. Some time later, Chapman and McLauchlan (1969) combined calculations of the motion of the water molecules with other measurements, notably dielectric constant and deuterium resonance experiments, to propose that the model shown in Figure 4.24(a) was the most probable. The following points may be noted about the model: (i) The water molecules are asymmetrically arranged with respect to the

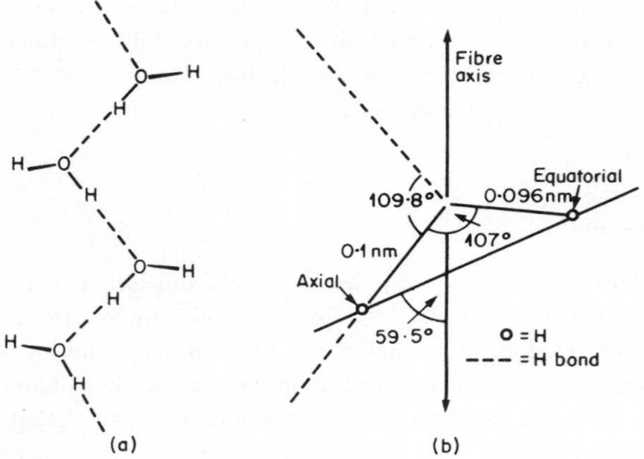

Figure 4.24 (a) Schematic diagram of the water chain model; (b) detail of (a). (From Chapman *et al.*, 1971. Reproduced by permission of the Royal Society)

chain axis, (ii) O—H bonds are different lengths because only one of the hydrogen atoms is involved in a hydrogen bond, (iii) If deuterium is substituted for hydrogen, the electric field at each deuterium nucleus will be different, and so the electric quadrupole coupling constants of the two deuterium nuclei will also differ.

To investigate further the structure of this water chain, Chapman *et al.* (1971) constructed a more detailed model (Figure 4.24b) based on dimensions and geometry known for water molecules in ice (hydrogen-bonded) and water vapour (non-hydrogen-bonded), and then calculated theoretical values for proton spin–spin and deuteron quadrupole splittings based on the new model. The values obtained were +10.5 kHz for the proton—proton splitting, and −232 kHz for the equatorial and 161 kHz for the axial deuteron. Since the two latter were rapidly exchanging, the average splitting of −35.5 kHz was predicted. The signs of these splittings and their ratio agreed closely with measured values, thereby lending support for the model.

Further data regarding the hydration structure of collagen were assembled by considering the effect of temperature and of water content on the NMR spectrum. Figure 4.25 shows the temperature dependence of the proton doublet at a 36% water content which is also seen to be superimposed on a broad peak from protein resonances. Even at −50 °C a quantity of water up to 55% by weight of collagen is sufficiently mobile to give a spectrum, implying that this amount of water is involved in the hydration structure to such an extent as to be unable to form ice. This is a large amount of water, and is more than would be expected in the primary hydration structure. Thus it was proposed that some water was associated with the chain other than that in the primary hydration structure. Since this water would presumably be less oriented than the primary chains, and would also exchange with the water in them, a study was made of the effect on the spectrum of increasing

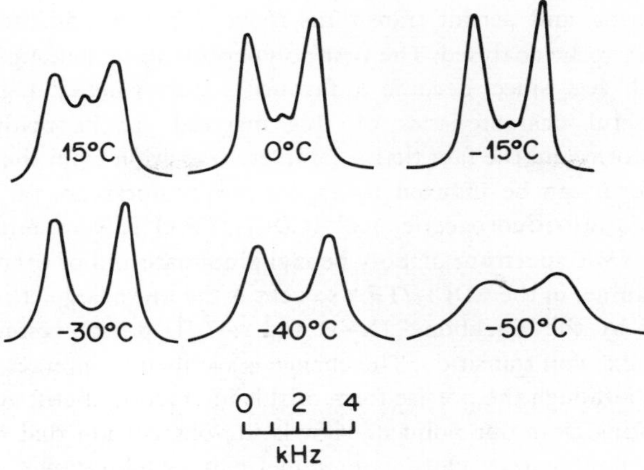

Figure 4.25 Proton NMR spectra of water adsorbed on collagen fibres at a water content of 36% per weight of dry collagen. (From Chapman *et al.*, 1971. Reproduced by permission of the Royal Society)

water content. The orientation, as measured by the spectral splitting, remained constant up to 24% hydration by weight, and decreased thereafter, fitting calculated values very closely.

There is therefore clear evidence for a primary hydration structure containing 24% of water by weight, arranged in chains as shown in Figure 4.24. These chains should fit into the interstices of the collagen triple helix; the alternative placing, between the collagen molecules, would require at least a 50% swelling of the collagen on hydration, which is not observed. Calculations of the activation energy for breaking the hydration structure, based on the temperature dependence of water orientation, gives results which are fully consistent with the water chain being attached to the collagen chain by hydrogen bonding. It appears probable that this hydrogen bonding contributes substantially to the stability of the collagen structure; measurements of the denaturation enthalpy and energy of collagen reveal that its stability is greater than could be accounted for by the interpolypeptide chain bonds alone. It thus appears that the regular water structure plays an essential role in stabilizing the structure of the macromolecule.

It is interesting that similar NMR phenomena have been observed for water adsorbed on oriented films of DNA.

4.10 Polypeptides: Helix—coil interconversion rates

Although synthetic polypeptides are not biological macromolecules they have been used extensively as models for proteins; they can provide spectroscopic characteristics of the simpler conformations in solution, notably the α-helical and random-coil forms, and permit transitions to be followed and the accompanying spectral changes to be analysed. The first polypeptide to be investigated in this way was one which has since become a favourite, poly-γ-benzyl-L-glutamate. Two particularly useful characteristics of this material are its ready solubility in deutero-chloroform and the fact that a complete transition from the random coil to the α-helical form can be induced by raising the temperature of a solution in a deutero-chloroform/trifluoroacetic acid ($CDCl_3$/TFA) solvent mixture. A major feature of the NMR spectrum of poly-benzyl glutamate and of other polypeptides, such as polyalanine, in the $CDCl_3$/TFA solvent is the quite large change in chemical shift exhibited by the 'backbone' (N—H and α—CH) proton resonances on going through the helix—coil transition. The change is ascribed to interaction of the chain with the TFA, although the precise form of this interaction is still under discussion. What is interesting from our point of view is the observation that the spectrum of partly helical poly-benzyl glutumate sometimes exhibits two separate peaks, corresponding to the helical and random-coil forms and varying in area as the percentage of helix varies (Figure 4.26) while at other times a single peak is observed, its position varying between the two extremes as the material passes through its transition, Figure 4.27. The situation appears to present a classical example of the exchange effects described in Chapter 2: the question is, how are the two different sets of results to be interpreted? The situation has been somewhat complicated by the fact that some workers have only seen one type of behaviour – for example Ferretti and Paolillo (1969) concluded that 'the observation of separate helix and random coil peaks is a completely general phenomenon which permits lower limits to the lifetime of the helix and random-coil portions of the polypeptide to be evaluated'. Since the separation of the two peaks is about 0.5 ppm (50 Hz at a measuring frequency of 100 MHz) for poly-benzyl glutamate, this would imply that the lifetime of a given backbone proton in either the helical or the random-coil form could not be less than 10^{-1}–10^{-2} s since exchange at a faster rate than this would cause coalescence of the peaks. This result would not then be in agreement with the result obtained from kinetic studies that the lifetime of a residue in one form or the other is very much shorter, of the order of 10^{-7}–10^{-8} s (see for example, Lumry *et al.*, 1964). When this is added to the observation of single peaks for some samples, notably those of higher molecular weight, it is clear that another explanation must be sought for the two peaks. The next line of enquiry was the attempted correlation of two-peaks/single peak with the molecular weight of the polymer. This was shown to be a false trail when two samples of poly-γ-benzyl-L-glutamate of nominally almost identical molecular weight were found to exhibit the two types of behaviour. Further investigation of these two samples revealed the vital clue – the nominal molecular weights, that is the number average molecular weights of the polymers, were almost identical, as were their sedimentation coefficients when centrifuged, but analysis by gel permeation chromatography showed that these averages concealed wide differences in polydispersity. In other words, the polypeptide which gave the two-peak transition had a very much wider *spread* of molecular weights than the one which gave an almost single peak.

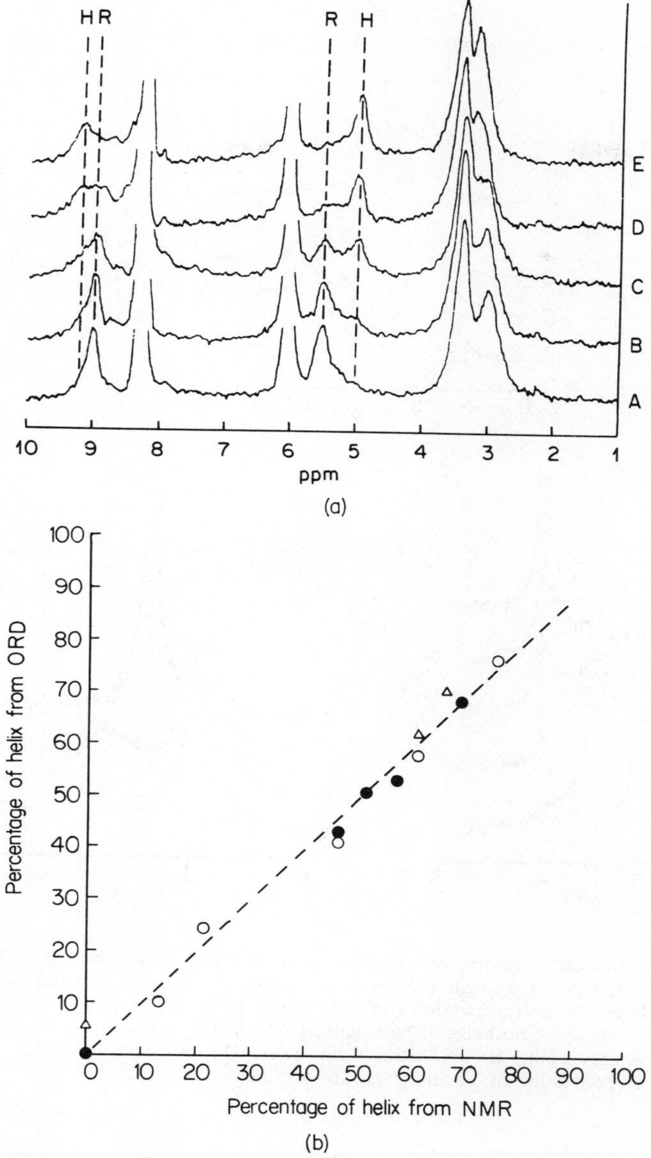

Figure 4.26 (a) Nuclear magnetic resonance spectra at 100 MHz showing the temperature induced helix-coil transition of poly-γ-benzyl-L-glutamate, dp 92, in 8 per cent trifluoroacetic acid/92 per cent deuterochloroform. H, helix; R, random. A no helix, B 16% helix, C 35% helix, D 54% helix, E 75% helix. (b) The correlation of NMR and ORD estimates of helix content for three samples; (○) degree of polymerization (dp) 92; (△) dp 21; (●) dp 13. (From Badbury *et al.*, 1968. Reproduced by permission of Macmillan (Journals) Ltd)

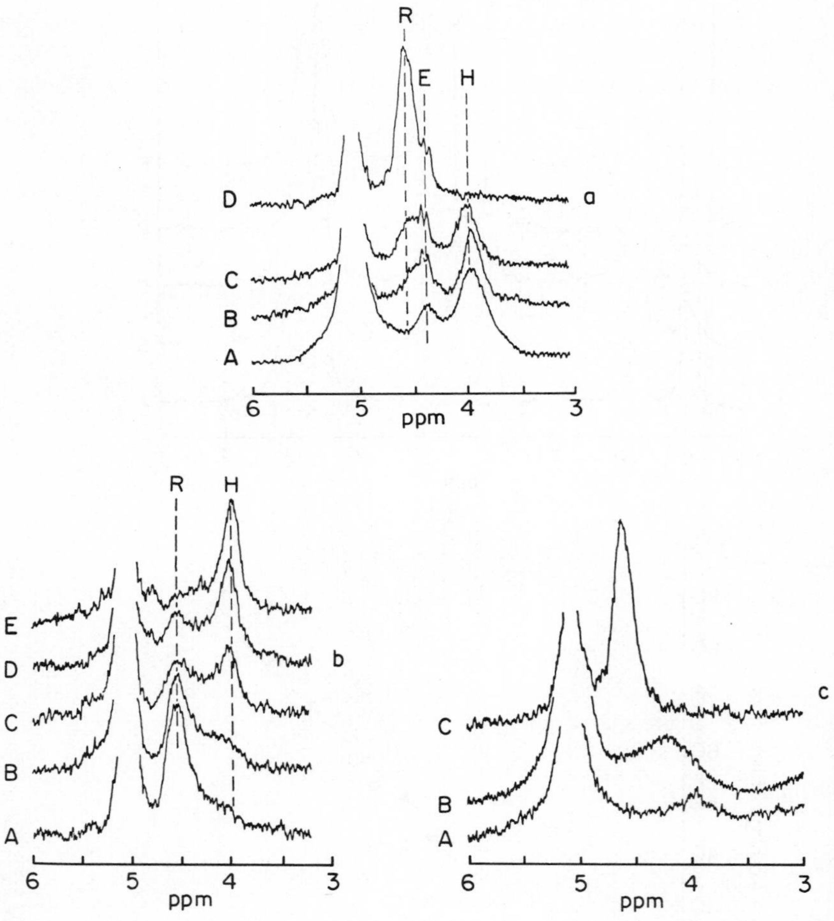

Figure 4.27 Nuclear magnetic resonance spectra of different polymers at 100 MHz showing the α CH peaks through the helix-coil transition. H, helix; R, random; E, end groups. (a) Degree of polymerization (dp) 13: A 58% helix, B 52% helix, C 35% helix, D no helix. (b) dp 92: A no helix, B 16% helix, C 35% helix, D 54% helix, E 75% helix. (c) dp 640: A 95% helix, B 65% helix, C no helix. (From Bradbury *et al.*, 1968. Reproduced by permission of Macmillan (Journals) Ltd)

An explanation now presents itself, and may be simply summarized as follows:

(1) We may assume the kinetic studies to be correct – the rate of helix-coil exchange in a partly helical polypeptide is very fast and would normally give one peak only for the α–CH or the NH resonance.

(2) In a given solvent, the amount of helix present is a function of the molecular weight of the particular molecule – large molecules tending to have a higher helix content than small ones.

(3) In a very polydisperse sample, when as a whole the sample is partly helical, most of the molecules are at one extreme or the other of the transition – very few molecules out of the total population are themselves partly helical. These partly helical molecules will give a single intermediate peak, but since there are few of them this peak will not contribute much to the total spectrum, which consists mainly of the separate peaks of the random-coil and the helical molecules.

(4) In a sample with a very narrow range of molecular weights, on the other hand, a partly helical state implies a high proportion of partly helical molecules; because of the rapid exchange between helix and random coil forms within any one molecule, which may be envisaged as a 'rippling' of helical segments up and down the molecule, the spectrum observed for α—CH or N—H resonances is a single time averaged peak whose position between two extreme positions depends on the degree of helicity of the molecules.

The overall molecular-weight effect, in which samples of low molecular weight show more tendency to give two peaks than those of high molecular weight, may be explained by saying that the correlation between helix content in a given solvent and molecular weight is less marked at high molecular weights. This does not appear unreasonable – one would expect the difference between, say, a 5-mer and a 10-mer to show up more than that between a 5000-mer and a 10,000-mer.

The biological significance of the above comes in the form of a principle and a warning: the backbone proton peaks of a polypeptide chain may act as sensitive indicators of different backbone conformations, but the presence of two separate peaks does not allow the automatic assumption of a low exchange rate between two forms until the possibility of the molecules of the sample being segregated in some way between them has been eliminated.

4.11 Observation of tissue metabolites using ^{31}P NMR (Hoult *et al.*, 1974)

Because of the low sensitivity of ^{31}P compared to protons for NHR detection, it is only recently that spectrometers capable of studying phosphorus resonances at biological concentrations have been developed. A very high field (7.5 tesla, corresponding to 129 MHz) machine has now been used to detect phosphorus-containing tissue metabolites in whole muscle and to monitor changes in the concentrations of the metabolites with time. The first stage was to assign chemical shifts to metabolites such as inosine monophosphate, fructose-1,6-diphosphate, inorganic phosphate, creatine phosphate and adenosine triphosphate by running their spectra both individually and as mixtures. This done, a spectrum was obtained from an intact, freshly excised muscle from the hind leg of a rat (Figure 4.28). The signals from this muscle, while broader than those of the isolated metabolites, could be assigned, and changes in them monitored as a function of time after excision (Figure 4.29). Many conclusions may be drawn from the results, for example that creatine kinase maintains the ATP level constant at the expense of creatine phosphate until the latter substrate has been used up, demonstrating the ability of the kinase to buffer the muscle ATP concentration. Another interesting observation

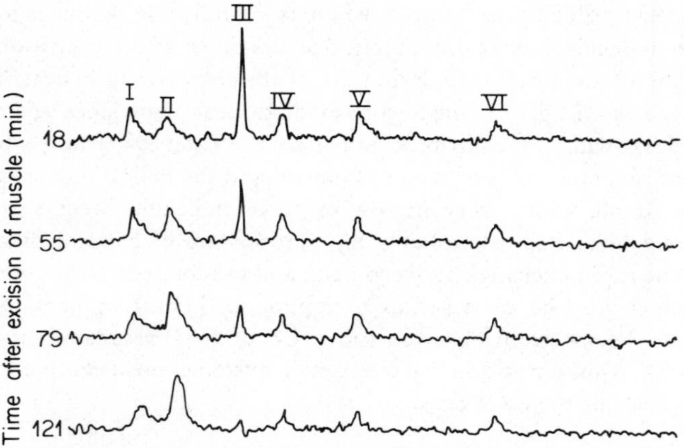

Figure 4.28 ^{31}P NMR spectrum of an intact muscle from the hind leg of the rat recorded at 129 MHz without proton irradiation. Temperature 20 °C and pulse interval 16 s. Peak assignments: I, sugar phosphate and phospholid; II, inorganic phosphate; III, creatine phosphate; IV, γ ATP; V, a ATP; VI, β ATP. The times are the midpoints of the 50 scan spectral accumulations (referred to excision time as zero). The muscle was bathed in a minimum volume of calcium-free Locke ringer. (From Hoult *et al.*, 1974. Reproduced by permission of Macmillan (Journals) Ltd)

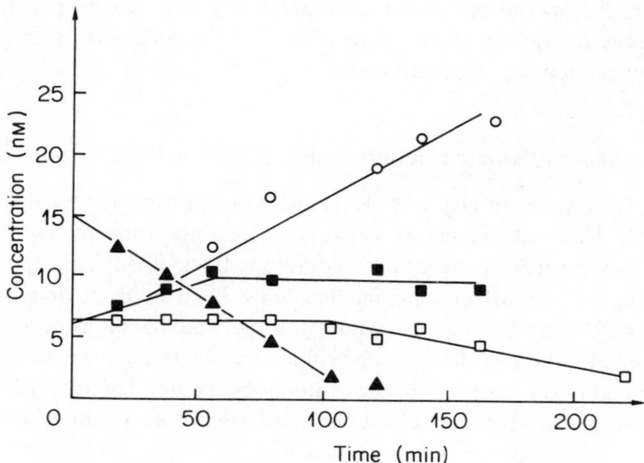

Figure 4.29 Variation of phosphorus metabolite levels in an intact rat leg muscle with time after excision. The integrals of spectra shown in Figure 4.28 are plotted in this graph. ○, Inorganic phosphate; ▲, creating phosphate; ■, sugar phosphate and phospholipid; □, ATP. An absolute concentration scale was established by running a standard sample of 10 mM phosphate in the same conditions as the muscle. (From Hoult *et al.*, 1974. Reproduced by permission of Macmillan (Journals) Ltd)

is that these results can only be obtained with intact muscle. Samples which are even slightly lacerated during handling have only an inorganic phosphate peak in the phosphorus spectrum. Breakdown of organic phosphates by phosphatases is assumed to have occurred in the damaged muscle. It appears that such studies of ^{31}P resonance in intact tissues will provide a wealth of information on metabolite levels, turnover, interaction and compartmentation, and further publications are awaited with interest.

4.12 Summary

(1) The complete structure of low molecular weight biomolecules in solution can be determined by NMR.

(2) Resolution and line broadening effects prevent complete structural information being obtained *directly* from protein NMR spectra.

(3) NMR evidence bearing on models for the cooperative binding of oxygen by haemoglobin has been presented.

(4) The iron centre in cytochromes can be used as an inherent paramagnetic shift probe for aiding spectral assignment and has lead to a proposed structure for cytochrome c_3.

(5) A plausible model for the structure of t-RNA has been proposed on the basis of high-resolution NMR studies.

(6) The structure of histones and the molecular basis for their interactions with nucleic acids can be investigated.

(7) Flexibility gradients and other motions in phospholipid membranes can be analysed from NMR relaxation time studies.

(8) The biological importance of bound water can be understood from NMR measurements and has contributed to our knowledge of collagen structure.

(9) Conclusions drawn from NMR on the rates of conformational interversions, e.g. polypeptide helix – random coil transitions, should be considered with caution.

References

Asakura, T. (1973). *Ann. N.Y. Acad. Sci.*, **222**, 68.

Berendsen, H. J. C. (1962). *J. Chem. Phys.*, **36**, 3297.

Birdsall, N. J. M., Lee, A. G., Levine, Y. K., and Metcalfe, J. C. (1971). *Chem. Comm.*, 1171.

Blake, C. C. F., Johnson, L. N., Mair, G. A., North, A. C. T., Phillips, D. C., and Sarma, V. R. (1967). *Proc. Roy. Soc.*, **B167**, 378.

Bradbury, E. M., Crane-Robinson, C., Goldman, H., and Rattle, H. W. E. (1968). *Nature*, **217**, 812.

Bradbury, E. M., Cary, P. D., Crane-Robinson, D., and Rattle, H. W. E. (1973). *Ann. N.Y. Acad. Sci.*, **222**, 266.

Bradbury, E. M., and Rattle, H. W. E. (1972), *Eur. J. Biochem.*, **27**, 270.

Bradbury, E. M., Cary, P. D., Chapman, G. E., Crane-Robinson, C., Danby, S. E., Rattle, H. W. E., Boublik, M., Palau, J., and Aviles, F. J. (1975a). *Eur. J. Biochem.*, **52**, 605.

Bradbury, E. M., Danby, S. E., and Rattle, H. W. E. (1975b). *Eur. J. Biochem.*, in press.

Brewster, A. I. R., Hruby, V. J., Spatola, A. F., and Bovey, F. A. (1973). *Biochemistry,* **12**, 1643.

Cassoly, R., Gibson, Q. H., Ogawa, S., and Shulman, R. G. (1971). *Biochem. Biophys. Res. Comm.,* **44**, 1015.

Chapman, G. E., and McLauchlan, K. A. (1969). *Proc. Roy. Soc. Lond.,* **B173**, 223.

Chapman, G. E., Danyluk, S. S., and McLauchlan, K. A. (1971). *Proc. Roy. Soc. Lond.,* **B178**, 465.

Deslauriers, R., Walter, R., and Smith, I. C. P. (1972). *Biochem. Biophys. Res. Comm.,* **48**, 854.

Dobson, C. M., Hoyle, N. J., Geraldes, C. F., Wright, P. E., Williams, R. J. P., Bruschi, M., and LeGall, J. (1974). *Nature,* **249**, 425.

Ferretti, J. A., and Paolillo, L. (1969). *Biopolymers,* **7**, 155.

Hoult, D. I., Busby, S. J. W., Gadian, D. G., Radda, G. K., Richards, R. E., and Seeley, P. J. (1974). *Nature,* **252**, 285.

Jardetzky, O., Thielmann, H., Arata, Y., Marsley, J. L., and Williams, M. N. (1971). *Cold Spring Harbour Symp. Quant. Biol.,* **36**, 257.

Jardetzky, O., and Wade-Jardetzky, N. G. (1971). *Ann. Rev. Biochem.,* **40**, 605.

Kearns, D. R., Lightfoot, D. R., Wong, K. L., Wong, Y. P., Reid, B. R., Cary, L., and Shulman, R. G. (1973). *Ann. N.Y. Acad. Sci.,* **222**, 324.

Kearns, D. R., Wong, Y. P., Hawkins, E., and Chang, S. H. (1974). *Nature,* **247**, 541.

Lee, A. G., Birdsall, N. J. M., and Metcalfe, J. C. (1972). *Biochem. Biophys. Acta.,* **255**, 43.

Lee, A. G., Birdsall, N. J. M., and Metcalfe, J. C. (1973). *Biochemistry,* **12**, 1650.

Lee, A. G., Birdsall, N. J. M., and Metcalfe, J. C. (1974). *Methods in Membrane Biology*, Vol. 2. (Plenum Publishing Corp.).

Levine, Y. K., Birdsall, N. J. M., Lee, A. G., and Metcalfe, J. C. (1972), *Biochemistry,* **11**, 1416.

Levine, Y. K., Partington, P., Roberts, G. C. K., Birdsall, N. J. M., Lee, A. G., and Metcalfe, J. C. (1972). *FEBS Lett.,* **23**, 203.

Lumry, R., Legare, R., and Miller, W. G. (1964). *Biopolymers,* **2**, 484.

McDonald, C. C., Phillips, W. D., and LeGall, J. (1974). *Biochemistry,* **13**, 1952.

Marsh, D., Phillips, A. D., Watts, A., and Knowles, P. F. (1972). *Biochem. Biophys. Res. Comm.,* **49**, 641.

Ogawa, S., Shulman, R. G., and Yamane, T. (1972a). *J. Mol. Biol.,* **70**, 291.

Ogawa, S., Shulman, R. G., Fujiwara, M., and Yamane, T. (1972b). *J. Mol. Biol.,* **70**, 301.

Ogawa, S., and Shulman, R. G. (1972c). *J. Mol. Biol.,* **70**, 315.

Smith, I. C. P., Deslauriers, R., Suits, H., Walter, R., Carrigon-Lagrange, C., McGregor, H., and Sarantakio, D. (1973). *Ann. N.Y. Acad. Sci.,* **222**, 597.

Suddath, F. L., Quigley, G. J., McPherson, A., Sneden, D., Kim, J. J., Kim, S. H., and Rich, A. (1974). *Nature,* **248**, 20.

Trauble and Sackmann (1972). *J. Amer. Chem. Soc.,* **94**, 4499.

Reading List

Bradbury, E. M., Cary, P. D., Crane-Robinson, C., and Hartman, P. G. (1973). 'Nuclear magnetic resonance of polypeptides', *Rev. Pure App. Chem.*, **36**, 63.

Cohen, J. S. (1972). 'Nuclear magnetic resonance investigation of the interactions of biomolecules', *Experimental Methods of Biophysical Chemistry*, Vol. 6, Chapter 12, 521.

Dwek, R. A. (1973). *NMR in Biochemistry: Application to Enzyme Systems*, Oxford, Clarendon Press.

Lee, A. G., Birdsall, N. J. M., and Metcalfe, J. C. (1974). *Methods in Membrane Biology*, Vol. 2. (Plenum Publishing Corp.).

McDonald, C. C., and Phillips, W. D. (1970). 'Proton magnetic resonance spectroscopy of proteins', *Fine Structure of Proteins and Nucleic Acids*, **Vol. 4, p. 1**, Fasman, G. D., and Timasheff, N. (Eds.), Dekker, New York.

Mildvan, A. S., and Cohn, M. (1970). 'Aspects of enzyme mechanism studied by nuclear spin relaxation induced by paramagnetic probes', *Advances in Enzymology,* **33**, 1 (Ed. F. F. Nord), Interscience, New York.

Rattle, H. W. E. (1974). 'NMR in the study of biopolymers', *Progress in Biophysics and Molecular Biology,* **28**, 1–40.

Roberts, G. C. K., and Jardetzky, O. (1970). 'Nuclear magnetic resonance spectroscopy of amino acids, peptides and proteins', *Advances in Protein Chemistry,* **24**, 448.

Sheard, B., and Bradbury, E. M. (1970). 'Nuclear magnetic resonance in the study of biopolymers and their interactions with ions and small molecules', *Progress in Biophysics and Molecular Biology,* **20**, 187.

Sykes, B. D., and Scott, M. (1972). 'NMR studies of the dynamic aspects of molecular structure and interaction in biological systems', *Ann. Rev. Biophys. and Bioeng.*, **1**, 27.

Wuthrich, K. (1970). 'Structural studies of hemes and hemoproteins', *Structure and Bonding,* **8**, 53.

Chapter 5
Advanced NMR Techniques

5.1 Introduction

Although 'normal' NMR spectra have found many uses in the study of biomolecules, the technique is capable of development in ways which overcome some of the limitations of the basic method and reveal much more information. Such advances draw heavily on advances in chemistry and physics. This chapter describes the main ways in which NMR can be extended in usefulness including one or two ways which have yet to find biological application; undoubtedly many techniques which will become important have been omitted, since change comes about very rapidly.

5.2 Resolution enhancement

In Chapter 3 the possibility of reducing the noise level of a spectrum obtained by Fourier transformation of a free induction decay pattern was described and illustrated; it consisted in 'convoluting' the FID, or in other words multiplying it by a factor which decreased exponentially. The improvement in signal-to-noise ratio was obtained at the cost of some line broadening, and this may be understood by considering that the rate of decay of the FID is the measure of T_2, from which linewidth information is obtained. Convolution has the same effect as shortening T_2, and produces broader lines. Clearly deconvolution, or multiplying by an exponentially increasing function, should produce artificially narrow lines, thereby improving the resolution of the spectrum; this is possible but carries with it the disadvantage of a considerable increase in noise level. The right-hand end of an FID as displayed contains mostly noise, and yet this is the part which is multiplied by the largest factor in deconvolution. A way of improving resolution without a large increase in noise level is found in the method of convolution difference described by Campbell *et al.* (1973a). The method may be summarized as follows:

(1) Take two copies (a) and (b) of the FID.

(2) Convolute (a) with a small exponential multiplier (this step may be omitted) – Figure 5.1(a).

(3) Convolute (b) with a larger exponential multiplier (Figure 5.1b).

(4) Subtract a fraction of (b) – say about 0.8 x (b) – from (a) Figure 5.1(c).

(5) Transform and phase correct the resultant FID in the usual manner.

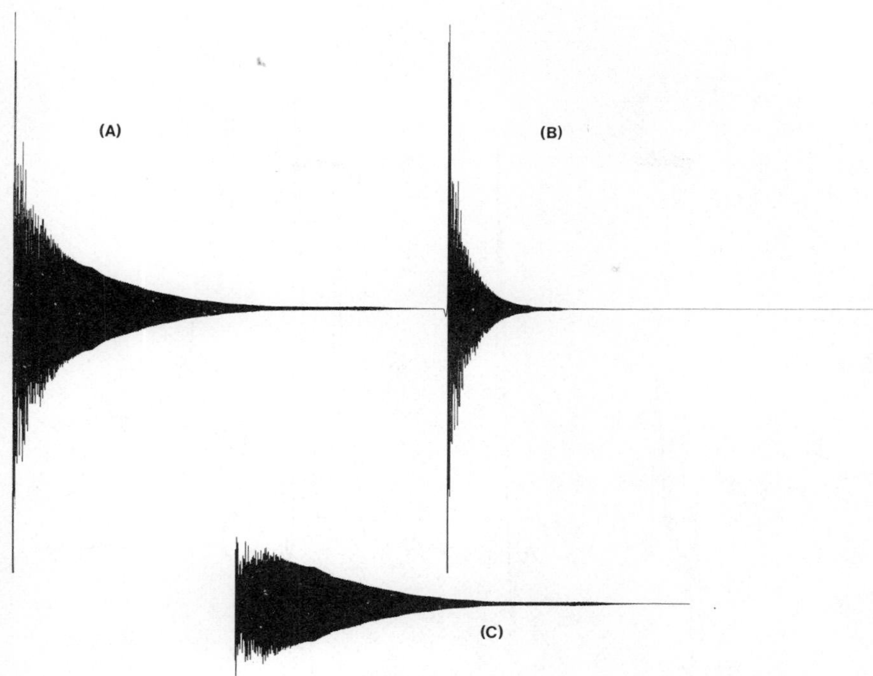

Figure 5.1 (a) Normal FID. (b) Same FID after convolution. (c) Difference FID produced by (c) = (a) − [0.8 × (b)] where (a) has exponential multiplier of −3 and (b) has exponential multiplier −12

The resultant enhanced spectrum is shown as Figure 5.2(c) together with the original spectrum (Figure 5.2a).

An alternative method is to follow steps 1, 2 and 3 above, then to transform the two FIDs, subject them to identical phase corrections to give a normal spectrum as Figure 5.2(a) and a broadened spectrum as Figure 5.2(b) and then to subtract fractions of the broadened spectrum from the original until the desired degree of resolution enhancement is obtained (Figure 5.2c). The maximum reduction of linewidth obtainable using the method is about a factor of 2; the lineshapes of the final spectrum are no longer Lorenzian, although this is of small importance in most applications. Loss of signal-to-noise is quite small using this method, although if the original spectrum is marginal in signal-to-noise, the deconvoluted version will certainly be unacceptable. Resolution enhancement by convolution difference is a most valuable tool in the hands of the biochemist who uses NMR.

5.3 Paramagnetic probes

The presence of a paramagnetic ion in a molecule can perturb the chemical shifts, the linewidths, or both, for resonances from the nuclei near the paramagnetic centre. When such a paramagnetic ion can be placed in a known position in a

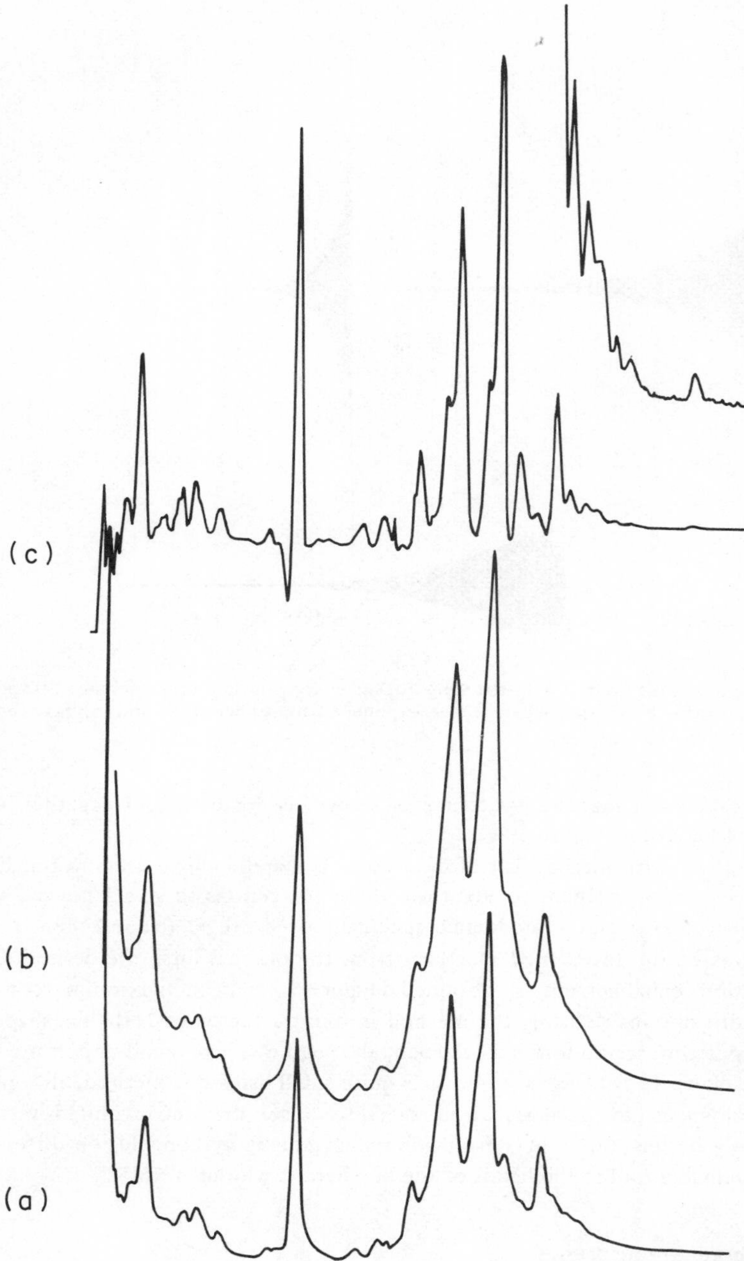

Figure 5.2 (a) Original spectrum (from FID (a) of Figure 5.1). (b) Broadened spectrum (from FID (b) of Figure 5.1). (c) Difference spectrum with resolution enhancement – obtained either from FID (c) of Figure 5.1 or by subtracting a fraction of spectrum (b) from spectrum (a)

molecule, then the region around it can be mapped by correlating the shift or broadening effects with distances from the perturbing ion. The most useful ions for this purpose are the lanthanides, which may usefully be divided into three classes (Barry *et al.*, 1971).

(1) Those such as Eu^{3+} which have very short electron relaxation times. These cause large chemical shifts but with negligible line broadening (~0.03 Hz per Hz of shift for Eu^{3+}).

(2) Those such as Gd^{3+} and Eu^{2+} which have long relaxation times and cause large isotropic broadening effects.

(3) Ions such as Ho^{3+} which both shift and broaden.

Since these ions are all part of a rare-earth series, they have identical chemical properties and so experiments may be carried out to compare the effects of groups (1), (2) and (3) ions under identical binding conditions. Lanthanum itself, as the lanthanide ion, is diamagnetic and can be used for control experiments.

The electron structure of the lanthanides is such that the shift effects which they produce can be considered to be entirely of pseudocontact origin, so that the equation

$$\frac{\Delta\nu_i}{\nu_0} = D\,\frac{(3\cos^2\chi_i - 1)}{r_i^3} \tag{5.1}$$

may be used, where r_i is the distance between the metal and the *i*th proton on the ligand, and χ_i is the angle between the vector r_i and the principal symmetry axis of the complex ion, averaged over motions rapid on the NMR time scale. D is a constant for a given metal but depends on temperature and the overall magnetic properties of the complex. Data obtained from the application of this equation can be confirmed using specific broadening probes from group (2). In this case the relevant equation has the form

$$\delta\nu_i(½) = fn\,\frac{(\gamma_i, \mu_{\text{eff}}, \tau_i)}{r_i^6} \tag{5.2}$$

where μ_{eff} is the effective magnetic moment of the paramagnetic species, γ is the nuclear magnetic moment and τ the correlation times for the magnetic perturbations.

Thus the use of shift probes yields distance and angle information, the effects changing from one ion to another, while broadening probes give distance information and over a shorter range, so that the use of a series of probes may yield a set of simultaneous equations whose solution gives unique positions and orientations for resonance near the paramagnetic ion. The method is particularly applicable to enzymes which contain one or more active-site metal ions which may be replaced by lanthanides. A series of general principles, mostly caveats, to be observed in performing such experiments has been given by Bleaney *et al.* (1971). These are:

(1) Reagents which shift to both high and low field must be used.

(2) The observed shifts must be corrected by observing shifts due to complex formation with diamagnetic lanthanides, La^{3+} and Lu^{3+}.

(3) Ratios of shifts at different proton sites should then be compared for different lanthanides. If the ratios are independent of the lanthanide cation then the shifts have their origin in dipolar coupling, and to a good approximation the anisotropy of the susceptibility has axial symmetry.

(4) In general the dependence of the shift ratios on the concentration of the lanthanide and its ligand must be followed so that the stoichiometry of the complex is proved.

The main practical difficulty in using lanthanide shift reagents is their reluctance to stay in aqueous solution at pH much above 5. For molecular species which may not directly complex with the ions, they are commonly available in two chelated forms: a tris (2,2,6,6 tetramethyl-hepto-3,5 dionato) or (DMP) complex, and a 1,1,1,2,2,3,3 heptafluoro-7,7 dimethyl,4.6 oxanedione (FOD) form which is superior for binding to weak Lewis bases such as ether and ester groups. The use of such chelated reagents will, of course, complicate the methods for calculating distances and angles from the lanthanide ion. A detailed account of the theory and use of paramagnetic probes in their application to enzyme systems is given by Dwek (1973). An example of their use will be found in Section 5.5.

5.4 Proton relaxation enhancement

The presence of paramagnetic ions in a molecular structure can give rise to contact shifts and may be of considerable value in the analysis of structure and structural changes. The presence of paramagnetic ions in a solution of macromolecules may also give valuable information through the relaxing effect that such ions have on the molecules of solvent. This effect has been of particular use in aqueous solutions, and we shall concentrate on these.

In an aqueous solution of a paramagnetic ion, for example Fe^{2+}, Co^{2+}, Ni^{2+}, Mn^{2+}, Cu^{2+}, Cr^{2+}, each ion is surrounded by a 'coordination shell' of water molecules; the water molecules in the shells are exchanging rapidly with free water molecules in the solution. While a water molecule is associated with a paramagnetic ion, its correlation time (and hence its relaxation times) may be determined by the tumbling motion of the whole complex, by chemical exchange, or by the relaxation of the unpaired electrons in the paramagnetic ion. In each case the relaxation will be more effective, due to the proximity of the large magnetic moment of the paramagnetic ion, than in the water alone. If, now, macromolecules are introduced into the solution, and these interact with the paramagnetic ions, binding them (and their coordination shells of water molecules) for times which may vary from very long to very short, the relaxation of the water protons will again be enhanced, since the hindering of free rotation caused by binding will increase the efficiency of spin relaxation. The presence of the macromolecules will thus be the cause of proton relaxation enhancement, and a parameter ϵ_1 may be defined for T_1, the spin–lattice relaxation time, as follows

$$\epsilon_1 = \frac{\text{Contribution of paramagnetic ions to spin–lattice relaxation rate of water in presence of macromolecules}}{\text{Contribution of same concentration of paramagnetic ions to spin–lattice relaxation rate in absence of macromolecules}}$$

The observed ϵ is a weighted average of the enhancement of relaxation in protons bound (via the paramagnetic ion) to the macromolecule and those not bound. The precise average depends on the length of time spent in the bound state and the number of sites available for binding. The mole fraction of the paramagnetic ions in the bound state may be determined analytically, or it may be found by measuring ϵ at different concentrations of the macromolecule (at infinite concentration of macromolecules, all the paramagnetics would be bound) and, once this is known, the enhancement parameter for bound paramagnetic ions may be found. Knowing this, it is possible to determine association constants, for example in enzyme–Mn^{2+}–substrate systems, to investigate the nature and structure of the binding site, and also to analyse changes in the binding site of enzymes. Of course, enzymes are not the only biological molecules to be associated with paramagnetic ions; for example, Sheard and coworkers (1967) have studied the nature of the binding of the Mn^{2+} ions which are necessary to the structural integrity of ribosomes. It was possible from this study to conclude that the Mn^{2+} ions were bound mainly to the RNA, in positions which were not deeply buried in the structure of the ribosome or in the 50s–30s interface. The method is reviewed and described in more detail by Sheard and Bradbury (1970) and Dwek (1973).

5.5 Paramagnetic and other difference methods

As has been stressed earlier in the book, one of the chief difficulties encountered in biological NMR is the overlap of data, in which vital information is often obscured beneath a mass of less relevant resonances. The computer interfaced to a Fourier-transform spectrometer makes possible the use of difference spectroscopy, in which small changes in the spectrum, induced by paramagnetic probes or by spin decoupling, or by chemical modification or other alternation of the sample, may be revealed by subtracting the changed from the original spectrum so that all resonances not so modified are subtracted out, leaving only the resonances of interest. Figure 5.3 illustrates the effect to be expected and Figure 5.4 gives an example of paramagnetic broadening difference spectra from the methyl region of hen egg-white lysozyme, both before and after resolution enhancement by convolution difference (Campbell *et al.*, 1973b). Once the resonances have been revealed to view by difference spectroscopy, they are of course amenable to assignment by spin–decoupling methods (i.e. performing difference spectroscopy with a second irradiating frequency present). Spin decoupling is described in Chapter 2. An example, again from the study of lysozyme, is shown in Figure 5.5. Spectra like this are not obtained without considerable effort, but such methods may be the only way of assigning resonances and getting to the biologically significant stage of an investigation. Paramagnetic difference spectroscopy may be

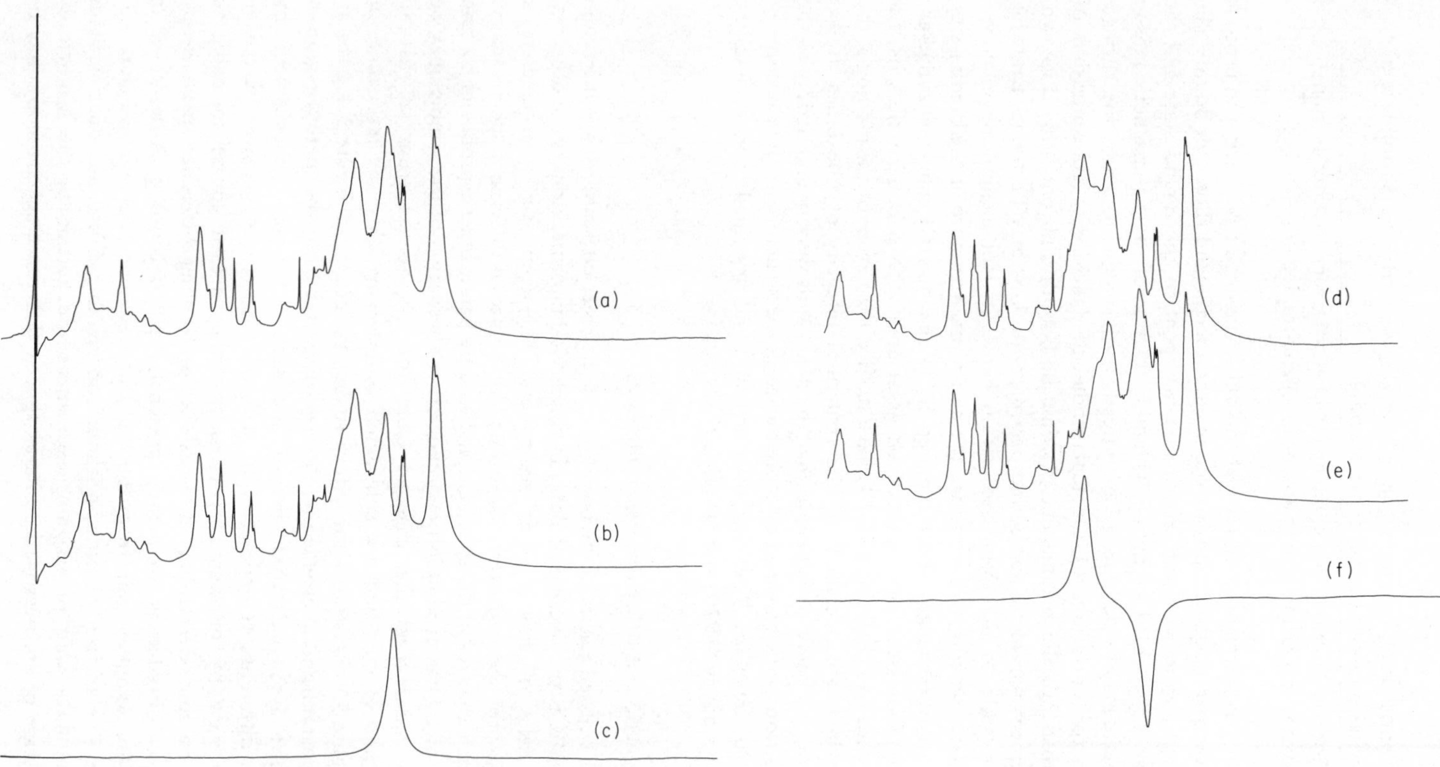

Figure 5.3 Simulated spectra: (a) unmodified spectrum; (b) spectrum (a) modified by broadening one peak (which effectively disappears); (c) difference spectrum (a)−(b); (d) another unmodified spectrum; (e) spectrum (d) modified by shifting one peak; (f) difference spectrum (d)−(e)

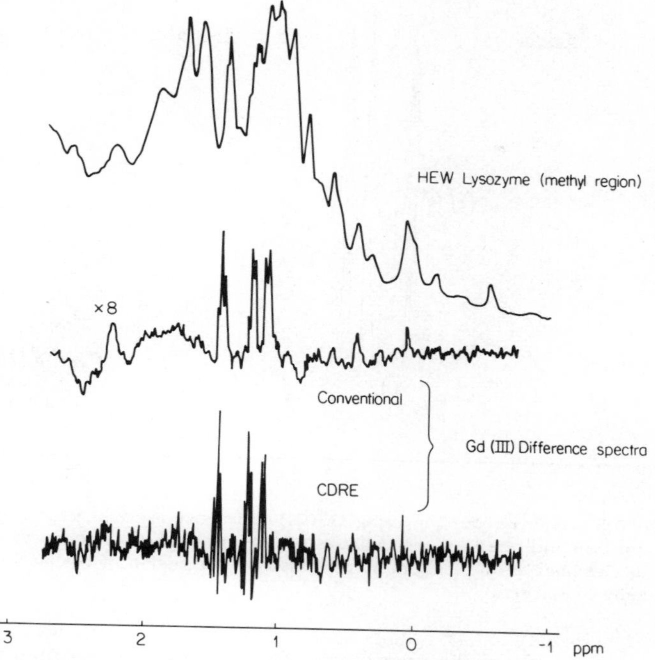

Figure 5.4 Paramagnetic difference spectra of HEW lysozyme (Lys) = 5.2 mM, (Gd) = 5 x 10^{-5} M, (La^{3+}) = 50 mM. The lower spectrum shows the convolution difference spectrum of the paramagnetic difference spectrum. This reveals the multiplet structure. Shift probes confirm the presence of three doublets. The other peaks in the spectrum respresent contributions from a number of more distant protons. (From Campbell *et al.*, 1973b. Reproduced by permission of the New York Academy of Sciences)

applied to shifting as well as broadening probes, and temperature dependence used to separate paramagnetically shifted (temperature-dependent) from ring-current shifted (temperature-independent) resonances. The permutations for the ingenious experimenter are almost endless. Figure 5.6 shows the radial distribution diagram for the active site region of lysozyme in solution; initial positions were obtained from the known crystal structure of the molecules and it was then possible to confirm that the structure in solution was the same by the correlation of paramagnetic probe data.

Difference spectroscopy need not be limited to paramagnetic probes; one approach used by one of the authors in investigating the interaction between two histone molecules suspected of interacting in a specific way which might produce small changes in the spectrum is as follows:

Run the spectrum of a mixture of the two histones under appropriate interaction-inducing solution conditions. Run the spectra of the individual histones under identical solution conditions. Add the latter spectra together. Subtract the

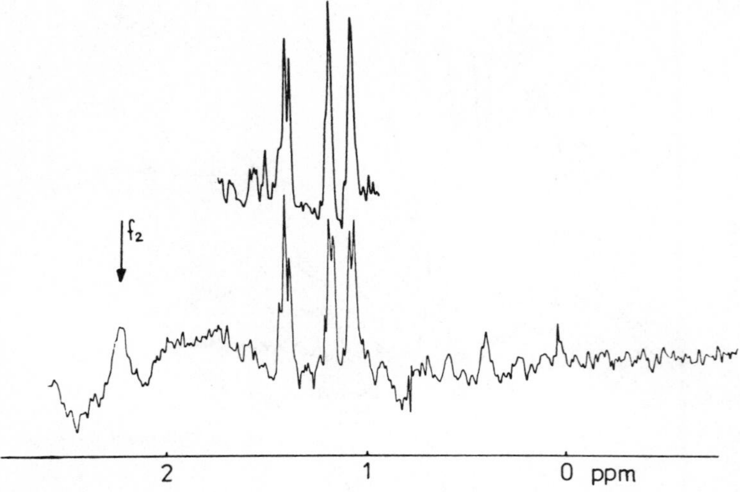

Figure 5.5 Spin-decoupling using Gd(III) difference spectra. Irradiation at the position indicated causes collapse of the two upfield resonances only. (From Campbell *et al.*, 1973b. Reproduced by permission of the New York Academy of Sciences)

sum of these spectra from the spectrum of the mixture. The result is a few clearly visible signals corresponding to those resonances shifted or broadened by the interaction.

A major problem with difference spectroscopy is to ensure that the only difference between the spectra to be subtracted is the desired one – in other words nominally identical parts of the spectrum must be identical. In particular they should be identical in phase, shift and area. Phase is relatively easy to manage by trial and error, but the lock frequency of a spectrum is liable to be changed by alterations in pH, ionic strength or temperature, and very small shifts of the whole spectrum give complex, uninterpretable and often irrelevant difference spectra. It is desirable that as far as possible spectra to be subtracted are run under identical solution conditions. The best way of ensuring equal areas for the spectra seems to be to integrate the difference spectrum and adjust the subtraction until the total integral is zero, i.e. until the levels of the integral are equal at both ends of the difference spectrum.

5.6 Solvent elimination

One of the major problems which has always faced the investigator of the proton magnetic resonance of biological molecules is the fact that water, which is the 'natural' solvent for such molecules, gives rise to an enormous resonance which can swamp the spectrum. The use of D_2O as a solvent alleviates the problem and also simplifies the spectrum by the removal of signals from exchangeable protons, which is desirable provided they are not the peaks of interest! However, the advent of FT

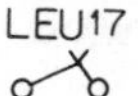

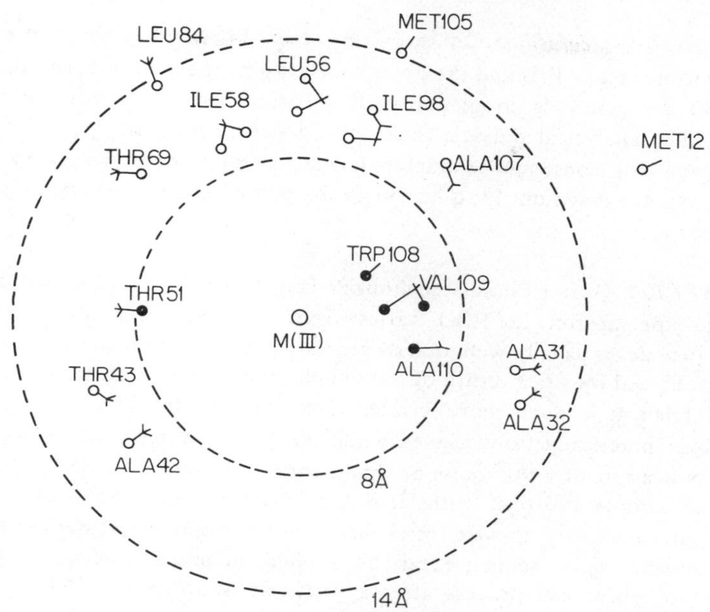

Figure 5.6 Radial distribution projection diagram for some of the residues of HEW lysozyme. These data were obtained from the crystal structure and the known Gd(III) binding position in the crystal. The paramagnetic shifts found in solution correlate exactly with this structure. (From Campbell *et al.*, 1973b. Reproduced by permission of the New York Academy of Sciences)

adds a new dimension to the problem; even in a well-deuterated sample, the HDO peak usually dominates in terms of height if not in total area, and since the whole height of the FID must be recorded, this water component, arising from the residual HDO molecules in the sample, uses up the available computer space and reduces the number of scans possible as well as cutting down the efficiency of digitization of the FID of the sample resonances.

The water signal may be reduced or eliminated in one of several ways; if it is really critical to reduce it to a minimum, it is often a good idea to dialyse the sample against good D_2O before starting, because much of the residual HDO is due to the protons from the exchangeable groups of the sample, and dialysis will largely get rid of these. The water resonance may then be reduced on an FT spectrometer by:

(a) Fast pulsing. This is very simple; if the sample has a fast relaxation time relative to the HDO, which is usual in proton spectroscopy of biomolecules, then

the spectrometer may be pulsed at a rate which does not allow the water to relax completely while still allowing the sample to relax. The water may be reduced to perhaps one-quarter of its normal height by this means.

(b) Selective saturation. A short time (say 0.3 s) is left between the end of accumulation of one FID and the pulse which begins the next one. During this time the HDO frequency is irradiated with sufficient power to saturate the water protons. The analytical pulse is then applied before the water can relax, and the water signal is in consequence much reduced. Using this method it is easy to get the water resonance down until it is no longer the tallest peak in a sample at, say, 1 mM concentration.

(c) WEFT. (Water-Eliminated Fourier Transform). The longitudinal relaxation time for the proton in HDO varies from 5–15 s, while T_1 for biological macromolecules is usually well under a second. Thus the application of a 180° pulse will be followed by a fast return of the sample spins to equilibrium, while the water protons relax at a much more leisurely rate, to such an extent that the sample protons are practically fully relaxed while the M_z for water is still passing through zero. Application of a 90° pulse at this point is followed by an FID coming only from the sample protons, with zero contribution from the water. It is then theoretically necessary to wait for a long time for the whole system to equilibrate before another pulse sequence can be applied; in practice, however, it is often possible to repeat the process after a relatively short time ($\sim 5T_{1(\text{sample})}$), in which case the production of a water-eliminated Fourier-transform (WEFT) spectrum need only take about twice as long as normal. The process requires a magnet with a heteronuclear lock.

Of the three methods selective saturation stands out as being uncritical and easy to use, although WEFT is in principle capable of eliminating the water completely if set up with care.

5.7 Long-term accumulation of spectral data

It is sometimes necessary to accumulate a large number of spectra in order to see clearly a small signal; in such cases the largest signals may overflow the memory capacity of the accumulating device. This presents no problem when a CAT is being used with a continuous-wave spectrometer, but in a Fourier-transform spectrometer the whole of the FID must be accumulated so that there is an absolute limit to the number of scans which are possible and hence to the available signal-to-noise ratio. For example, if the input signal is digitized using 12 bits (i.e. its maximum value is assigned a value of 2^{12}) and it fills this accurately, the maximum number of pulses possible using a 20-bit computer is $2^{20}/2^{12} = 2^8 = 256$. If more scans than this are required, special provision must be made. There are two ways of dealing with the problem: the more common is known as 'block averaging' and is performed by accumulating FIDs until the memory is nearly full, transforming the result and transferring it to another section of the memory. Although the solvent peak still dominates the transformed spectrum, it no longer matters that the top of it overflows the memory. The whole process is then repeated as often as necessary, accumulating transformed spectra in the same way as a CAT accumulates normal continuous-wave spectra. The procedure may be performed manually (a very tedious business) or may be programmed into the computer for automatic block averaging. A disadvantage of this method is that it requires the conditions of Fourier transformation, and particularly the exponential multiplier, to be set up before accumulation starts, and cannot be used for any techniques involving manipulation of the FID. This may be overcome by using a method of accumulation in which the FID is accumulated as before until the memory is nearly full, then converted into a double-precision form (i.e. using twice as many bits of store per spectral point) and storing in the double-precision form in another part of the memory. In this way a very large number of scans may be accumulated without fear of over-filling the memory. After accumulation, the FID is divided down until it again fits single-precision locations and is then transformed in the usual way. The method requires that at least three times as much computer store space is available as is being used for the single-precision FID.

5.8 Inter-nuclear double resonance (INDOR)

The INDOR (inter-nuclear double resonance) technique is not new; however, there have recently been published two papers (Gibbons *et al.*, 1972a, 1972b) which indicate that, properly applied, the method may have considerable uses in conformational studies, particularly of the smaller proteins. The major problem connected with the proton spectra of such materials is, of course, the overlap of resonances which obliterates much of the information which is present. One form of double resonance experiment, spin decoupling, is often used in assigning the resonances in such a spectrum, but suffers from the disadvantage that it produces a perturbation of only a few resonances in a spectrum containing many other lines which may obscure the effect. A homonuclear INDOR spectrum, on the other hand, contains only a few lines, corresponding only to transitions which are directly coupled to the one being monitored. In an INDOR experiment, a single frequency f_1 (which usually corresponds to a single transition) is observed, while the perturbing (decoupling) frequency, f_2, is swept through a selected range of frequencies. Signals only appear in the INDOR spectrum when f_2 passes through a transition which has an energy level in common with the transition at f_2. The INDOR signal may be either positive or negative according to the precise connection between the transitions. Because each amino acid in a polypeptide is an isolated spin system, the INDOR method can be used to identify mutually coupled protons in a single amino acid residue without interference from the transitions of the other amino acids. It is thus possible to determine chemical shifts and coupling constants which would otherwise be completely inaccessible. Figure 5.7 shows an example. The top spectrum is that of a small region of the proton spectrum of gramicidin S–A. The region contains the C_β and C_γ protons of leucine, the C_β and C_γ methylene protons of ornithine and proline, and the C_β proton multiplets of

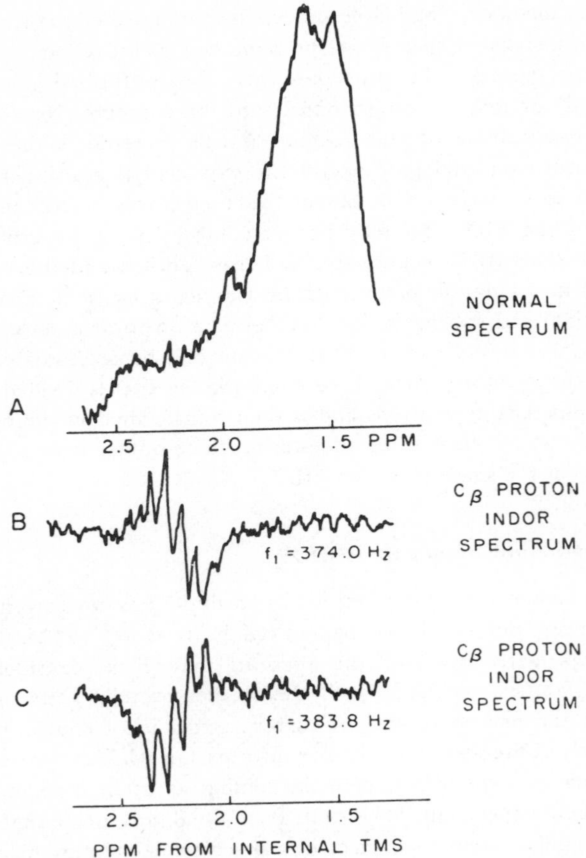

Figure 5.7 A comparison of the normal (A) and indor (B and C) proton spectra of gramicidin S-A in CD_3OD at 90 MHz. The temperature was 27°C and the internal standard was TMS. Spectrum A is the normal PMR spectrum of only those protons whose chemical shift is between 1.0 and 2.5 ppm. INDOR spectra B and C were obtained by monitoring the intensity of C_α proton transitions with f_1 at 374.0 and 383.8 Hz, respectively, while sweeping the decoupling field (f_2) from 240.0 to 120.0 Hz (2.67–1.33 ppm, respectively) through the C_β proton region. (Reprinted with permission from Gibbons, W. A., Alms, H., Bockman, R. S., and Wyssbrod, H. R. (1972). *Biochemistry*, 11, 1721. Copyright by the American Chemical Society)

valine. By monitoring at the appropriate α–CH frequencies (determined by trial and error or from model compounds), only the valine C_β resonance appears in the INDOR spectrum, revealing at once its precise chemical shift and spin–spin splittings. The experiment further confirms the precise resonance frequencies of the C_α resonances. By applying the appropriate relationships between bond angles and coupling constants and extending the measurements to the other protons in the residue, it clearly becomes possible to define the conformation of each individual residue, at least for cases where there is only one of that type of residue present in the molecule, or where the same conformation is shared by all such residues.

5.9 Nuclear Overhauser enhancement (NOE) (Figure 5.8)

For ^{13}C NMR, the combination of low natural abundance and the small gyro magnetic ratio ($^{13}C = \frac{1}{4}\gamma' H$) results in a sensitivity which is 6000 times lower than for ^{1}H NMR. Thus any improvement in sensitivity for ^{13}C, no matter how small, will reduce the number of scans necessary to produce a spectrum with the required signal-to-noise ratio. An enhancement in signal-to-noise by a factor of three can be achieved through nuclear Overhauser enhancement. We have seen that for continued resonance absorption from the irradiating field, nuclei in their higher energy spin state must dissipate this energy. Fluctuating fields at the Larmor frequency in the lattice provides a mechanism for return from the upper spin state to the equilibrium condition. If the dominant relaxation process is through dipolar coupling to an adjacent nucleus (B), then the irradiating at the Larmor frequency for this second nucleus (ω_B) results in improved relaxation of the nucleus under consideration (nucleus A) and effectively allows more RF power to be absorbed at frequency ω_A, resulting in improved signal-to-noise. The maximum enhancement is given by $\epsilon = \frac{1}{2}(\gamma_A/\gamma_B)$ which for $^{13}C/^{1}H$ coupling gives $\epsilon = 2$ and an improvement in signal-to-noise of $1 + \epsilon = 3$. There is also an enhancement for like nuclei in different chemical environments where $\epsilon \simeq \frac{1}{2}$; a 50% signal-to-noise improvement results.

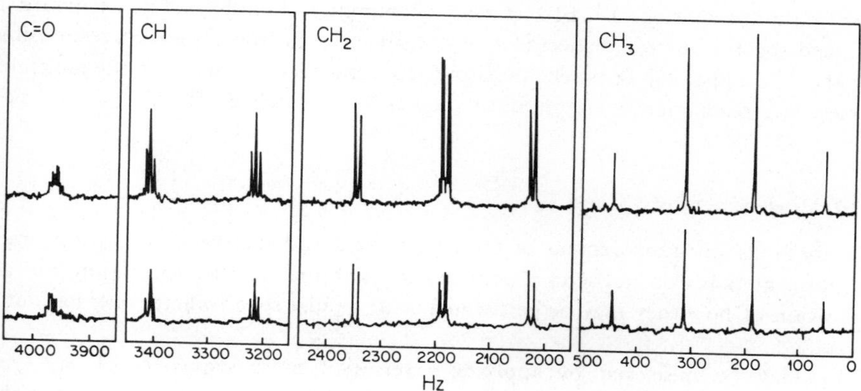

Figure 5.8 The carbon-13 spectrum of vinyl acetate observed by Fourier-transform methods without decoupling the proton resonances. The upper trace was obtained with a pulse-modulated decoupling field which was gated off whenever the carbon-13 free induction signals were being acquired. These intensities are to be compared with those in the lower trace where the decoupler was not used at all. The relative intensities may be taken as measures of the nuclear Overhauser enhancements. Note that in the spectrum of the methylene carbon, the two direct couplings have different magnitudes: 159 ± 1 Hz and 163 ± 1 Hz. The carbonyl resonance is a quartet of doublets with J(COCH) = 3 ± 1 Hz and J(CCH) = 7 ± 1 Hz (Freeman and Hill, 1971)

However, in practice these enhancements are achieved in only a limited number of cases since other criteria must also be satisfied.

(a) The rotational correlation time should be short relative to the proton resonance frequency, i.e. $\tau_R \omega_H \ll 1$.

Whilst this is true for small molecules it is not true for macromolecules unless τ_R happens to be dominated by fast internal reorientations. It is perfectly reasonable, therefore, that increased Overhauser enhancements might be observed on denaturation of a protein and this might be used as a way of monitoring sequential unfolding of a protein.

(b) Nuclear Overhauser enhancement proceeds normally by a dipole–dipole mechanism. Those carbons which do not have directly bonded hydrogens will show zero enhancement obviously but there will also be varying enhancements according to the chemical environment in which the nuclear pair resides. This prevents comparison of integrated areas, an important feature of structure determination by high resolution NMR. It is possible to short-circuit the nuclear dipole–dipole interactions through addition of paramagnetic ions which would also result in large Overhauser enhancements, but in view of the chemical shift and line broadening which also can result from addition of paramagnetic ions this must be approached with caution.

It would seem as though the wealth of spectral information in the hyperfine structure must be sacrificed in order to achieve NOE. Techniques have been developed whereby the structure can be retained whilst still gaining enhancement.

The second irradiating field (H_2) may be pulse modulated or better still switched off before the B_1 excitation pulse and restored just after the ^{13}C receiver has finished acquiring the FID (Gated decoupling). Full hyperfine structure is retained together with enhancement of ~2 since the proton saturation responsible for the ^{13}C signal enhancement persists for several seconds, whereas the multiplet coalescence phenomenon disappears as soon as B_2 is switched off.

5.10 Measurement of T_1 and T_2

The methods for measurement of the longitudinal and transverse relaxation times by pulse methods do not lend themselves to brief and simple explanation, but an indication of how they may be performed using a pulse spectrometer may be found useful.

T_1 may be measured by applying a series of pulse sequences of the type $180°$, τ, $90°$, where τ is a small time which is varied from one pulse sequence to the next. The first, $180°$, pulse inverts M_z, which then proceeds to decay back towards its original value. After a time τ the magnetization will have reached a value M which may be measured by applying a $90°$ pulse, thus tipping it into the xy plane where it may be detected. M will vary, as τ is increased, from a negative value, through zero, to its original positive value, and it may be shown that the value of τ for which M passes through zero is given by $\tau = 0.69T_1$.

Given a Fourier-transform facility, the 180–τ–90 method may be extended to

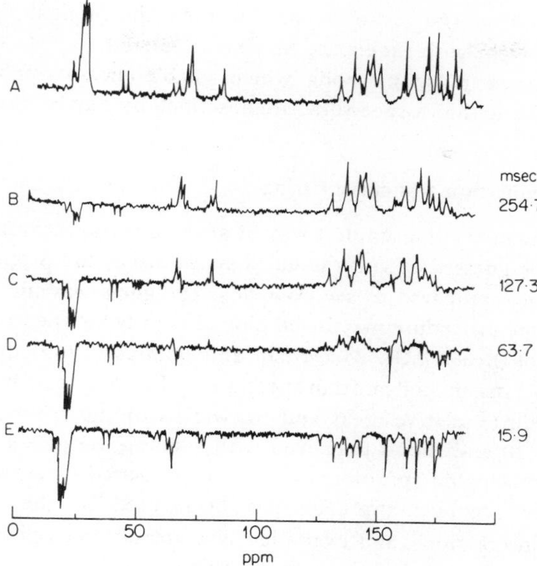

Figure 5.9 Set of partially relaxed natural abundance ^{13}C NMR spectra of RNase A, pH 2.12, 15 nM. The delay times τ in the 180°, τ, 90° sequence are shown by the spectra. The normal spectrum is shown as A (Glushko, Lawson and Gurd, 1972)

give measurements of the T_1 for the individual resonances in the spectrum. A series of FIDs, corresponding to different values of τ, are accumulated and transformed. In the resulting 'partially relaxed' spectra, the size of each individual peak is a function of its own T_1 value. Figure 5.9 shows a series of such partially relaxed spectra obtained by Glushko, Lawson and Gurd (1972) for the ^{13}C resonances of ribonuclease A. Clearly the different peaks pass through zero intensity at different delay times τ; as with the ordinary pulse method, the time at which any peak passes through zero is given by $\tau = 0.69T_1$. Given access to spectrometers of different frequencies, it is possible, using these techniques, to detect frequency dependence of T_1. Analysis of this frequency dependence may then give quite important information on the motion and separation of relaxing groups in the molecules.

T_2 may be measured by 'spin-echo' experiments, which may take one of several forms. Basically a 90° pulse, which tips the magnetization into the xy plane, is followed by a decay of M_{xy} (a) by loss of phase coherence of the nuclei through transverse relaxation and (b) by loss of phase coherence through magnetic-field inhomogeneities. At a time τ after the 90° pulse, a 180° pulse (or a series of 180° pulses) is applied. The change of 180° means that the spins which were originally dephasing are now regaining their phase coherence, and when they come together again a signal (a spin-echo) is detected. But only the systematic dephasing (b) is reversible by this process; true transverse relaxation (a), which is a random process, is not reversed and so the 'echo' is smaller than the original signal. From the variation of echo height with time τ, T_2 may be calculated.

More sophisticated pulse methods which enable measurements to be made selectively on peaks within a spectrum, are described by Farrar and Becker (1971).

5.11 Spectrum simulation and curve fitting

Occasionally in chemistry the simplest way of analysis is to synthesize; an unknown compound may be guessed at and the guess synthesized, the properties of known and unknown being compared to see how close the guess was and how it might be improved. The same procedure may be employed with NMR spectra, and has found application in biological NMR. McDonald and Phillips (1969) describe a simple method by which random-coil protein spectra may be computed from a knowledge of the chemical shift, relative areas and linewidths of the spectra; an example is given as Figure 5.10 and shows that even with a simple triangle approximation to the lineshape, a reasonable approximation to the measured spectrum is obtained. A similar but more accurate approach has been used in the investigation of histone—histone interactions, and examples have already been given as Figures 2.3 and 4.18. Simulation has also proved of value in analysing complex spin—spin splittings in the investigation of small molecules. A simple example is found in Figure 5.11, where side-chain orientation of a polypeptide was found by using an analogue curve generator to analyse a multiplet structure.

The more complex and accurate procedure of curve-fitting, in which a computer performs a least-squares (as distinct from 'by-eye') fitting of components to an envelope, has found limited use in the precise placing of histidine peaks (Sachs *et al.*, 1971) during titration experiments, but in general too many assumptions are involved in any situation more complex than this.

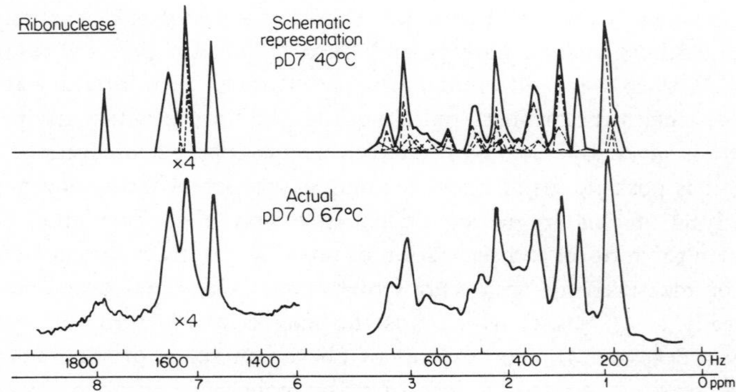

Figure 5.10 PMR spectra of denatured bovine pancreatic ribonuclease at 220 MHz, together with spectrum simulated by adding together 'resonances' at chemical shifts corresponding to amino acid residues of the protein. (Reprinted with permission from McDonald, C. C., and Phillips, W. D. (1969). *J. Amer. Chem. Soc.*, **91**, 1519. Copyright by the American Chemical Society)

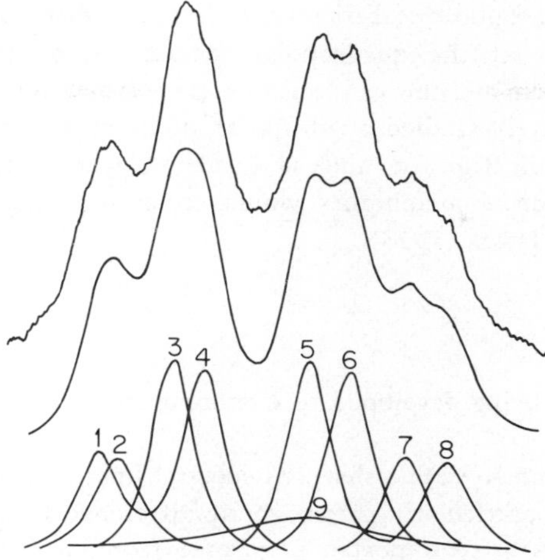

Figure 5.11 Spectrum (100 MHz) of the β-CH_2 group of poly (β-benzyl-L-aspartate) in chloroform at 100° together with a curve resolver readout and analysis. (Reprinted with permission from Bradbury, E. M., Carpenter, B. G., Crane-Robinson, C., and Goldman, H. (1971). *Macromolecules,* 4, 557. Copyright by the American Chemical Society)

5.12 Nuclear quadrupole resonance

For nuclei with $I > ½$, the distribution of positive charge over the nucleus may be aspherical and give rise to a nuclear electric quadrupole moment. Modulation of the electric field gradient of the surrounding electron cloud can, through coupling with the quadrupole moment, provide an additional mechanism for nuclear relaxation. The relevant correlation time for this modulation may be rotational or diffusional in a liquid.

In ESR, it is customary to think of nuclear quadrupole effects as being much smaller than nuclear dipolar effects. However, it should be realized that the electric field gradients produced by chemical bonds are strong and electric quadrupole interaction may completely dominate the relaxation time of the nucleus. For example, the large electric field gradient produced by tumbling of CCl_4 molecules results in a ^{35}Cl NMR spectrum which has a linewidth of 10 kHz; contrast this with the 15Hz linewidth of the ^{35}Cl resonance in aqueous solutions of NaCl.

The variation of relaxation times due to nuclear quadrupole effects are of importance in biological systems. The binding of ions or ligands having quadrupolar moments to macromolecules can produce dramatic changes in the relaxation times of a quadrupolar nucleus. Due to the low concentration of biological macromolecules (10^{-3}M) and the low NMR sensitivity of quadrupolar nuclei, the complex between the macromolecule and the ion or ligand cannot be detected directly; observation of the NMR of the free ion of ligand which is in fast exchange with the complex is the way around this difficulty. Even with a fast exchange situation, very high concentrations of the quadrupolar species are needed to overcome the low-sensitivity problem and this can lead to non-specific binding.

The most extensively studied quadrupolar nuclei in biological systems are ^{23}Na and ^{35}Cl. The application of nuclear quadrupolar resonance to the study of transport of ions across membranes would seem to be plausible. The matter is discussed further by Dwek (1973).

5.13 Summary

(1) Methods are being developed to overcome some of the basic limitations of the NMR method.

(2) Resolution enhancement sharpens spectral lines and reduces overlap whilst difference methods, particularly paramagnetic difference spectroscopy, and double resonance techniques isolate important resonances from the rest of the spectrum.

(3) Accumulation of very large numbers of spectra to improve signal-to-noise ratios becomes possible using block averaging or double-precision accumulation methods.

(4) Relaxation times may be measured directly using pulsed NMR spectrometers.

(5) Line assignments are facilitated by spectral curve fitting and simulation techniques.

(6) The importance of nuclear Overhauser effects and nuclear quadrupole resonance are briefly discussed.

References

Barry, C. D., North, A. C. T., Glasel, J. A., Williams, R. J. P., and Xavier, A. V. (1971). *Nature,* **232**, 236.

Bleaney, B., Dobson, C. M., Levine, B. A., Martin, R. B., Williams, R. J. P., and Xavier, A. V. (1972). *J. Chem. Soc. Chem. Comm.,* 791.

Bradbury, E. M., Carpenter, B. G., Crane-Robinson, C., and Goldman, H. (1971). *Macromolecules,* **4**, 557.

Campbell, I. D., Dobson, C. M., Williams, R. J. P., and Xavier, A. V. (1973a). *J. Magn. Res.,* **11**, 172.

Campbell, I. D., Dobson, C. M., Williams, R. J. P., and Xavier, A. V. (1973b). *Ann. N.Y. Acad. Sci.,* **222**, 163.

Dwek, R. A. (1973). *NMR in Biochemistry: Application to Enzyme Systems*, Oxford, Clarendon Press.

Farrar, T. C., and Becker, E. D. (1971). *Pulse and Fourier Transform NMR*, Academic Press, New York.

Freeman, R., and Hill, H. D. W. (1971). *J. Magn. Res.,* **5**, 278.

Gibbons, W. A., Alms, H., Bockman, R. S., and Wyssbrod, H. R. (1972a). *Biochemistry,* **11**, 1721.

Gibbons, W. A., Alms, H., Sogn, J., and Wyssbrod, H. R. (1972b). *Proc. Nat. Acad. Sci.,* **69**, 1261.

Glushko, V., Lawson, P. J., and Gurd, F. R. N. (1972). *J. Biol. Chem.*, **247**, 3176.
McDonald, C. C., and Phillips, W. D. (1969). *J. Amer. Chem. Soc.*, **91**, 1513.
Sachs, D. H., Schechter, A. N., and Cohen, J. S. (1971). *J. Biol. Chem.*, **246**, 6576.
Sheard, B., and Bradbury, E. M. (1970). *Progress in Biophysics and Molecular Biology* (Ed. J. A. V. Butler). **20**, 187, Pergamon Press.
Sheard, B., Miall, S. H., Peacocke, A. R., Walker, I. O., and Richards, R. E. (1967). *J. Mol. Biol.*, **28**, 389.

Chapter 6
The ESR Spectrum

6.1 Introduction

As was mentioned in Chapter 1, electron spin resonance is extremely specific in its application; it looks only at the paramagnetic centres in the system under study. Only those systems which contain an electron whose spin is not paired with the oppositely directed spin of another electron (pairing would give zero net spin) will give an ESR signal. Since the paired spin system is an energetically favourable configuration, chemical bonding normally results in molecules which have no unpaired electrons and hence no ESR signal. The exceptions to this rule are transition-metal ions, free radicals and free electron centres such as might be produced by X-irradiation of macromolecules. By virtue of their unpaired electrons these systems will have ESR signals which are extremely specific and often capable of giving direct information about the centre of biochemical activity in the system.

For instance, transition-metal ions participate directly in the mechanism of action of the metalloproteins (cytochromes) in electron transfer chains, are also involved in the active sites of metalloenzymes such as catalase and superoxide dismutase, and also in the physiological site of action of the liganding of haemoglobin and myoglobin by oxygen. Further it is to be expected that free radicals will appear as intermediates in various biochemical reactions. Indeed Michaelis has postulated that all biological oxidations might proceed in one-electron steps, hence giving rise to free radicals. Free electrons generated by X-irradiation will clearly report on the irradiation damage centres in their host macromolecules.

The application of ESR in biological systems has been extended to include structural and dynamic studies, and also made more versatile in the study of biochemical activity by the introduction of the spin-label probe method. Spin labels are stable free radicals whose ESR spectra are environmentally sensitive and which can be covalently attached to macromolecules, can be intercalated in macromolecular systems such as membranes, or can be present as spin-labelled ligands, substrates, inhibitors, etc. The selectivity of the ESR method can be retained if the spin label can be attached to a specific group on a macromolecule, or if a biologically active analogue of a particular small molecule, e.g. enzyme substrate, can be synthesized.

Having mentioned the types of biological systems to which ESR investigations can be applied, we now go on to consider the sort of information which can be obtained from such investigations. The interpretation of ESR spectra falls into two parts, the second rather more difficult than the first. The first part consists basically of assigning the lines in the spectrum to specific molecular groupings, if possible, and relating the line positions and splittings to the energy-level splittings from which they arise, i.e. to particular *g*-values, hyperfine splitting constants, etc. The second part consists of interpreting the measured parameters in terms of the basic electronic and structural properties of the molecule or molecular grouping – such properties as molecular orientation and motion, free electron densities, degree of covalent binding, etc.

In the following, the details of the assignment and straightforward spectral interpretation are discussed in the sections headed: *g*-values, hyperfine splittings, isotropic hyperfine splittings and spectral anisotropy. These sections can be concentrated on at a first reading. The sections on spin-label spectra, spin densities and transition-metal ions deal with interpretation of the spectra in terms of molecular properties. This, of course, is the main part of the chapter and leads directly to the applications in Chapter 8. A section is included on spin Hamiltonians at an appropriate juncture in the chapter, since these so often occur in the discussion of ESR spectra. However, since this requires at least a slight quantum-mechanical background for full understanding, the rest of the chapter has been written without recourse to the spin Hamiltonian formalism and this section may be omitted if desired.

The treatment of the various types of ESR spectra has been split roughly into three sections: free radicals, spin labels and transition-metal ions. The ESR spectra from free radicals in solution are considered first, since under these conditions the molecules tumble rapidly and all anisotropic interactions are averaged out. In this case the spectra are relatively easy to interpret because the hyperfine splittings are proportional to the free-electron spin densities, although the hyperfine patterns may be rather complicated if the nuclei of a large number of atoms in the molecule are involved. In this type of spectra, relatively little information is obtained from the *g*-values (absolute positions) of the spectra, but the hyperfine splittings can be used to determine the electron-spin densities in the various regions of the molecule. These results may be compared with calculations using molecular-orbital theory.

The anisotropy of ESR spectra with respect to the orientation of the magnetic field is considered next. This topic is essential for an understanding of the spectra of spin labels and transition-metal ions. It is the spectral anisotropy of the nitroxide free-radical group which gives structural sensitivity to the spin-label ESR spectrum. The 'partial motional averaging' of this anisotropy gives information about the nature and the amplitude of molecular segmental motion, and the linebroadening and lineshapes give a measure of the rate of motion and degree of conformational restriction of the spin-labelled group.

The final sections show how anisotropy of transition-metal ion ESR spectra can give information about the metal ion–ligand symmetry, and if single crystals are available can help to define the orientation of the ligand site relative to the rest of the molecule. The magnitude of the anisotropy can also provide detailed insight into the electronic configuration of the metal ion–ligand complex.

6.2 g-Values

The absolute magnetic field position of the lines of an ESR spectrum is characterized by the g-value (see Chapter 1)

$$h\nu = g\beta H_0 \tag{6.1}$$

where H_0 is the magnetic field at which the centre of the line occurs and ν is the microwave (klystron) frequency used. h and β are fundamental atomic constants as explained in Chapter 1; β, the Bohr magneton, being the natural atomic unit for electron magnetic moments, and h is Planck's constant. A useful number when calculating g-values is $h/\beta = 0.71444$ when ν is expressed in GHz and H_0 in kgauss. Recall from Chapter 1 that gauss are the commonly used units for expressing the magnetic field and spectral splittings in ESR spectroscopy. 1 kG = 10^3 G, and the SI equivalent is 1 tesla = 10^4 G.

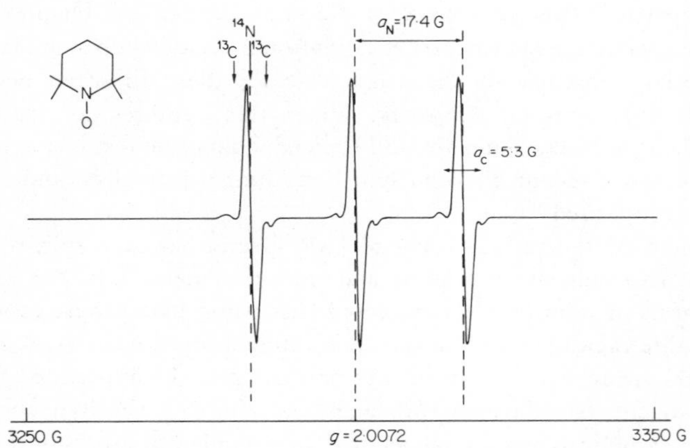

Figure 6.1 ESR spectrum of the TEMPO nitroxide spin label in aqueous solution. The three main lines arise from nitrogen hyperfine structure, and small satellite lines from the ^{13}C hyperfine structure

In the case of lines which are split, for instance by hyperfine interactions, the pattern is centred about H_0. This is illustrated in Figure 6.1 which gives the ESR spectrum of TEMPO, a small spin-label molecule, in aqueous solution. The lines are split by the hyperfine interaction of the free electron with the nucleus of the nitroxide nitrogen atom. H_0 is given by the centre of the middle line which is also the mid-point of the two outer lines.

In free radicals, the unpaired electron is often delocalized over the whole molecule and behaves like an almost totally free electron. In these cases the g-value of the free radical approaches very closely to the theoretical value for a free electron of $g_e = 2.0023$. Resonances in the $g = 2$ region are thus ones characteristic of free radicals, although this is not exclusively a property of free radicals. Deviations from the free-electron g-value can give some information about the

Table 6.1
Typical *g*-values for paramagnetic species in biological systems

	g-value
Fe^{3+} (low spin)	1.4–3.1
(high spin)	2.0–9.7
Cu^{2+}	2.0–2.4
Flavin semiquinone, ubiquinone, etc.	2.0030–2.0050
S–S, –SH	2.02–2.06
Spin label nitroxide	2.0020–2.0090

degree of orbital restriction of the free-radical wavefunction. The *g*-values of nitroxide spin labels, for instance, tend to be somewhat higher than for radicals in which the unpaired electron is extensively delocalized. In nitroxides the unpaired electron is essentially localized in a *p*-orbital on the nitrogen atom. Typical *g*-values are given in Table 6.1 for the paramagnetic species which are most commonly found in biological systems. The table indicates that *g*-values can be of some help in identifying the magnetic species, but in most cases not uniquely.

From Table 6.1 it is clear that the transition metal ions have *g*-values which differ quite significantly from $g= 2$, and in some cases are totally different from $g = 2$. One of the reasons for this is that there is a well-defined orbital motion associated with the transition-metal-ion wavefunction. This orbiting motion of the charged electron gives rise to an additional magnetic moment (just as the electric current in a solenoid gives rise to a magnetic moment) which changes the *g*-value and also causes the *g*-values to be extremely anisotropic. Transition-metal-ion *g*-values are discussed in detail later below. For the present we turn to the consideration of hyperfine splittings.

6.3 Hyperfine Splittings

As was explained in Chapter 1, the lines in an ESR spectrum can be split by interaction of the paramagnetic electron with the magnetic moments of neighbouring nuclei. These splittings arise from the magnetic field associated with the nuclear moment. Not all atoms have nuclei which have magnetic moments, and in some cases the isotope with a magnetic moment has only a low natural abundance, as will be clear from the discussion of nuclear magnetic resonance in the previous chapters. Table 6.2 lists the nuclei which are likely to give rise to ESR hyperfine splittings in biological systems. The natural abundance of the magnetic isotopes is given, together with the nuclear spin, the number of hyperfine lines which this gives rise to, and typical values of splittings for this particular nucleus.

The natural abundance indicates which species are likely to be of importance in the hyperfine splitting pattern. For instance, ^{13}C hyperfine structure will be of little significance in most biological systems. This can be seen from Figure 6.1 where the small humps in the wings of each of the main nitrogen hyperfine lines of the nitroxide free radical spectrum arise from the hyperfine interaction with the 1.1% of adjacent carbon nuclei which have a magnetic moment. (The common ^{12}C

Table 6.2
Typical hyperfine splittings for magnetic nuclei commonly found in biological systems

Nucleus	Natural abundance (%)	Spin	No. of lines	Splitting (gauss)
^{1}H	100	½	2	0–6
^{14}N	99.6	1	3	0–20[a]
^{19}F	100	½	2	0–30
^{63}Cu	69.1	3/2	4	20–200
^{65}Cu	30.9	3/2	4	
^{95}Mo	15.8	5/2	6	40
^{97}Mo	9.6	5/2	6	
^{55}Mn	100	5/2	6	95

[a]6–32 gauss for nitroxides (spin labels).

isotope has no nuclear moment.) For most free radicals in solution the proton hyperfine splittings are most important (see, e.g., Figure 6.2a) since hydrogen nuclei are extremely abundant in nearly all biological molecules and have large nuclear moments. For nitroxide spin labels, the nitrogen hyperfine splitting is dominant (Figure 6.1), since the free electron is essentially localized on the nitrogen atom. For transition-metal ions the dominant hyperfine splitting comes from the nucleus of the paramagnetic ion, and smaller 'superhyperfine structure' may come from the ligands, the most common being nitrogen as illustrated in Figure 6.2(b). The equally spaced lines at low field come from the copper nucleus and the very small, sharp splittings of the line to high field of these come from nitrogen ligands. The spectrum is complicated because both the *g*-values and hyperfine splittings are anisotropic, as is characteristic of transition-metal ions.

The number of hyperfine lines from a particular nucleus depends on the nuclear spin, I; this number is given by $(2I + 1)$ and is listed for the various nuclear species in Table 6.2. For $I = ½$, e.g. protons, each nucleus gives rise to two hyperfine lines as was shown in Chapter 1, Figure 1.10. For $I = 1$, e.g. nitrogen, each nuclear spin is quantized and has three equally probable allowed orientations corresponding to the spin projections: $I_z = 1, 0, +1$ relative to the magnetic field as is indicated diagrammatically in Figure 6.3. In this case each nucleus gives rise to three hyperfine lines as indicated in Figure 6.4 and as illustrated by the nitroxide spectrum in Figure 6.1.

The hyperfine splitting of the energy levels is given by $½A$ in Figure 6.4, where A is known as the hyperfine splitting constant. This factor of a half arises because the hyperfine interaction energy is conventionally given as $AI_z \,.\, S_z$, since the local magnetic field from the nucleus (see Chapter 1) is directly proportional to the nuclear magnetic moment, I_z. In the case of hyperfine structure, Equation (6.1) can thus be replaced by

★ $$h\nu = g\beta H \pm ½A m_I \qquad (6.2)$$

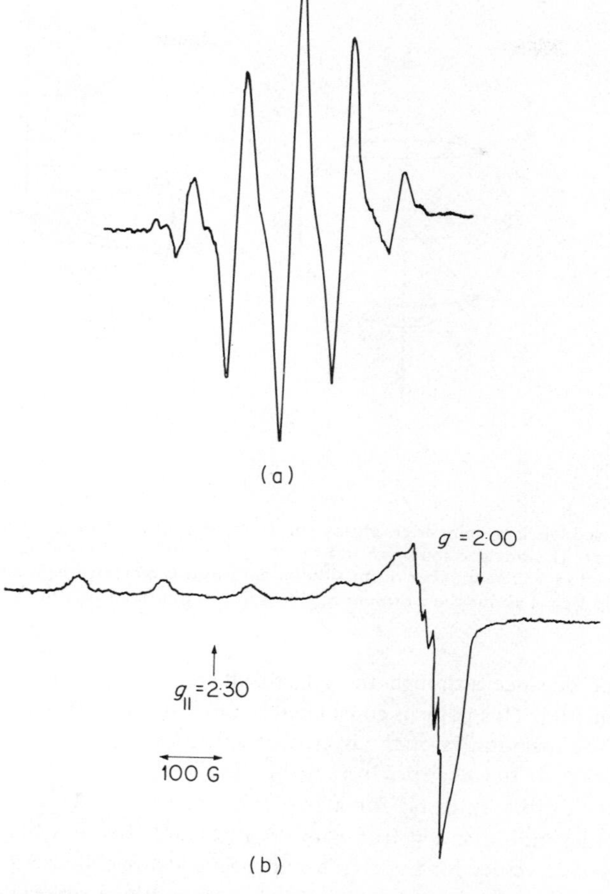

Figure 6.2 Hyperfine structure. (a) Proton hyperfine structure of an enzymatically generated free radical: oxidation of benzoquinone by laccase. (From Nakamura, 1961). (b) Copper and nitrogen hyperfine structure in a copper protein: copper conalbumin. (Reprinted with permission from Windle, J., Wiersema, A., Clark, J., and Feeny, R. (1963). *Biochemistry*, **2**, 1341. Copyright by the American Chemical Society)

where m_I are the various values of I_z. The hyperfine splitting between ESR lines is then A, in energy units (cm^{-1}), or $A/g\beta$ in magnetic field units (gauss). In general a nuclear spin, I, has the allowed spin projections given by: $m_I = -I$, $-I + 1, \ldots, I, -1$, x + I, as illustrated in Figure 6.3, giving rise to $(2I + 1)$ equally spaced hyperfine lines.

The number of hyperfine lines can thus assist in identifying the nucleus which gives rise to the hyperfine splittings of the ESR spectrum. Multiple lines from a single nucleus can be distinguished from the multiple lines arising from several

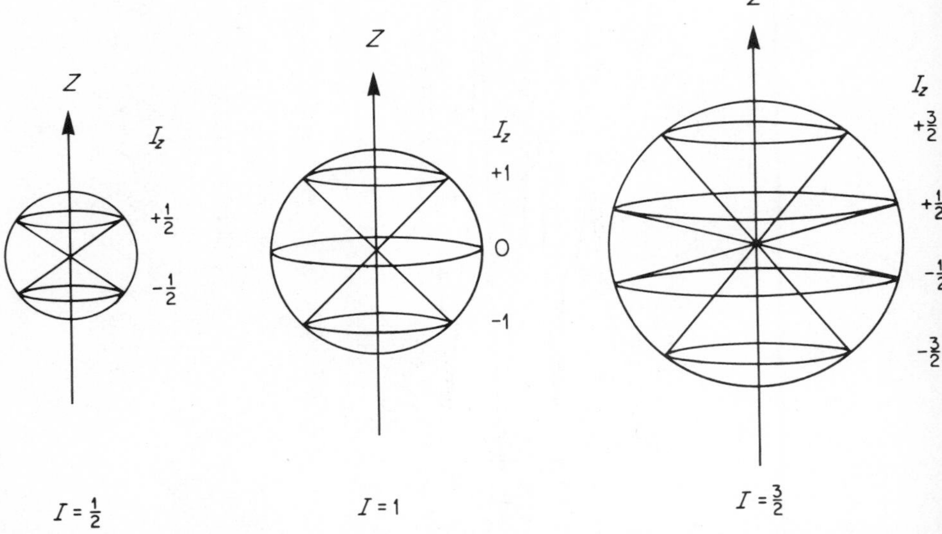

Figure 6.3 Allowed nuclear spin orientations for $I = ½$ (e.g. hydrogen), $I = 1$ (e.g. nitrogen) and $I = 3/2$ (e.g. copper). The nuclear spins can only take up certain allowed orientations relative to the magnetic field direction, z. The number of possible orientations is greater, the larger the nuclear spin. The spins precess in a cone about the z-direction, giving rise to the fixed spin projections, I_z

equivalent nuclei, since although the latter will be equally spaced they will have different intensities. This point is considered in more detail in the following section. In principle, the magnitudes of the hyperfine splittings can also be used to help in the identification of the nucleus. In fact this is not such a useful criterion because the magnitude of the splitting for a particular nucleus varies considerably with environment, depending on electron spin densities and chemical bonding. For this reason the typical values for hyperfine splittings given in Table 6.2 are subject to considerable variation, and the quoted ranges are sometimes rather large, especially in the case of transition-metal ions which can have highly anisotropic hyperfine splittings.

6.4 Isotropic Hyperfine Splittings (radicals in solution)

Free radicals in aqueous solution produce characteristically sharp ESR spectra, often with complex hyperfine splittings arising from interaction of the free electron with the numerous hydrogen nuclei in the radical. Typical splitting patterns are indicated in Figure 6.5; the spectra are characteristic of a free electron interacting with none, one and four equivalent hydrogen atoms in (a), (b) and (c) respectively. The hydrogen nuclei giving rise to these hyperfine splittings are easily identified in Figure 6.5. In the case of the radical derived from fumarate, the carboxyl hydrogens are ionized (or too remote) and therefore do not interact with the free electron; no hyperfine structure is seen. In the case of the ascorbate radical, the free

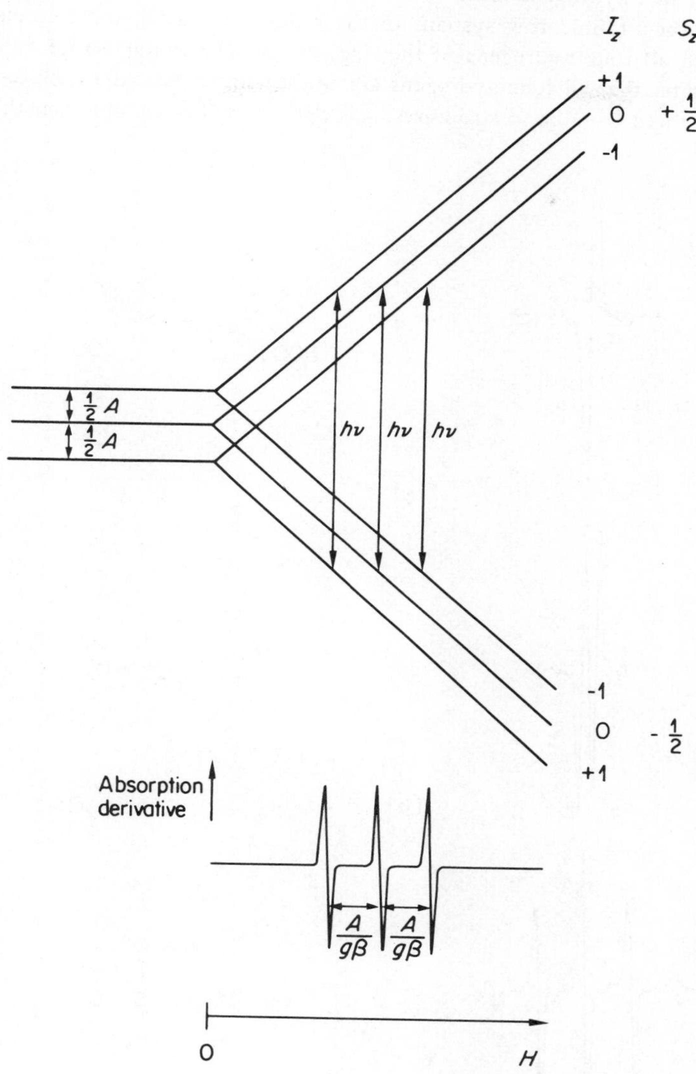

Figure 6.4 Hyperfine energy-level splittings for nuclear spin $I = 1$ (e.g. nitrogen). The ESR transitions for a single electron, $S = ½$, are indicated (constant frequency; selection rules: $\Delta S_z = \pm 1$, $\Delta I_z = 0$). The hyperfine splittings in the ESR spectrum clearly mirror the energy-level splittings and the number of lines is characteristic of the value of the nuclear spin, I (see also Figure 1.10)

electron interacts with the single ring hydrogen, producing a single splitting. In this case the sidechain hydrogens must be too remote, showing that the free electron is confined to the olefinic ring system. In the reductate radical, the free electron interacts with all four hydrogens of the ring system. The characteristic hyperfine pattern indicates that all four hydrogens are equivalent, i.e. that there is isomerism between the three C—O bond structures. It is clear from this example that the ESR

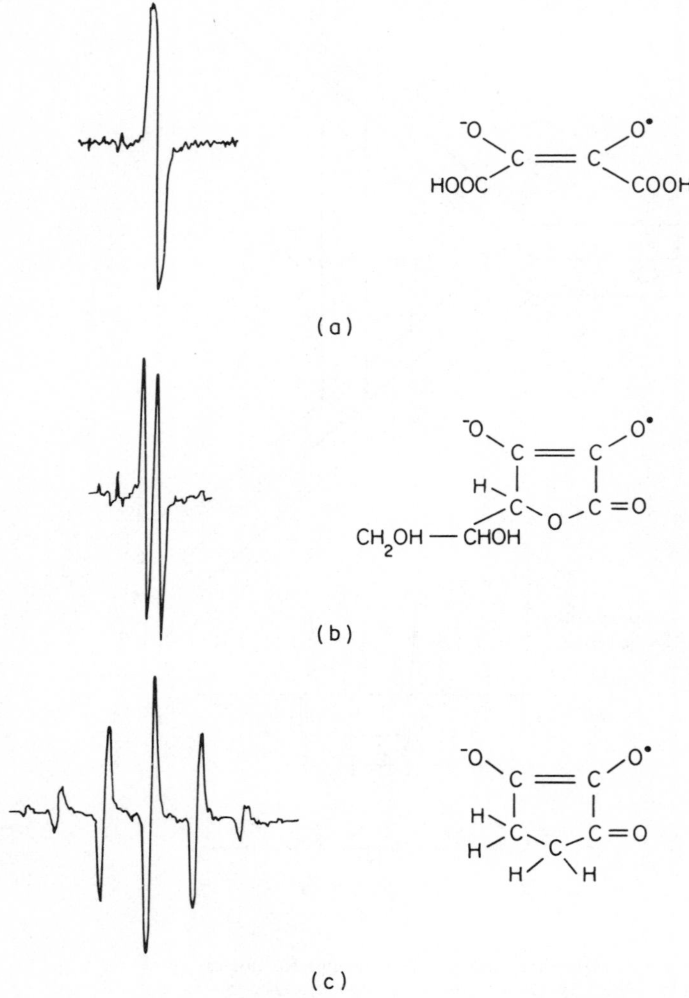

Figure 6.5 Free radicals generated by the enzymatic oxidation of substrates by peroxidase-hydrogen peroxide. Proton hyperfine structure of free radicals derived from the following substrates: (a) fumarate, (b) ascorbate, (c) reductate. (From Yamazaki and Piette, 1961. Reproduced by permission of ASP Biological and Medical Press)

spectrum is capable of giving information about the chemical structure of the free radical generated, or conversely can help in the identification of the radical.

The spectrum of Figure 6.5(c) has both a uniform splitting and a highly distinctive intensity pattern. The intensity pattern indicates that the hyperfine structure arises from several nuclei rather than from a single nucleus with $I = 2$ $(2I + 1 = 5)$ in which case all lines would be of equal intensity. The constancy of the splitting indicates that all the nuclei are equivalent. In general the hyperfine splitting pattern for n equivalent nuclei consists of $(n + 1)$ lines which are equally spaced and has an intensity pattern given by Table 6.3. The relative intensities of Table 6.3 are the so-called binomial coefficients obtained in the expansion of the expression $(1 + x)^n$. The splitting patterns for multiple, equivalent nuclei, of the type shown in Figure 6.5(c) can be readily understood from Figure 6.6. This figure gives the energy-level splittings arising from the hyperfine interaction of the free electron with various numbers of protons. From consideration of Figure 6.4 and also Figure 1.10, it is clear that both the intensity and the splitting pattern of the ESR spectrum will be identical with this energy-level splitting pattern.

Table 6.3
Relative intensities of the hyperfine lines from n equivalent nuclei

n													
0							1						
1						1		1					
2					1		2		1				
3				1		3		3		1			
4			1		4		6		4		1		
5		1		5		10		10		5		1	
6	1		6		15		20		15		6		1

In the case in which the nuclei are not equivalent, the hyperfine splitting pattern can become rather complicated. However, if the hyperfine splitting from one type of nucleus is much smaller than from the other type of nucleus, a simple pattern will result. Each of the lines in the larger hyperfine splitting pattern will have its own hyperfine structure governed by the smaller splitting. This can be seen in Figure 6.1, where a ^{13}C hyperfine structure is superimposed on each line of the much larger ^{14}N hyperfine structure. The ^{13}C lines are not very strong, however, because most of the 'nitrogen lines' comes from the ^{12}C isotope (99%) which has no nuclear spin.

Spin Densities in Free Radicals

It is clear from Figure 6.5(b) that not all the protons in the ascorbate free radical contribute to the doublet hyperfine structure; the aliphatic side-chain protons do not contribute. This is because the radical free electron is primarily localized in the ring system. In fact the free radical proton hyperfine splittings are a sensitive

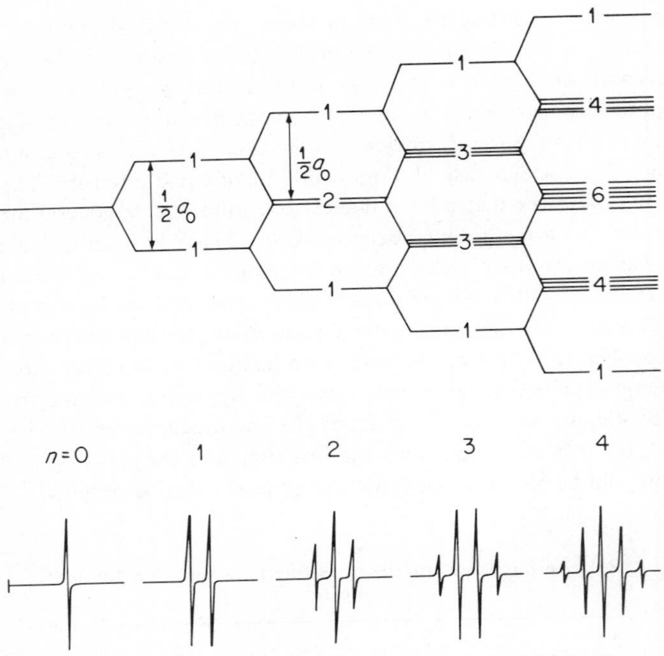

Figure 6.6 Hyperfine energy-level splittings for increasing numbers, n, of equivalent protons. The splitting pattern of the ESR spectrum is the same, with splittings, a_0, and intensities given by the numbers of coincident levels

monitor of the distribution of the free electron density throughout the molecule. The relative hyperfine splittings are a direct measure of the time which the free electron spends in the region of the particular proton. This is illustrated in Figure 6.7 which gives the spectrum of the ascorbate radical at higher resolution, revealing a small hyperfine splitting of each of the two main hyperfine lines resulting from the hyperfine interaction with protons of the aliphatic side chain.

The interpretation of the hyperfine splittings in terms of the free electron spin densities in the various parts of the molecule is complicated by the fact that nearly all free radicals are conjugated π-electron systems in which the free electron is centred on the carbon atom framework of the molecule and spends no time directly on the hydrogen atoms. The hydrogen hyperfine splittings arise from so-called spin polarization of the valence electron on the hydrogen atom by the free electron of the π-electron system. Under these conditions the hyperfine splitting a_H due to a particular proton is proportional to the free electron density ρ_π of the π-electron system on the adjacent carbon atom

★ $$a_H = Q\rho_\pi \tag{6.3}$$

The proportionality constant Q has values varying from 22 to 30 gauss, depending on the particular system. (Q-values can be calculated from the experimental

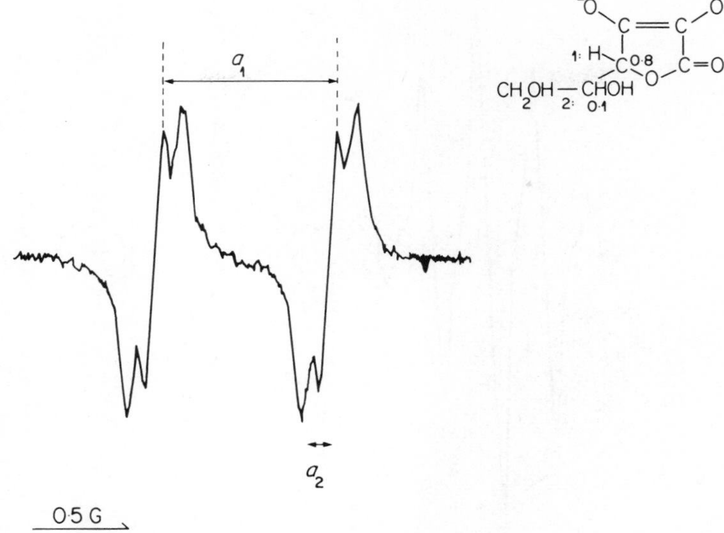

Figure 6.7 ESR spectrum of the ascorbate free radical in steady state concentration formed by ascorbate oxidase during continuous flow. The spectrum is recorded at higher resolution than that in Figure 6.5. (From Ohnishi *et al.*, 1969. Reprinted by permission of ASP Biological and Medical Press).

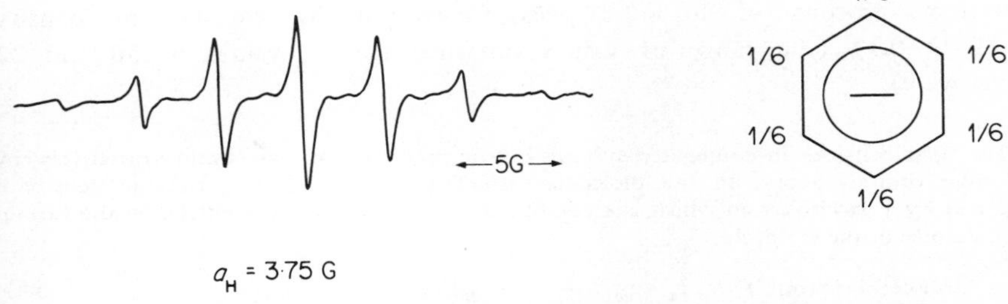

Figure 6.8 ESR spectrum of the benzene negative ion radical (from Wertz and Bolton, 1972), with the free π-electron spin densities on the ring carbon atoms. (From Bolton, 1963. Reproduced by permission of Taylor and Francis, Ltd)

hyperfine splittings in symmetrical systems in which the spin densities are obvious. For instance, in the benzene radical ion (Figure 6.8) all six carbon atoms are equivalent and hence the spin density on each will be equal: $\rho_\pi = 1/6$. The experimental hyperfine splitting is $a_H = 3.75$ gauss, thus $Q = 3.75 \div 1/6 = 22.5$ gauss.) Given the value of Q, spin densities in other situations can be calculated from the experimental hyperfine splittings. For example, the *p*-benzosemiquinone anion, which can be produced by enzymatic oxidation of the hydroquinone (see Figure 6.9), has a hyperfine splitting for each of its four

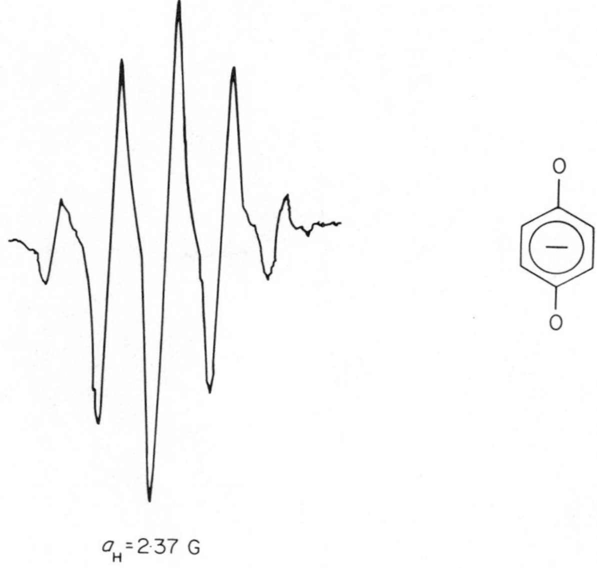

Figure 6.9 ESR spectrum of the benzosemiquinone free radical generated in continuous flow by the oxidative action of the enzyme laccase. (From Nakamura, 1961)

equivalent protons of $a_H = 2.37$ gauss, corresponding to a spin density $\rho_\pi = 0.08-0.11$ (the range of values obtained from Q-values of 30 and 22 respectively).

The Spin densities in conjugated systems can be predicted, at least semiquantitatively, by molecular orbital theory. In the molecular orbital treatment the free electron density is described by a wavefunction which is a combination of wavefunctions centred on the various carbon atoms of the molecule

$$\psi\,(\text{molecular orbital}) = c_1\phi_1 + c_2\phi_2 + \ldots + c_n\phi_n \tag{6.4}$$

where $\phi_1, \phi_2, \ldots, \phi_n$ are the various atomic wavefunctions and the c-coefficients represent the proportion of its time that the unpaired electron spends on each of the n carbon atoms. Since the electron density is given by the square of the wavefunction $|\psi|^2$, the free electron densities on the various carbon atoms are given by $c_1^2, c_2^2, \ldots, c_n^2$, respectively. An instructive example is the benzene negative radical ion and its substituents. The free electron in the benzene radical ion can go into either of two antibonding molecular orbitals which are of equal energy. The electron densities in these two molecular orbitals, as predicted by Hückel molecular orbital theory, are given in Figure 6.10. In the benzene radical ion the free electron will spend equal lengths of time in the A- and in the S-orbital, hence the net electron densities will be the average of the two, i.e. 1/6 on each carbon atom. As already mentioned, this is the result one would expect from the symmetry of the benzene molecule. However, this symmetry is destroyed by substitution in the benzene ring, and either the A- or the S-orbital will be favoured depending on the electron withdrawing or releasing properties of the substituent. For example, consider the p-benzosemiquinone radical ion shown in Figure 6.9. The electron withdrawing properties of the semiquinone oxygens will favour the orbital with the high electron density in the para position, i.e. the S-orbital. Hence, one would expect the electron

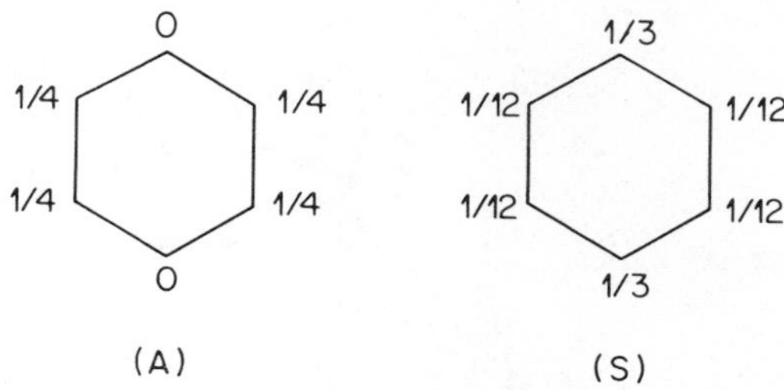

Figure 6.10 Electron densities in the free electron molecular orbitals of the benzene radical ion. (A) is the so-called antisymmetric orbitals and (S) the symmetric orbital. In the benzene radical, the two orbitals are of equal energy, but one or other of the orbitals will be favoured in substituted benzene radicals

density on the four ring protons to approach the value $\rho_\pi = 0.083$ given for the S-orbital in Figure 6.10. This is in reasonable agreement with the value deduced above from the hyperfine splittings.

It is thus clear that molecular orbital theory is capable of some degree of success in interpreting the spin densities measured from hyperfine splittings, or conversely can be of help in identifying which groups of protons give rise to particular hyperfine splittings, and hence of giving information about the structure of the free radical. More complicated theories exist which are able to predict the measured spin densities more accurately. The reader is referred to the books by Stretweiser, and Wertz and Bolton, quoted in the references, for a more detailed account of the application of molecular orbital theory. Of particular relevance is the general method of deriving the free electron molecular orbitals for configurations other than the benzene ring system quoted above in Figure 6.10.

6.5 Spectral Anisotropy

One of the unique features of ESR spectra is that in many cases the positions and splittings of the lines (specified by the *g*-values and hyperfine constants) depend on the direction of the magnetic field relative to the molecular axes. This spectral anisotropy was not encountered in the free radical spectra considered above since in these systems the free electron is extensively delocalized and therefore the anisotropy is small, and also because the rapid random rotation of these (relatively small) radicals in free solution averages out all the remaining, small anisotropic splittings and shifts. As was seen in the two previous sections, this rapid averaging yields spectra which can be interpreted in a relatively simple manner and also gives rise to the characteristically narrow linewidths in which the hyperfine splittings are well-resolved.

The spectral anisotropy is very important in interpreting the spectra of transition-metal ions and is also the fundamental basis of the usefulness of the spin-label method. The effects of anisotropic splittings and *g*-values is most easily understood by considering the spectra from single crystals. Figure 6.11 gives the spectra of a nitroxide spin label oriented in a single crystal host. The spectra are given for the magnetic field oriented relative to the single crystal axes such that the

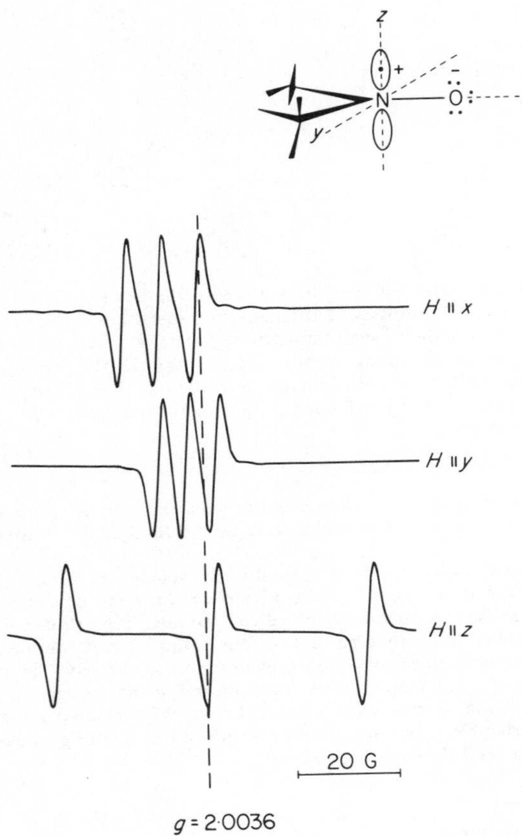

Figure 6.11 Spectral anisotropy of tert-butyl nitroxide spin label oriented in a single crystal host. The principal axes of the nitroxide moiety are indicated. (Spectra reprinted with permission from Griffiths, O. H., and Waggoner, A. S. (1969). *Acc. Chem. Res.*, **2**, 17. Copyright by the American Chemical Society)

field direction is parallel to the principal molecular axes of the spin-label group, as indicated in the figure. The nitroxide radical unpaired electron is principally localized in the $p\pi$ orbital on the nitrogen atom, unlike most of the extensively delocalized free radicals considered above. The anisotropy of the spectra between the three principal directions is clearly seen, both in the hyperfine splittings and in the g-value positions about which the lines are centred. Intermediate spectra are obtained for the orientations between the principal directions. The spectral anisotropy is normally completely specified by the three g-values and hyperfine constants obtained parallel to the principal axes: A_{zz} = 32 gauss, A_{xx} = 6 gauss, A_{yy} = 6 gauss and g_{zz} = 2.0027, g_{xx} = 2.0089, g_{yy} = 2.0061. These are known as

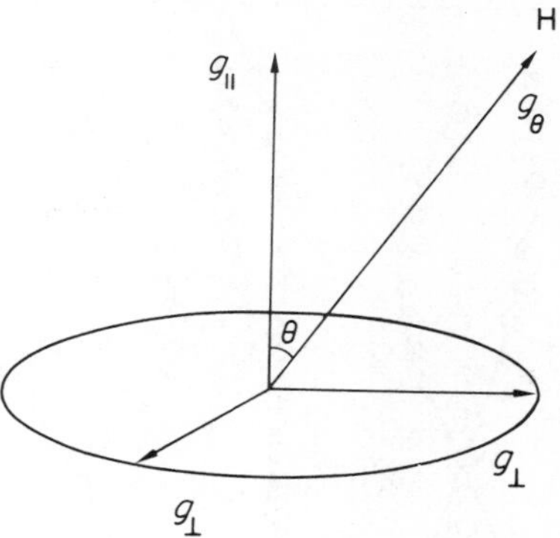

Figure 6.12 Variation of g-value with magnetic field orientation, θ, in an axially symmetric system

the principal values of the hyperfine constants and the principal g-values, respectively. In many cases the molecular system is axially symmetric and the principal values are designated as: $A_\parallel = A_{zz}$; $A_\perp = A_{xx} = A_{yy}$, and similarly for the g-values: $g_\parallel = g_{zz}$; $g_\perp = g_{xx} = g_{yy}$.

For intermediate orientations, the g-values and hyperfine splittings depend on the angle which the magnetic field makes with the principal axes. For an axially symmetric system as shown in Figure 6.12, the g-values and hyperfine splittings vary with magnetic field orientation in the following manner

★ $$g_\theta^2 = g_\parallel^2 \cos^2 \theta + g_\perp^2 \sin^2 \theta \tag{6.5}$$

and similarly

★ $$A_\theta^2 = A_\parallel^2 \cos^2 \theta + A_\perp^2 \sin^2 \theta \tag{6.6}$$

where g_θ, A_θ are the g-value and hyperfine constant found with the magnetic field at an angle θ to the ($\parallel$) axis of symmetry. The magnetic field positions, H, of the ESR transitions are then given by the corresponding equation to equation (6.2)

$$h\nu = g_\theta \beta H + \tfrac{1}{2} A_\theta m_I \tag{6.7}$$

If single crystal samples are available, angular orientation studies can give important information regarding the orientation of the principal axes of specific molecular groupings. A notable example is the determination of the orientation of the haem ring in myoglobin, which is discussed in Chapter 8. A typical angular variation of an ESR spectrum is given in Figure 6.13. More usually single crystals are not available and the so-called polycrystalline powder spectrum is obtained (Figure 6.14). In this case spectra from all the different directions are obtained superimposed and a much more complicated spectrum is obtained. Instead of the characteristic three-line spectra obtained for a nitroxide free radical (see Figure 6.1, 6.11), one gets a powder spectrum which has much broader lines and a considerably distorted lineshape, as indicated in Figure 6.14(a). In principle all the g-value and

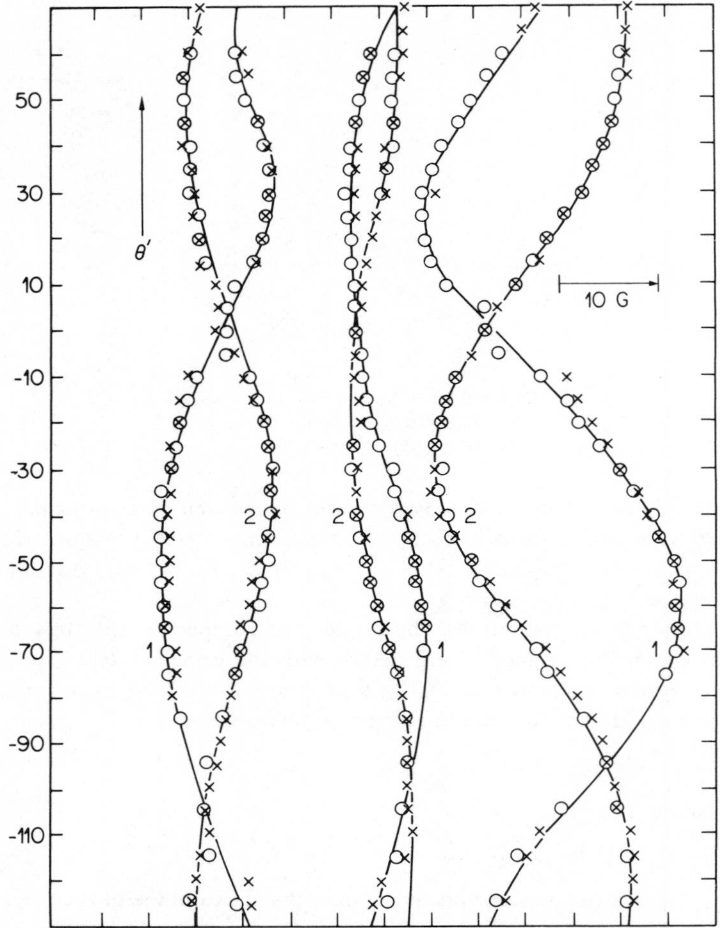

Figure 6.13 Typical angular variation of the ESR spectrum of spin-labelled horse carbonmonoxyhaemoglobin (o) and methemoglobin (x). The positions of the lines are plotted as a function of the orientation, θ', of the magnetic field relative to a specific crystal axis. (From McConnell and McFarland, 1970. Reproduced by permission of Cambridge University Press)

hyperfine splitting information is contained in this spectrum and since the principal values of the hyperfine splitting constant correspond to the maximum and minimum extent of the hyperfine splitting, and similarly the principal *g*-values correspond to the maximum and minimum field positions, these principal values should be obtainable from the outer and inner extrema in the powder spectra. However, because of spectral overlap, much of this detail is often lost and not all the principal hyperfine and *g*-values can be determined from the spectrum. For example, in the powder spectrum of a nitroxide spin label, only the largest

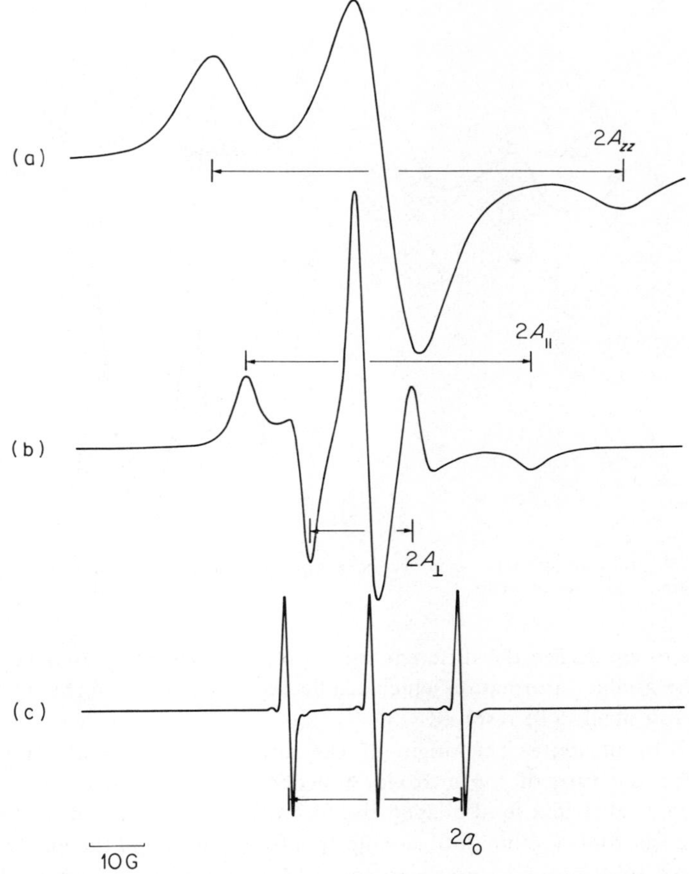

Figure 6.14 Anistropy of a nitroxide spin-label ESR spectrum under various conditions of motion. (a) Powder spectrum, from a nitroxide randomly and rigidly oriented in frozen solution. (b) Lipid dispersion spectrum, from a nitroxide spin label undergoing anisotropic motion in a randomly oriented lipid dispersion. (c) Isotropic spectrum, nitroxide randomly tumbling in a non-viscous solution

hyperfine splitting can be measured, A_{zz}, as illustrated in Figure 6.14(a). The two smaller splittings are lost because of the broadening by spectral overlap in the central region of the spectrum. This can be contrasted with the spectrum, Figure 6.14(b), of a nitroxide spin label in a randomly oriented lipid dispersion. In this case the spin label has a limited axial motion which partially averages the splittings (as explained in the sections on spin-label spectra below) so that $A_{\parallel}$ is smaller than the principal value A_{zz}, and, more importantly, $A_{\perp}$ is larger than the principal axis values A_{xx} and A_{yy}. In this case the increase in the smaller splitting means that $A_{\perp}$ can be measured as well as $A_{\parallel}$. Figure 6.15 gives the powder spectrum of a frozen aqueous solution of a copper protein, which has an axially symmetric copper site.

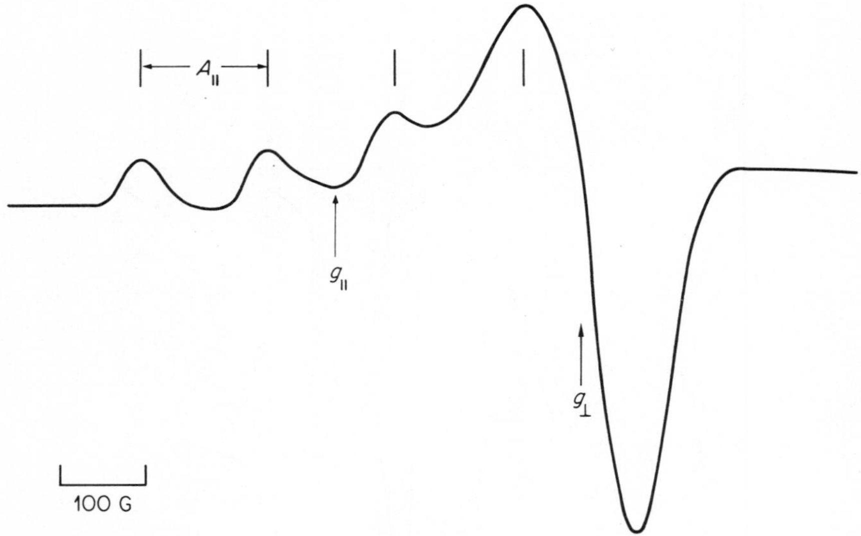

Figure 6.15 Powder spectrum of a typical copper protein in frozen solution. Spectrum of benzylamine oxidase at $-150\ ^{\circ}\mathrm{C}$

This serves to emphasize the different types of lineshapes which may be obtained, and also the *g*-value information which can be derived. Here again the $A_{\perp}$ hyperfine splitting is too small to be resolved.

Figure 6.16 illustrates the origin of the rather strange lineshapes which are obtained for the case of the nitroxide powder spectrum, and for the case of a nitroxide spin label in a lipid bilayer dispersion. Emphasis is given to the spectral splittings (anisotropic *g*-value shifts are omitted for clarity), and the justification for the measured splittings in Figures 6.14 and 6.15 is given. The two upper absorption spectra in Figure 6.16 indicate the envelopes of the individual absorption lines formed by the extreme principal values A_{zz} and A_{xx}, and all the intermediate orientations, $A(\theta)$. The central line is given as a single, large peak from all directions, because *g*-value differences are neglected. The A_{xx} splitting is not resolved in the powder spectrum because it falls under the central peak, whereas the corresponding $A_{\perp}$ splitting in the lipid dispersion spectrum is larger and can be resolved. The derivative lines, the normal form of recording ESR spectra, are then given by the slopes of the absorption envelopes, as indicated in the figure. Further examples of powder spectra involving *g*-value shifts are discussed in the following chapter, Chapter 7, with reference to *g*-value and hyperfine splitting measurements.

Returning from solid crystalline samples and frozen solutions to small molecules (free radicals) in non-viscous solutions, one finds that all anisotropic effects are lost, as in Figure 6.14(c). The small molecule tumbles in a random manner which averages out all anisotropic effects. The spectra are the same, independent of the magnetic field orientation, and the *g*-values and hyperfine splittings are in fact the mean of the principal-axis values. These values are known as the *isotropic* hyperfine

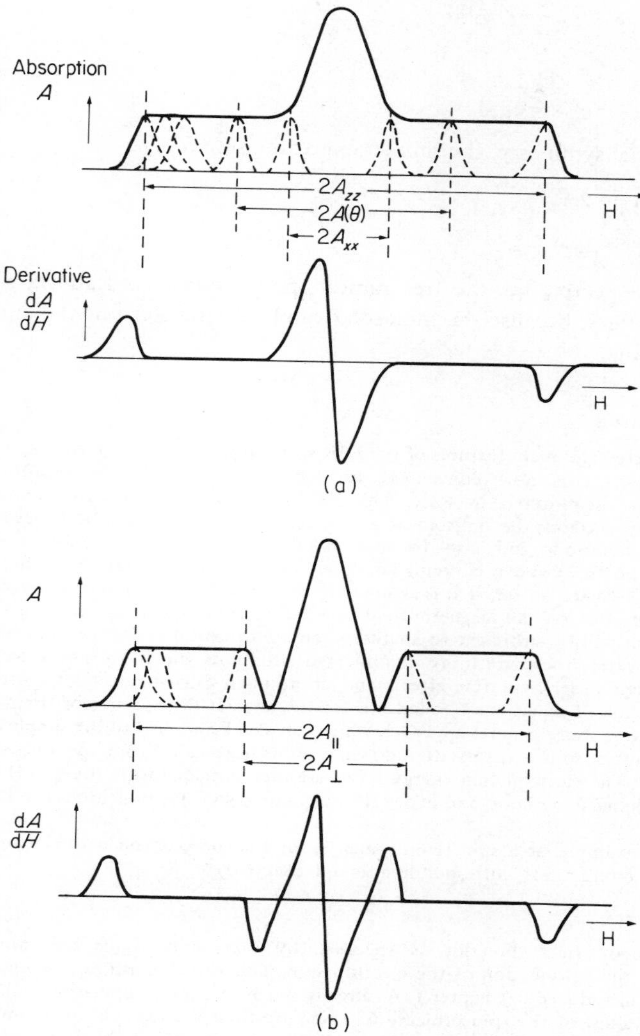

Figure 6.16 Schematic diagrams of absorption and first-derivative spectra of randomly oriented nitroxide spin labels, showing anisotropy in the three-line nitrogen hyperfine structure. Dotted lines indicate the component spectral lines at specific orientations; full lines indicate the envelope from all the random orientations. (a) The polycrystalline powder spectrum. (b) The lipid dispersion spectrum

splitting constant, a_0, and the isotropic g-value, g_0, and are given by

★ $$a_0 = {}^1/_3(A_{zz} + A_{xx} + A_{yy}) \tag{6.8}$$

and similarly

★ $$g_0 = {}^1/_3(g_{zz} + g_{xx} + g_{yy}) \tag{6.9}$$

In the case of axial symmetry, the simpler expressions hold

$$a_0 = {}^1/_3(A_{\parallel} + 2A_{\perp}) \tag{6.10}$$

$$g_0 = {}^1/_3(g_{\parallel} + 2g_{\perp}) \tag{6.11}$$

These isotropic spectra, i.e. the free radical spectra considered above, also have much narrower lines, because the molecular tumbling averages out the anisotropic dipolar broadening.

6.6 Spin Hamiltonians

Having considered the main features of the ESR spectrum: g-values, hyperfine splittings and spectral anisotropy, it is now convenient to digress and explain the spin-Hamiltonian formulation often encountered in ESR. This section doesn't introduce many really new concepts, and may certainly be omitted at a first reading. It is included both because it is a commonly used notation, and also because it becomes necessary in more complicated situations. Equation (6.2) above contains nearly all the information required to interpret the spectral features discussed so far, if it is assumed that the g-values and A-values are anisotropic, i.e. their value depends on the magnetic field orientation as indicated in equation (6.7). This simple formulation will be sufficient to analyse a large proportion of the spectra which will be encountered. However, there are more complicated situations which are not accounted for; these include second-order hyperfine effects and situations involving zero-field splittings, (and indeed the derivation of equations 6.5 and 6.6 for the angular dependence of simple spectra). These cases require a more general approach which can also be applied to the simple cases. The energy of the electron spin is first written down in terms of so-called spin operators—this is the spin Hamiltonian. The electron spin energy levels are then obtained from the spin Hamiltonian by quantum-mechanical methods, and hence the magnetic resonance transitions can be deduced as in Figure 6.4.

The simplest example of a spin Hamiltonian is for a single electron with isotropic g-value and no hyperfine interactions, corresponding to equation (6.1)

$$\mathcal{H} = g\beta H_z S_z \tag{6.12}$$

where the magnetic field direction is specified by the z-axis. S_z is the spin operator corresponding to the z-projection of the electron spin. This spin Hamiltonian is exactly of the form: $E = -\boldsymbol{\mu}\cdot\mathbf{H}$ introduced in Chapter 1. As already suggested, the S_z operator can be replaced by the allowed values of the spin projection. These are the so-called spin quantum numbers: $m_s = \pm 1/2$, corresponding to the spin-up and spin-down z-projections of the single electron spin. (For more than one electron the total spin, S, can be greater than ½, the spin quantum number can then take the values: $m_s = -S, (-S+1), \ldots, (S-1), +S$. For example, for two electrons the total spin is $S = 1$ or 0 depending on their relative orientations; for $S = 1$ the spin quantum numbers are: $m_s = -1, 0, +1$. This is similar to the situation encountered in the hyperfine structure of nuclei with $I > 1/2$.) For this reason the z-axis is called the spin quantization axis. The spin energy levels of equation (6.12) are then $E = \pm 1/2 g\beta H$, as found before.

For a single electron with anisotropic g-values, the spin Hamiltonian is more complicated because different spin-projection operators enter. For axial symmetry as indicated in Figure 6.12

$$\mathcal{H} = g_{\parallel}\beta H_z S_z + g_{\perp}\beta H_x S_x \tag{6.13}$$

where H_z is the component of the magnetic field along the $\parallel(z)$ direction of the molecular axes and H_x is the magnetic field component along the $\perp(x)$ direction. If the magnetic field is directed along the $\|$ molecular axis direction (in a single crystal), then the situation is identical to equation (6.12) and the energy levels are $\pm\frac{1}{2}g_{\|}\beta H$. For off-axis orientations the situation is not so simple; this is because there is no quantum number corresponding to the S_x spin operator. From the geometry of Figure 6.12 the components of the magnetic field are: $H_z = H \cos\theta$, $H_x = H \sin\theta$, hence equation (6.13) may be written

$$\mathcal{H} = g_{\|}\beta H \cos\theta\, S_z + g_{\perp}\beta H \sin\theta\, S_x \tag{6.14}$$

This spin-Hamiltonian problem may be solved either by a rotation of axes or by the more general method of quantum-mechanical matrix diagonalization. By an axis rotation the spin-Hamiltonian equation (6.14) can be transformed to

$$\mathcal{H} = (g_{\|}^2 \cos^2\theta + g_{\perp}^2 \sin^2\theta)^{\frac{1}{2}}\, \beta H\, S_z \tag{6.15}$$

This is the same form as the simple spin Hamiltonian of equation (6.12), with an angularly dependent g-value given by equation (6.5). The diagonalization procedure would yield energy levels equivalent to those of equation (6.15).

This discussion should have served to illustrate both the use and the implications of the spin-Hamiltonian formalism. A few more commonly encountered examples will be presented, and their complications discussed. The spin Hamiltonian for an axially symmetric system with hyperfine structure is as follows

$$\mathcal{H} = g_{\|}\beta H_z S_z + A I_z S_z + B(I_x S_x + I_y S_y) \tag{6.16}$$

For simplicity the magnetic field has been taken to be along the $\|$ molecular axis. The g-value (magnetic field) term specifies the direction of the z-quantization axis because it is much larger than the hyperfine term; this is clear from the fact that the hyperfine interaction causes splittings of up to 100 gauss in a resonance which occurs at a field of about 3000 gauss. The z-axis hyperfine term presents no problems; its values are $\pm{}^1\!/_2 A m_I$, obtained simply by replacing the I_z, S_z spin operators by their quantum numbers, m_I being the nuclear spin quantum number. This term is the dominant hyperfine term, and the treatment so far corresponds to energy levels and transitions defined by equation (6.2). The B-terms make only a small contribution because they correspond to off-axis spin operators and can be treated by the approximate quantum-mechanical perturbation theory. They add terms of the order of $B^2/g_{\|}\beta H$ to the energy in equation (6.16). This is approximately 3 gauss (i.e. (100 gauss)^2/ 3000 gauss) relative to a hyperfine splitting of $A \simeq 100$ gauss, i.e. approximately 3% of the total hyperfine splitting. The second-order corrections are thus often not of very great importance in ESR, but are of importance in the analysis of spin–spin splittings in NMR; indeed complete diagonalization of the spin Hamiltonian rather than perturbation theory is required in the analysis of the spin–spin splittings of AB systems.

An important feature of the spectra of systems which have more than one unpaired electron, such as the transition-metal ions, is the possibility of zero-field splittings caused by the surrounding ligand ions (and also by electron–electron interactions in triplet-state molecules). The spin Hamiltonian for an axially symmetric system with zero-field splitting can be written

$$\mathcal{H} = g_{\|}\beta H\, S_z + D[S_z^2 - {}^1\!/_3 S(S+1)] \tag{6.17}$$

where D is the zero-field splitting constant. The term in $S(S+1)$ is not a spin operator, but merely a constant term which is conventionally included: it shifts the energy zero level but does not affect the splittings (or ESR transitions). Clearly for $S = \frac{1}{2}$ the second term in equation (6.17) is zero and there is no zero-field splitting for a single unpaired electron. For $S = 1$ as in triplet-state molecules there is a splitting D between the $m_S = \pm 1$ and $m_S = 0$ levels. Since the ESR transitions take place between these levels, this leads to a splitting of $\Delta H = 2D/g\beta$ as illustrated in Figure 6.17. The axial zero-field splitting, D, is a very important feature of the Fe^{3+} ESR spectra of haem proteins, as is discussed in Chapter 8. Non-axial zero-field splittings are also possible, though these are frequently less important than the axial component. For example, an additional term of the form $E(S_x^2 + S_y^2)$ represents a rhombic component of the zero-field splitting. Small rhombic splittings are also found in haem proteins.

6.7 Spin-Label Spectra

Many molecules have no intrinsic paramagnetic centres, but ESR can give useful information about these molecules if a structurally sensitive 'spin label' is attached.

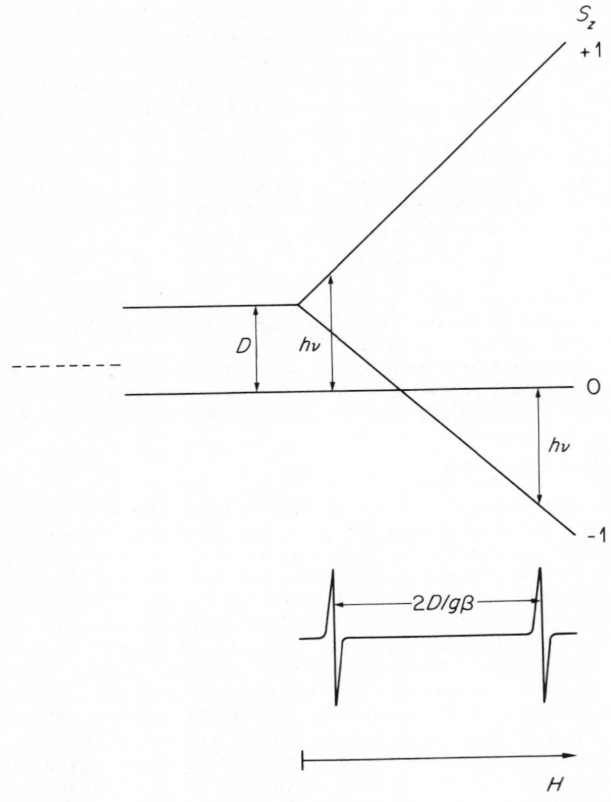

Figure 6.17 Axial zero-field splitting, D, in an $S = 1$ state. The ESR transitions ($\Delta M_S = \pm 1$) are seen to have a splitting of $2D/g\beta$

It is the purpose of the following sections to show how the ESR spectra can be interpreted to give information about the structure and dynamics of the labelled molecule. The spin-label group almost exclusively used is the nitroxide moiety introduced by McConnell.

The nitroxide group can be introduced in a spin-label analogue, e.g. as substrate, coenzyme, inhibitor or spin-labelled lipid, in which case the spin label will give information about the molecular mobility and the structure of the binding site or membrane. Alternatively, the nitroxide may be directly attached to the protein or other macromolecule, and in this case the spin label can give information about the structure of the macromolecule and its conformational changes, particularly in allosteric systems.

Several aspects of the ESR spectrum of the nitroxide group have already been discussed, particularly with respect to spectral anisotropy. The free electron is localized in a $2p\pi$ orbital of the nitrogen–oxygen bond, and interaction of the free electron with the nitrogen nuclear spin gives rise to the characteristic three-line hyperfine structure of the spin-label spectrum (see, for example, figures 6.1, 6.11). It is the anisotropy of this hyperfine splitting with respect to the magnetic field direction, as illustrated in Figure 6.11, which confers the structural and motional sensitivity on the spin-label method.

Spin-Label Immobilization – protein spin labels

When the nitroxide group is moving rapidly and isotropically the ESR signal consists of three narrow lines of equal heights. This high degree of mobility is obtained for small spin labels freely tumbling in non-viscous solutions, as indicated in Figures 6.1 and 6.14(c). Increasing immobilization of the spin label leads to a differential line broadening in the spectrum. This is illustrated in Figure 6.18 which gives the spectra of a small molecule nitroxide in glycerol–water mixtures of increasing viscosities. The various spectra are labelled with a correlation time, τ, for rotational reorientation, which can be thought of as being the average time for which the molecule moves in any one given direction. As the label becomes more immobilized, the motion becomes slower and the correlation time increases. The correlation times of Figure 6.18 have been derived from the viscosity, η, assuming a spherically symmetrical molecule (radius, a) and Stokes law viscosity

$$\tau = \frac{4\pi\eta a^3}{3kT} \tag{6.18}$$

Extremely marked and characteristic changes are seen in the nitroxide spectra as the correlation time for spin-label motion increases. In the weakly immobilized situation the high-field line is somewhat broadened relative to the other two. This broadening which is a relaxation-time effect arising from the modulation of the spectral anisotropies by the molecular motion, is most easily seen from the decreased lineheight of the high-field line. As the rate of spin-label motion decreases, there is a progressive differential broadening of the spectrum, up to the so-called moderately immobilized spectrum. Beyond this the spectra broaden out considerably and the lineshape begins to change with lines appearing to low field and high field in the spectrum. This is because the rotational reorientation is no longer sufficiently fast to average out the spectral anisotropies. The resulting spectra are referred to as 'strongly immobilized'. The limit of the strongly immobilized spectrum is the polycrystalline powder spectrum, already considered in Figure 6.14(a), in which the nitroxides are rigidly fixed in random orientations.

Spectra of the type shown in Figure 6.18 are found in the case of nitroxide spin labels covalently bound to proteins, and the concepts introduced above are used in

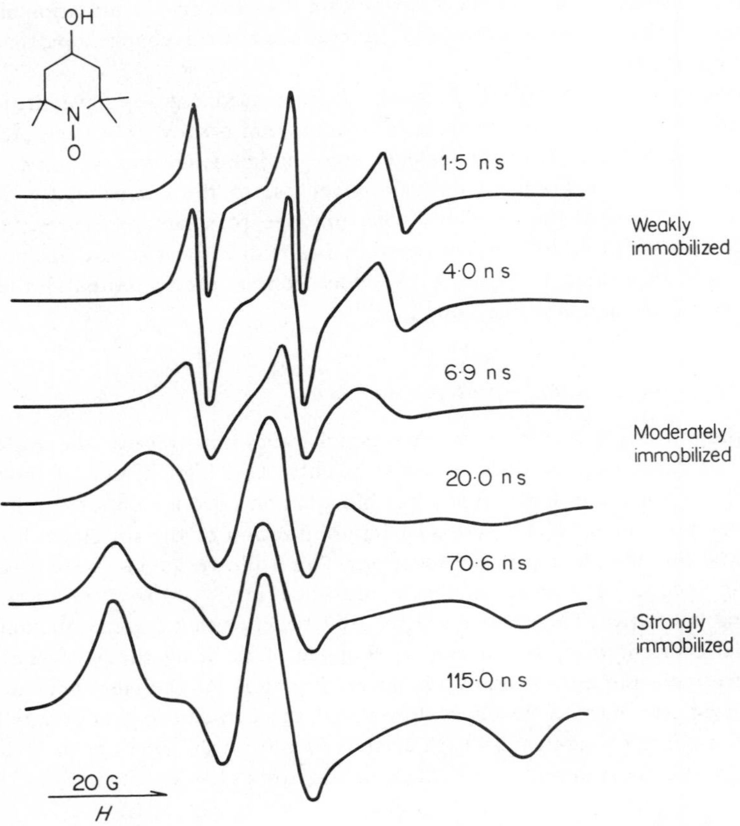

Figure 6.18 ESR spectra of a small molecule spin label in solutions of increasing viscosity. The extent of immobilization is indicated by the rotational correlation, time. (From Hsia and Piette, 1969. Reproduced by permission of Academic Press, Inc.)

interpreting the spectra of spin-labelled proteins. The motion of the protein as a whole is too slow to produce much significant effect on the spin-label spectrum (i.e. this would correspond to a completely immobilized spectrum, on the spin-label time scale). Consequently the degree of immobilization of the label depends on the flexibility of the covalent linkage, which will be very sensitive to the environment at the point of attachment. Very different states of spin-label immobilization can thus be obtained from different spin-labelled proteins, as indicated in Figure 6.19, and this reflects the protein structure at the site of labelling. The spectrum of the spin-labelled membrane ATPase (Figure 6.19a) corresponds to a very strongly immobilized spin label, with the sharp lines of some mobile spin label superimposed. The phosphofructokinase spectrum (Figure 6.19b) consists of a superposition of a moderately strongly immobilized spectrum and a weakly immobilized spectrum, and the phosphorylase-*b* spectrum (Figure 6.19c) is entirely

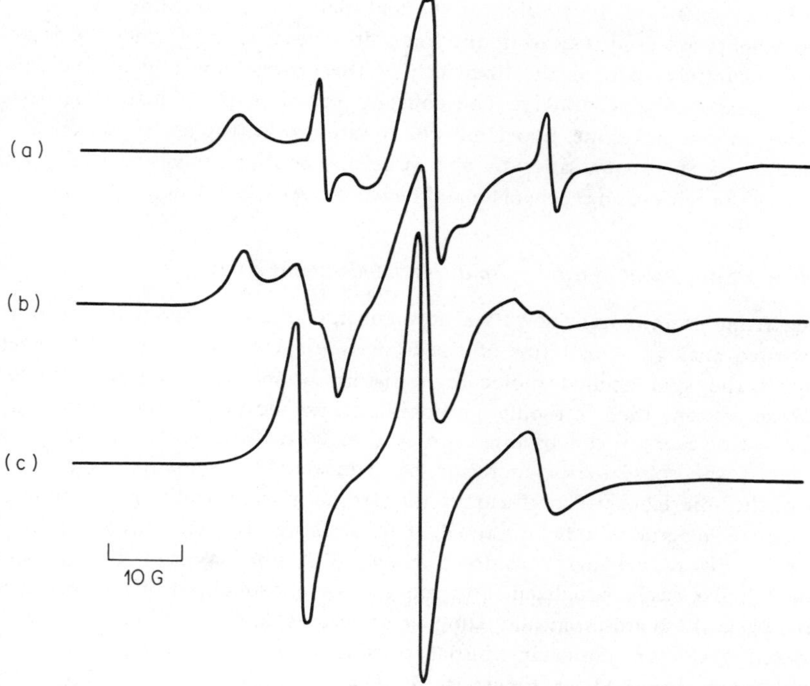

Figure 6.19 ESR spectra of a nitroxide spin label covalently bound to different enzymes. (a) A membrane-bound ATPase (from Marsh *et al.*, 1974). (b) Phosphofructokinase (see Jones *et al.*, 1972). (c) Phosphorylase-*b*. (See Dwek *et al.*, 1972)

weakly immobilized. Different conformations of a protein may well have different spin-label mobilities, hence the spin-label spectrum can be used in detecting conformational changes and carrying out ligand binding titrations. This has been done in the case of the phosphofructokinase and phosphorylase systems indicated in Figure 6.19(b) and (c), indeed the two superimposed spectra in Figure 6.19(b) correspond to different conformations of the enzyme (see Chapter 8). To some extent favourable conditions of spin-label mobility and sensitivity to conformational change can be chosen by varying the attaching group and chain length of the spin label. Intermediate situations of weak to moderate immobilization are probably best, since these are most sensitive to small changes. The mobility of a protein spin label can be quantitated in terms of a rotational correlation time, determined by comparison with model spectra, or in the case of weakly to moderately immobilized labels ($\tau = 10^{-9}-10^{-10}$ s) from the relative linewidths, using relaxation theory (see Chapter 1 for a discussion of relaxation). In this case the correlation time is given by

$$\star \quad \tau(\mathrm{s}) = 6.5 \times 10^{-10}\, \Delta H_0 \left(\sqrt{\frac{h(0)}{h(-1)}} - 1 \right) \qquad (6.19)$$

where $h(-1)$, $h(0)$ are the heights of the high-field and central lines respectively. The lineheights are used instead of the linewidths because the former are easier to measure accurately; ΔH_0 is the linewidth of the central line in gauss and can be measured reasonably accurately. The constant factor in this equation is derived from the known nitroxide hyperfine and g-value anisotropies. It is the rate of modulation of these quantities by the molecular motion, specified by τ, which determines the relaxation mechanism and hence the relative lineheights.

Anisotropic Spin-Label Motion – lipid spin labels/membranes

Turning from protein spin labels we now consider the analysis of the motion of spin-labelled analogues, in terms of the hyperfine splittings in their ESR spectra. Clearly if the spin-labelled molecule is rigidly bound to a macromolecule or membrane system then a rigidly immobilized, pseudopowder spectrum will be obtained. However, if the binding site is somewhat flexible, or the membrane fluid, or if the spin-labelled molecule has considerable segmental flexibility of its own, the spin label will perform an anisotropic motion, and more complicated, intermediate spectra will be obtained. This situation is well illustrated by the spectra of Figure 6.14(b) considered above. The interpretation of anisotropic motion is most easily visualized in membranes or phospholipid bilayer membrane models, since these are essentially lamellar structures, and it is these which will be considered here. An important initial consideration is the orientation of the nitroxide axes specified in Figure 6.11 relative to the molecular axes of the spin-labelled molecule. It is necessary to know this in order to determine the orientation of the spin-labelled molecule relative to the surface of the membrane in which it is incorporated. The orientation of the nitroxide axes in a spin-labelled stearic acid molecule is indicated in Figure 6.20. This is a lipid spin label which is commonly used in the study of phospholipid bilayers and membranes. It is seen from Figure 6.20, that the principal z-axis, which is the direction of the largest hyperfine splitting, is directed along the long axis of the stearic acid molecule. The two other, 6 gauss, hyperfine splittings are in a plane perpendicular to the long axis of the molecule. When the label is intercalated into a membrane its long axis will be oriented preferentially along a direction parallel to the normal to the membrane.

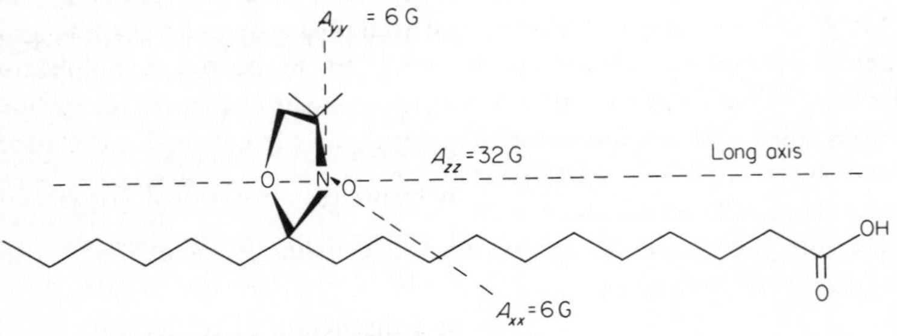

Figure 6.20 Orientation of the nitroxide axes in a stearic acid lipid spin label

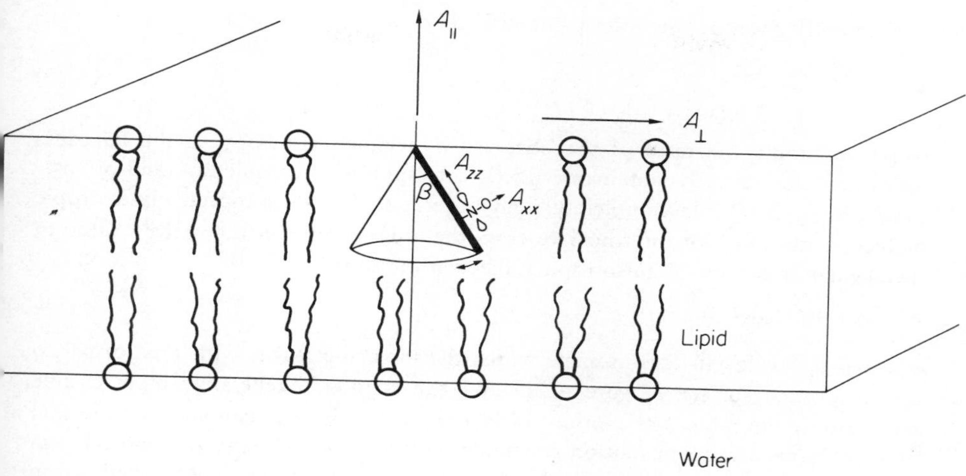

Figure 6.21 Anisotropic motion of a structural lipid spin label intercalated in the lipid region of a membrane. The nitroxide principal z-axis (A_{zz} = 32 gauss) is directed along the length of the lipid molecule. The axis of motional averaging is the normal to the membrane surface (∥ direction), and an axial spectrum, splittings $A_{\parallel}$, $A_{\perp}$ results

Thus the maximum hyperfine splitting will be obtained with the magnetic field in a direction parallel to the membrane normal (the ∥ direction) and the minimum splitting obtained when the magnetic field is in the plane of the membrane surface (the ⊥ direction), as indicated in Figure 6.14(b). This is a fortunate situation and contributes to the usefulness of this particular spin label; it is this type of structural spin label which is considered below. If the spin-labelled molecule undergoes rapid anisotropic motion of a limited amplitude, then part, but not all, of the anisotropy of the hyperfine splitting will be averaged. For a structural lipid spin label such a motion could be visualized as a type of conical motion of the lipid molecule about an axis perpendicular to the membrane surface, as indicated in Figure 6.21. The hyperfine splitting, $A_{\parallel}$, obtained with the magnetic field directed along the normal to the membrane surface will thus be less than the principal hyperfine value, A_{zz}, which would be obtained if the spin label were rigidly oriented along the membrane normal. (Recall that the z-axis of the hyperfine splitting is directed along the long axis of the structural lipid spin label as shown in Figure 6.21 and as is the case for fatty acid and phospholipid spin labels). Similarly the hyperfine splitting, $A_{\perp}$, with the magnetic field directed along the membrane surface will be larger than A_{xx}, the principal value which would be obtained for rigid orientation. This is because part of the maximum hyperfine anisotropy ($A_{zz} - A_{xx}$,= 25 gauss) is averaged out by the limited (anisotropic) molecular motion, in just the same way that the whole of the anisotropy is averaged out by isotropic molecular tumbling. This situation is again rather well illustrated by the nitroxide spectra in Figure 6.14(b), which also indicates the way in which $A_{\parallel}$,and $A_{\perp}$ can be deduced from the spectra of randomly oriented membrane dispersions. The extent of the limited motional averaging is conveniently given by the order parameter, S

★ $$S = \frac{A_{\parallel} - A_{\perp}}{A_{zz} - A_{xx}} \tag{6.20}$$

which is simply the ratio of the observed hyperfine anisotropy to the 25 gauss maximum theoretically obtainable which corresponds to completely rigid orientation. Clearly $S = 1$ for completely rigid order, and $S = 0$ for completely isotropic molecular motion. For intermediate cases the order parameter is directly related to the angular amplitude of anisotropic molecular motion:

★ $$S = \tfrac{1}{2}(3\langle\cos^2 \beta\rangle - 1) \tag{6.21}$$

where β is the instantaneous angle which the molecule makes with the normal to the membrane surface (Figure 6.21) and the angular brackets represent a time average over the molecular motion. If as a simple model it is assumed that the spin label performs a random motion restricted within a cone of angle γ, as indicated in Figure 6.22, then the angular amplitude of motion can be calculated directly from the measured order parameter

$$S = \tfrac{1}{2}(\cos \gamma + \cos^2 \gamma) \tag{6.22}$$

Clearly other more complicated motional models are possible which relate the experimentally observed order parameter to the amplitude of motion, hence giving information about the way in which the environment limits the motion of the spin-labelled molecule. The analysis can also be extended to include the intrinsic flexibility of the spin-label molecule as is done for the 'fluidity' of lipid spin labels in membranes in Chapter 8.

A modification of the ESR lineshapes resulting from anisotropic motion also arises from immobilization effects as already discussed for isotropic motion in the previous section. A differential broadening is obtained depending on the rate of

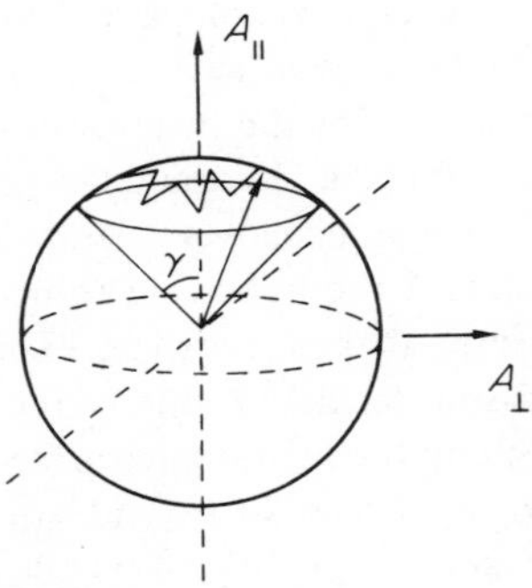

Figure 6.22 Restricted random walk of a lipid spin label in a membrane, within a cone of angle γ about the normal to the membrane surface

anisotropic motion, and a correlation time approach can again be applied. The correlation time is then the correlation time for the *anisotropic* motion.

Finally it is clear that this type of consideration is also applicable to the motion of spin-label molecules in protein binding sites, e.g. the motion of spin-labelled haptens in antibody combining sites.

Isotropic Hyperfine Splitting and Environment Polarity

The anisotropy of the spin-label hyperfine splitting (i.e. the difference between the splittings with the magnetic field in the parallel and perpendicular directions) gives the amplitude of the anisotropic motion, but the overall size of the hyperfine splittings can also vary and is an index of the polarity of the environment in which the spin label is situated. This latter is clearly an extremely useful parameter, since it can reveal whether the spin label is attached at the surface or in a hydrophobic pocket in the interior of a protein, or the depth at which a lipid spin label is situated within a membrane. The overall size of the hyperfine splitting is given by the average of the principal hyperfine splittings, i.e. by the isotropic hyperfine splitting constant given in equations (6.8) and (6.10) above. We recall that this is the hyperfine splitting which is measured for small molecules tumbling isotropically in solution. Table 6.4 gives the isotropic hyperfine splitting constants which are measured for a stearic acid spin label tumbling isotropically in solvents of different polarities. Clearly the isotropic splitting constant is high in highly polar solvents such as water and decreases as the polarity of the solvent decreases, to low values in hydrophobic solvents. The application of this polarity sensitivity of the spin label is neatly demonstrated in Table 6.5 which gives the isotropic splitting constant for stearic acids spin-labelled at various points down the chain. It can be seen that a_0 calculated from the measured $A_{\parallel}$ and $A_{\perp}$ splittings decreases the further the spin-label group is situated down the stearic acid chain, corresponding to deeper penetration into the hydrophobic interior of the phospholipid bilayer membrane. The higher values at the top of the chain are caused by the proximity to the aqueous-membrane interface.

Table 6.4
Isotropic hyperfine splitting constants for a stearic acid spin label in various solvents. (From Seelig, 1970)

Solvent	a_0 (gauss)
Water	15.6
Ethanol	15.2
Decanol	14.2
n-Decane	13.9

Table 6.5
Isotropic hyperfine splitting constants for stearic acid spin labels in aqueous phospholipid bilayers. The nitroxide label is attached to different C-atoms down the stearic acid chain. (From Seelig and Hasselbach, 1971)

Nitroxide position	a_0 (gauss) $= 1/3(A_{\parallel} + 2A_{\perp})$
C–4	15.1
C–5	14.9
C–8	14.8
C–9	14.8
C–10	14.6

6.8 Transition-metal Ions

The ESR spectra from transition-metal ions are, in many ways, more complex than those considered previously from free radicals and spin labels. The electrons with unpaired spins which give rise to the ESR spectrum, are primarily localized in d-orbitals on the transition-metal ion. This localization results in a strong contribution to the net electron magnetic moment from the orbital angular momentum of the d-electron. This in turn gives rise to anisotropic spectra with g-values which are frequently very different from the free-electron value of $g_e = 2.0023$, and to fast relaxation times, which sometimes means that the spectra can only be observed at low temperatures. The strong angular nature of the d-orbitals gives rise to very strong and very specific interactions with the ligands of the transition-metal ion, which can also dramatically affect the ESR spectra.

A further complication is the fact that the transition-metal ion may have more than one unpaired electron. The five possible d-orbitals which an unpaired electron can occupy are indicated in Figure 6.23. Each orbital can contain two oppositely directed electron spins. This gives a possibility of 10 different electron configurations from d^1, e.g. Mo^{5+}, to d^{10}, e.g. Cu^+. The electron configurations of the biologically important transition-metal ions are given in Table 6.6. With increasing numbers of d-electrons the orbitals are filled up with one electron each, all of the same spin (spin up, ↑). When all five orbitals contain one electron, the spins are

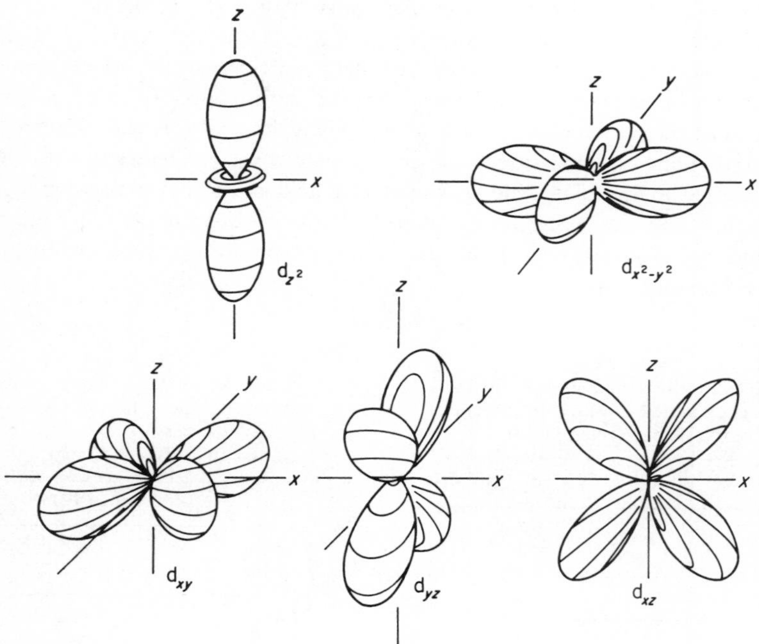

Figure 6.23 The five d-orbitals of transition-metal ions. Each orbital can contain two electrons with opposite spins. The subscripts indicate the angular form of the orbital

Table 6.6
Electron configurations for transition-metal ions of importance in biological ESR

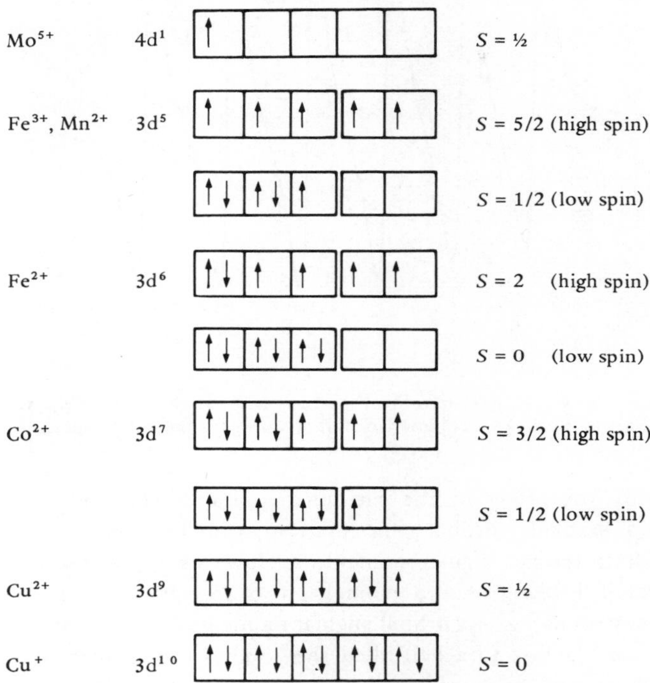

then paired, by putting spin-down, ↓, electrons into each of the singly occupied orbitals in turn. Table 6.6 lists the resultant spins obtained in this way. Thus Mo^{5+} has one d-electron with spin-up and a total spin of $S = ½$; Mn^{2+} has five d-electrons normally all with spin-up and a total spin of $S = 5/2$; and Cu^{2+} has nine d-electrons: five with spin-up and four with spin-down and hence a net spin of $S = ½$. Cu^+ has ten d-electrons and a net spin of zero, hence no ESR signal is observable. This forms a basis for the quantitation of the different oxidation states of copper: Cu^{2+} gives an ESR signal and Cu^+ does not. A complication to the spin-pairing system immediately arises, depending on the way in which the ligands cause energy-level splittings between the d-orbitals. If this splitting is small then a high spin derivative is obtained as already outlined, but if the splitting is large the order of spin pairing is altered and a low spin derivative is found, as indicated in Table 6.6. This high-spin, low-spin effect is discussed in more detail below, but at the moment it serves to show one of the ways in which the ligands can crucially determine the nature of the ESR spectrum.

The orbital angular momentum of the d-orbitals would be expected to contribute strongly to the total magnetic moment of the electron and hence to the g-value splitting. In fact the orbital magnetic moment is wholly or partially

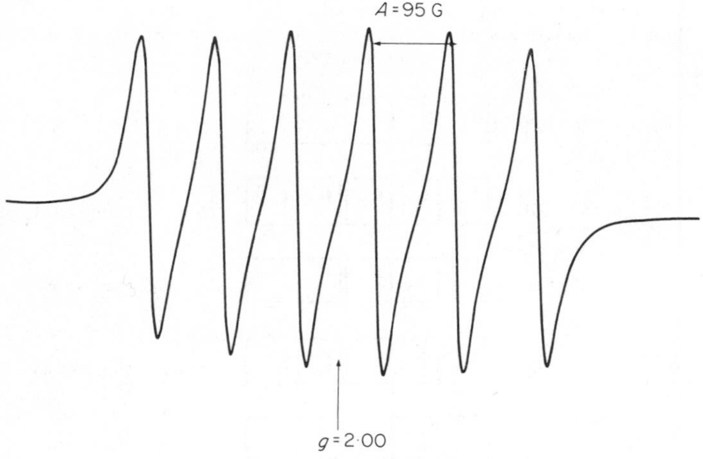

Figure 6.24 ESR spectrum of aqueous Mn^{2+} at room temperature. The spectrum is split by the hyperfine interaction with the Mn nucleus ($I = 5/2$)

'quenched' by the effect of the surrounding ligands (they effectively trap the electron in a particular orbital configuration), thus the spins of Table 6.6 are a reliable guide to the net angular momentum. How this quenching arises is discussed in some detail below; for the moment it is interesting to note that the d^5 (high-spin) system has no net orbital angular momentum, irrespective of the ligands, because it corresponds to a half-filled shell and is thus spherically symmetrical. These configurations are the so-called S-state ions, of which Mn^{2+} is a good example since it is normally found in the high-spin situation. This ion has a *g*-value very close to 2, and a long spin–lattice relaxation time in aqueous solution, the spectrum being readily observable at room temperature (Figure 6.24). For Fe^{3+}, which is also $3d^5$, the situation is much more complicated because of the zero-field splittings between the levels, giving rise to high-spin and low-spin derivatives; this is treated in some detail in Chapter 8 for haem proteins.

As already indicated, the ligand environment has a large effect on the ESR spectrum of a transition-metal ion, or conversely the ESR spectrum contains a considerable amount of information about the liganding and spin state of the transition-metal ion. This is because the electrostatic and covalent bonding interactions of the ligands with the metal ion produce large energy splittings between the different metal-ion orbitals of Figure 6.23, which affects the distribution of electrons between these configurations and hence the ESR properties of the ion.

Cu^{2+} g-values

We will consider the case of Cu^{2+} as an illustrative example for two main reasons. Firstly copper proteins are very important in biology as oxidative enzymes, or

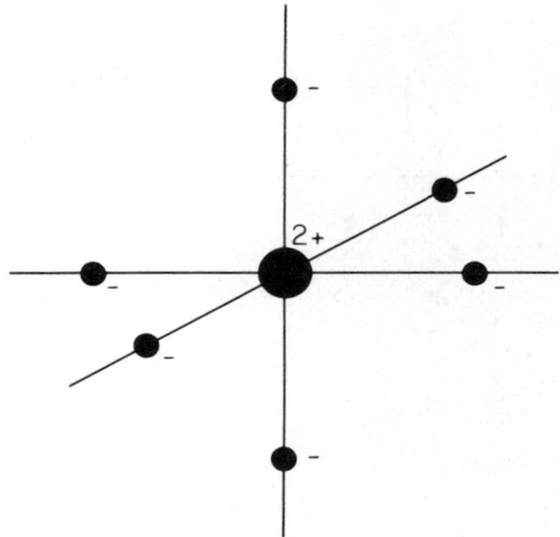

Figure 6.25 The six-fold octahedral co-ordination of ligand atoms about a central Cu^{2+} ion

fulfilling other redox functions, e.g. in electron transport chains. The second reason is that Cu^{2+} has a relatively simple electron configuration. Having 9 d-electrons, one less than for a completely filled shell, the Cu^{2+} ion can be considered simply as a single 'd-hole', as opposed to single d-electron, with a spin of a half and having the wavefunctions illustrated in Figure 6.23. Since these orbitals are strongly directional in nature, they will clearly interact differently with different ligand bonding structures. The simplest structure is the octahedral ligand coordination illustrated in Figure 6.25, in which six identical ligands are bonded at equal distances from the Cu^{2+} ion, along perpendicular x-, y- and z-axes. The interaction of such an octahedral ligand arrangement with the d-orbitals of the Cu^{2+} 'hole' is indicated in Figure 6.26. The ligands will be either negatively charged or have a high electron density, thus the 'positively charged' hole (i.e. absence of Cu^{2+} electron density) will interact more strongly with the ligands (with a net lowering of energy) in the case of orbitals $d_{x^2-y^2}$ and d_{z^2} than in the case of d_{xy}, d_{yz} and d_{xz}. This is illustrated in Figure 6.27 in which the two groups of orbitals are split by an energy, Δ, in an octahedral environment. The two sets of orbitals are conventionally labelled e_g and t_{2g}, a group-theoretical nomenclature which need not concern us here (alternative names are $d\gamma$ and $d\epsilon$ orbitals respectively). Clearly, less symmetrical ligand structures or changes in ligand type can produce further energy splittings in exactly the same way. This is illustrated for a tetragonal arrangement of ligands in Figure 6.27. Tetragonal distortions from octahedral symmetry occur when the ligand separations along the z-axis are elongated (or diminished). The axial type of ligand symmetry is commonly found in practice, and it can be seen from Figure 6.27 that in this case a single orbital, the $d_{x^2-y^2}$, is left with lowest energy. In this situation the orbital angular momentum of the Cu^{2+} ion is said to be quenched, because the electron hole resides solely in this orbital configuration and cannot interchange with the others (e.g. d_{z^2}, etc.).

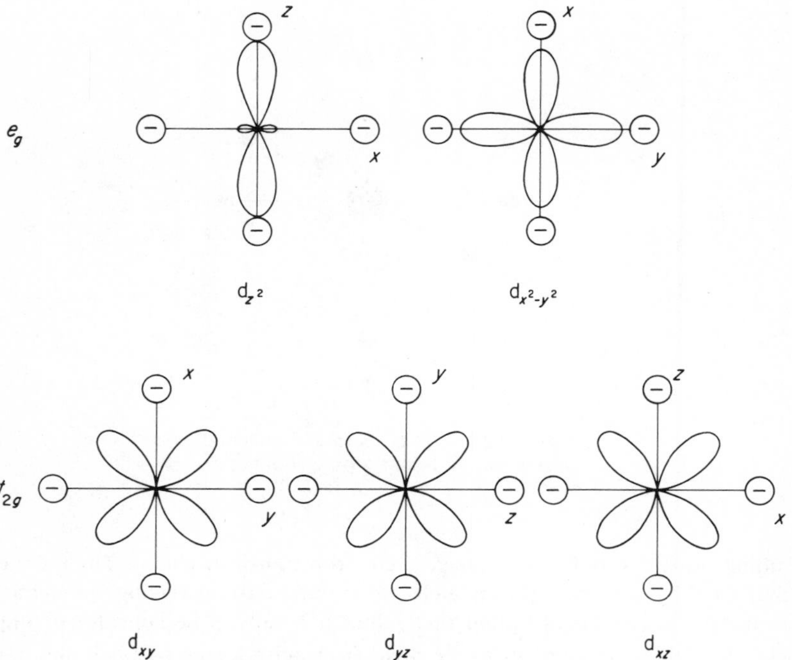

Figure 6.26 The angular disposition of the 3d orbitals in Cu^{2+} relative to an octahedral arrangement of negatively charged ligands. The Cu^{2+} hole has lower energy when occupying one of the e_g orbitals

In such a case of 'orbital quenching' the Cu^{2+} hole only has angular momentum (and hence magnetic moment) associated with the electron spin, $S = ½$. Under these circumstances the g-value of the Cu^{2+} ion approaches fairly closely to the free electron g-value of $g_e = 2.0023$, and g-values in the region of 2 are observed for copper proteins. Nevertheless, the Cu^{2+} hole may spend a very small amount of its time in the higher-energy orbitals, and this gives rise to so-called perturbations of the g-value which depend on the energy-level splittings, Δ, and thus on the nature of the copper ligands as indicated in Table 6.1. The g-values are then given by

★ $$g = g_e \left(1 + \frac{r\lambda}{\Delta}\right) \qquad (6.23)$$

where r is a constant which depends on the ligand coordination, λ is the spin–orbit coupling constant which is a measure of how strongly the spin and orbital angular momenta are associated together in the absence of ligands, i.e. in the free ion. The deviations from the free-spin g-value are thus smaller, the larger the ligand orbital energy splitting, Δ, is compared with λ. For octahedral symmetry the g-value will be isotropic, but in tetragonal symmetry the g-value is anisotropic. Depending upon whether the magnetic field is directed along the tetragonal (z) axis or perpendicular

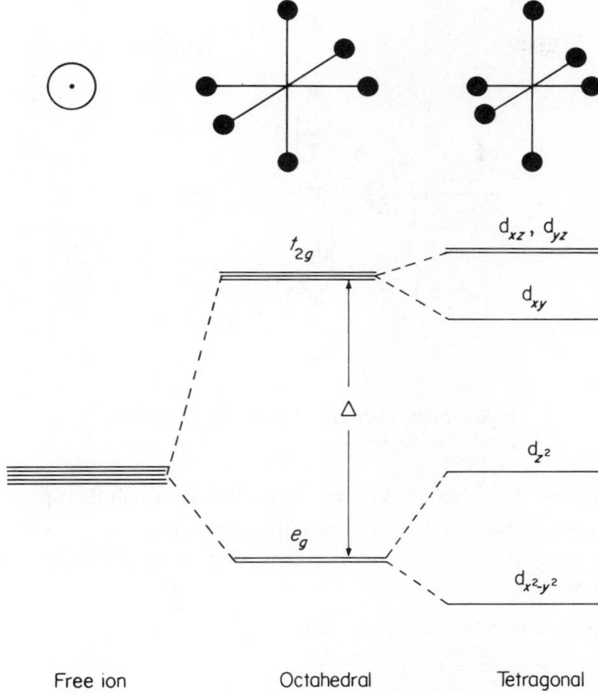

Figure 6.27 The energy splittings between the d-orbitals of a Cu^{2+} ion in octahedral and tetragonal ligand environments

to it, one gets the following *g*-values

$$g_{\parallel} = g_e \left(1 - \frac{4\lambda}{\Delta_1}\right)$$
$$g_{\perp} = g_e \left(1 - \frac{\lambda}{\Delta_2}\right) \tag{6.24}$$

where Δ_1 is the ligand splitting between the $d_{x^2-y^2}$ and d_{xy} orbitals and Δ_2 is the splitting between $d_{x^2-y^2}$ and d_{xz}, d_{yz}. Thus the *g*-values clearly give information about both the strength of the ligand interaction and the geometry of the metal–ligand complex. Similar perturbations are also found in the hyperfine splitting constants of the Cu^{2+} ion.

The treatment so far has really only considered electrostatic interactions between the metal ion and the ligands – this is the so-called crystal field approach. In fact, some degree of covalent bonding, i.e. partial transfer of electrons from metal ion to ligand and vice versa, will take place between the metal-ion d-orbitals and the ligand orbitals. This is indicated schematically in Figure 6.28 by the degree of overlap between a $d_{x^2-y^2}$ metal-ion orbital and the p-orbitals of its surrounding

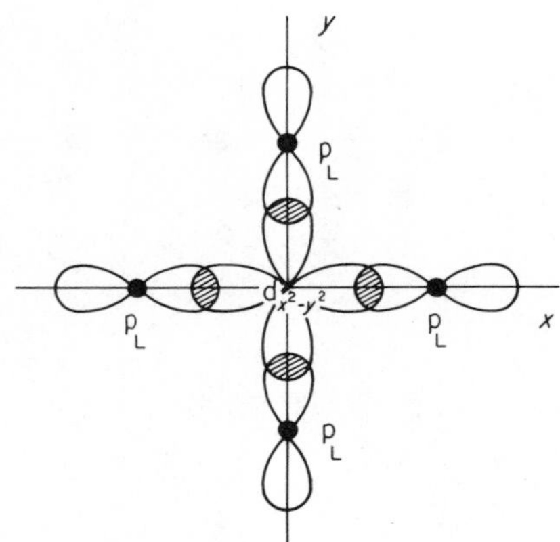

Figure 6.28 Covalent bonding of ligand p-orbitals to the $d_{x^2-y^2}$ orbital of Cu^{2+}

ligands. To account for this covalency, a molecular orbital approach known as ligand field theory is required. Covalency modifies the $d_{x^2-y^2}$ orbital which the unpaired electron occupies, admixing a certain fraction of the ligand orbital to form the molecular orbital

$$\text{M.O.(unpaired spin)} = \alpha d_{x^2-y^2} + \beta p_L \qquad (6.25)$$
$$\alpha^2 + \beta^2 = 1$$

Where α is a measure of the extent to which the unpaired electron is moved off the Cu^{2+} ion (α is somewhat less than one), and β is correspondingly the extent to which it is transferred to the ligand (β is somewhat greater than zero).

The effect of this covalent admixture is to modify the Cu^{2+} ion g-values of equation (6.24) to give

★
$$g_{\parallel} = g_e \left(1 - \frac{4\alpha^2 \lambda}{\Delta_1}\right)$$
$$g_{\perp} = g_e \left(1 - \frac{\alpha^2 \lambda}{\Delta_2}\right) \qquad (6.26)$$

and the hyperfine constants are similarly modified. Clearly the g-values and hyperfine splittings are also capable of giving information about the degree of covalency, α, of the metal-ion–ligand site. Typically α^2 is in the region of 0.6 to 0.9 in copper proteins.

The existence of covalent transfer between metal ion and ligand means that some of the unpaired electron spin density will be transferred from the metal ion to the ligand, as indicated by the molecular orbital of equation (6.25). Thus if the ligand has a nuclear spin, one would expect to see ligand hyperfine structure, just as one sees different hyperfine splittings from the spin densities on the various nuclei in free radicals, as discussed in a previous section of this chapter. In this case the spin densities on the ligands will be of order β^2, hence the ligand hyperfine structure will also give a measure of the degree of covalency. This ligand hyperfine structure is the most direct demonstration of covalent binding between metal ion and ligand, and can help in the identification of the ligands. Nitrogen is the most common ligand giving rise to hyperfine structure in the ESR spectra of copper proteins. A typical example has been given in Figure 6.2(b); in some cases the structure is too small or too complex to be resolved at all.

High-spin and Low-spin Fe^{3+}

To finish this discussion of transition-metal ions, we will briefly consider one aspect of an ion with a more complicated electron configuration than Cu^{2+}. This is the high- and low-spin states previously referred to in ferric iron, which is important in the analysis of the ESR spectra of haem proteins. The Fe^{3+} ion has five d-electrons, and the way these are arranged in the various d-orbitals depends on the relative values of the repulsive spin pairing energy in a particular orbital and the ligand field splitting, Δ. In the absence of ligand interactions the electrons would prefer to go one into each orbital with parallel spins until each orbital contains one electron, then spin pairing within orbitals would take place. When ligand interactions are present, two cases can be distinguished: the high- and the low-spin situations. This is illustrated in Figure 6.29 for an octahedral complex. If the pairing energy is greater than the ligand field splitting, Δ, one gets the normal, high-spin, situation and $S = 5/2$. If the pairing energy is less than Δ, then the low-spin state obtains and one gets $S = 1/2$. This example serves to indicate the more complex effects which can

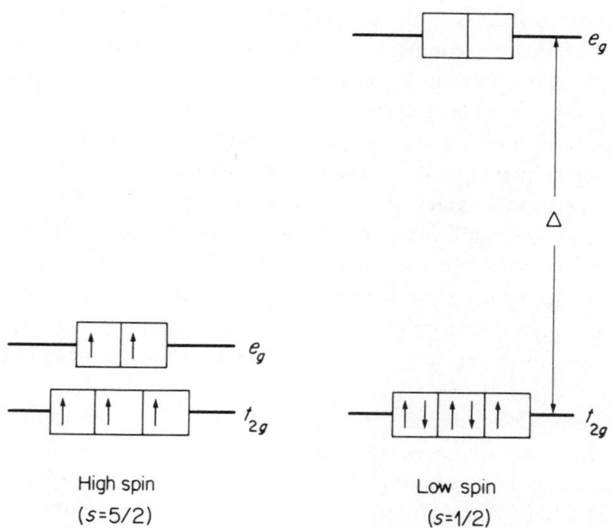

Figure 6.29 Electron occupancy of the d-orbitals of the $3d^5$ ion, Fe^{3+} in octahedral ligand symmetry. Occurrence of the high- or low-spin state depends on the magnitude of the ligand field splitting, Δ

be obtained with more than one electron or hole. The high-spin and low-spin states in octahedral coordination for other 3d ions of biological significance are indicated in Table 6.4. In ligand systems with coordination other than octahedral the situation may be different and 'intermediate' spin states can be obtained.

6.9 Summary

(1) The magnetic field about which an ESR spectrum is centred is specified by the g-value, which is dependent on the electron configuration, environmental polarity and bonding. The g-value is close to $g = 2$ for free radicals, but can be considerably different from $g = 2$ for transition-metal ions.

(2) The ESR spectrum is split by the hyperfine interaction of the unpaired electron(s) with the surrounding nuclei. The number of hyperfine lines depends on the nuclear spin of the nucleus and on the number of nuclei. Splittings by a single nucleus can be distinguished from those arising from several nuclei, because all lines are of equal intensity in the former case, whereas a characteristic intensity pattern is obtained with several nuclei.

(3) The hyperfine splittings are determined by the spin density at or near the particular nucleus, and thus give information on the electron densities in free radical molecular orbitals and on covalent bonding in transition-metal-ion–ligand complexes.

(4) Both line splittings and the magnetic field at which the spectrum occurs (specified by the g-value) depend on the orientation of the magnetic field with respect to the molecular axes. This spectral anisotropy yields information about the local symmetry of the environment of a transition-metal ion, and also about the orientation of the transition-metal ion site or of a spin-labelled group relative to the rest of the macromolecule (as specified by the single crystal axes).

(5) The spin-label method depends on the degree of motional averaging of the spectral anisotropy (principally of the 3-line nitrogen hyperfine structure) of a nitroxide reporter group attached to a biological molecule. The line-broadening gives the extent of immobilization of the spin label, which both depends on the macromolecular structure at the point of attachment and is sensitive to the conformation of the protein, or nucleic acid, to which the spin label is attached. The line splittings give the amplitude of motion of the spin-labelled molecule, and are particularly useful in the analysis of the motion of lipid molecules in membrane systems.

(6) Transition-metal ions are more complicated than free radicals since they contain more than one unpaired electron. The ESR spectrum then depends very strongly on the redox state of the metal, and can also be very sensitively influenced by the ligand bonding: high-spin and low-spin derivatives. g-values are often highly anisotropic, and hyperfine splittings consist of very large splittings from the transition-metal ion nucleus and much smaller splittings from the ligand nuclei. Both g-values and hyperfine splittings give information on the covalent bonding of the metal ion.

References

Bolton, J. R. (1963). *Mol. Phys.*, **6**, 219.

Dwek, R. A., Griffiths, J. R., Radda, G. K., and Strauss, U. (1972). *F.E.B.S. Lett.*, **28**, 161.

Griffith, O. H., and Waggoner, A. S. (1969). *Acc. Chem. Res.*, **2**, 17.

Hsia, J. C., and Piette, L. H. (1969). *Arch. Biochem. Biophys.*, **129**, 296.

Jones, R., Dwek, R. A., and Walker, I. O. (1972). *F.E.B.S. Lett.*, **26**, 92.

McConnell, H. M., and McFarland, B. G. (1970). *Quart. Rev. Biophys.*, **3**, 91.

Marsh, D., Radda, G. K., and Ritchie, G. A. (1974). Unpublished.

Nakamura, T. (1961) In *Free Radicals in Biological Systems* Blois, M. S., *et al.* (Eds.), Academic Press, New York.

Ohnishi, T., Yamazaki, H., Iyanagi, T., Nakamura, T., and Yamazaki, I. (1969). *Biochim. Biophys. Acta,* **172**, 357.

Seelig, J. (1970). *J. Am. Chem. Soc.*, **92**, 3881.

Seelig, J., and Hasselbach, W. (1971). *Eur. J. Biochem.*, **21**, 17.

Stretweiser, A. (1961). *Molecular Orbital Theory for Organic Chemists*, J. Wiley, New York.

Wertz, J. E., and Bolton, J. R. (1972). *Electron Spin Resonance*, McGraw–Hill, New York.

Windle, J., Wiersema, A., Clark, J., and Feeney, R. (1963). *Biochemistry,* **2**, 1341.

Yamazaki, I., and Piette, L. (1961). *Biochim. Biophys. Acta,* **50**, 62.

Reading List

Carrington, A., and McLachlan, A. D. (1969). *Introduction to Magnetic Resonance*, Harper Row, New York.

Ingram, D. J. E. (1969). *Biological and Biochemical Applications of Electron Spin Resonance*, Hilger, London.

Knowles, P. F. (1972). *Essays in Biochemistry,* **8**, 79–106, 'The application of magnetic resonance methods to the study of enzyme structure and action.' Academic Press, London.

Marsh, D. (1975). *Essays in Biochemistry,* **11**, 'Spectroscopic studies of membrane structure.' Academic Press, London.

Smith, I. C. P., Schreier-Muccillo, S., and Marsh, D. (1975). In *Free Radicals in Biology*, Vol. 1, Ch. 4, 'Spin labelling', W. A. Pryor, (Ed.). Academic Press, New York.

Swartz, H. M., Bolton, J. R. and Borg, D. C. (Eds.) (1972). *Biological Applications of Electron Spin Resonance*, Wiley, New York.

Wertz, J. E. and Bolton, J. R. (1972). *Electron Spin Resonance*, McGraw–Hill, New York.

Chapter 7
Practical Biological ESR

7.1 Introduction

The purpose of this chapter is to explain spectrometer operation, illustrate practically how to go about obtaining a spectrum and to discuss techniques of sample handling, particularly of biological materials. The function of the various units of the spectrometer is described only in so far as it is necessary to an understanding of the operator's manipulation of the spectrometer controls. It is thus hoped that this chapter will furnish the reader with information on sample handling which will enable him to prepare his problem in a manner suited for investigation by ESR and will give operational details enabling him to run the spectra on this sample.

7.2 Sample Requirements

Most samples of interest will be aqueous, and because of dielectric absorption (see below) there is a very restrictive limit on the total amount of water which can be put in the ESR cavity. Thus the minimum volume of aqueous sample required would be in the region of 20 μl. If a flat cell (see below) is used rather than a capillary, then the requirement is somewhat larger because of dead-volume effects. The minimum detectable concentration depends on how broad the spectra are. Thus for a small spin label in aqueous solution the lines are very sharp and concentrations in the range 0.1–1.0 μM should be detectable. A similar situation holds for free radical intermediates in enzymic reactions. For a moderately mobile spin label attached to a protein, concentrations in the region of 5 μM will be required to give adequate spectra, whereas for an immobilized protein spin label, concentrations of the order of 50 μM will be needed.

In the case of spin-labelled proteins, the spin label and the protein sample concentrations are equivalent. However, for lipid spin labels in phospholipid bilayers or membranes this is not the case. To prevent interaction broadening which would distort the spectrum, the spin-labelled lipid concentration should not be more than 1 mole % of the total lipid concentration. Since lipid spin-label spectra are moderately strongly immobilized, this means that a concentration of 3–5 mM of lipid is required, of which 1% is spin label.

Transition-metal ions pose different problems. For sensitivity reasons, and sometimes even just to see the spectra at all, metalloproteins are normally examined at low temperatures. Since the sample is frozen, more of it can be introduced into the cavity and a typical requirement is 200 μl. The transition-metal ion lines are much broader than any spin-label spectra, and the minimum concentration of metalloprotein required is about 0.3 mM. The ESR spectra of some small complexes of transition-metal ions can be observed in aqueous solution at room temperature. Concentrations of 5 mM would be required for copper complexes. Aqueous manganese (Mn^{2+}) is an exception and can be readily detected in concentrations down to 5–10 μM at room temperature.

Biological tissue handling is discussed below, but will have the attendant problems of aqueous samples if it is not frozen or freeze-dried. Minimum detectable quantities will be those quoted above for the various components, but it must be remembered that these components may be quite dilute relative to the total sample size. In these cases some form of signal averaging (see below) may be helpful.

7.3 Overall Spectrometer Features

Like any other form of absorption spectroscopy the ESR spectrometer consists basically of a radiation source, sample absorption cell and a detector, as indicated in Figure 7.1 in which these units are identified in a simple form of ESR spectrometer. The radiation source is a microwave klystron valve which requires a high-voltage DC power supply and may be tuned electronically over a small frequency range or

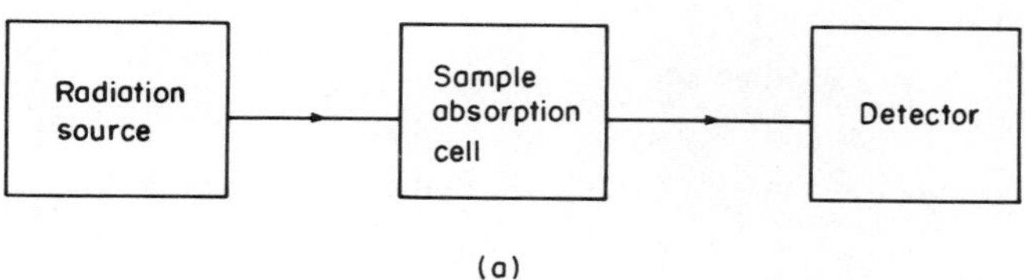

(a)

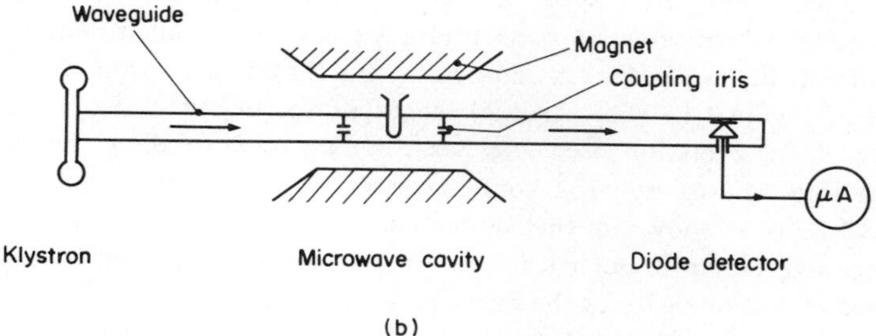

(b)

Figure 7.1 (a) Schematic layout of an absorption spectrometer. (b) Simple form of an ESR absorption spectrometer

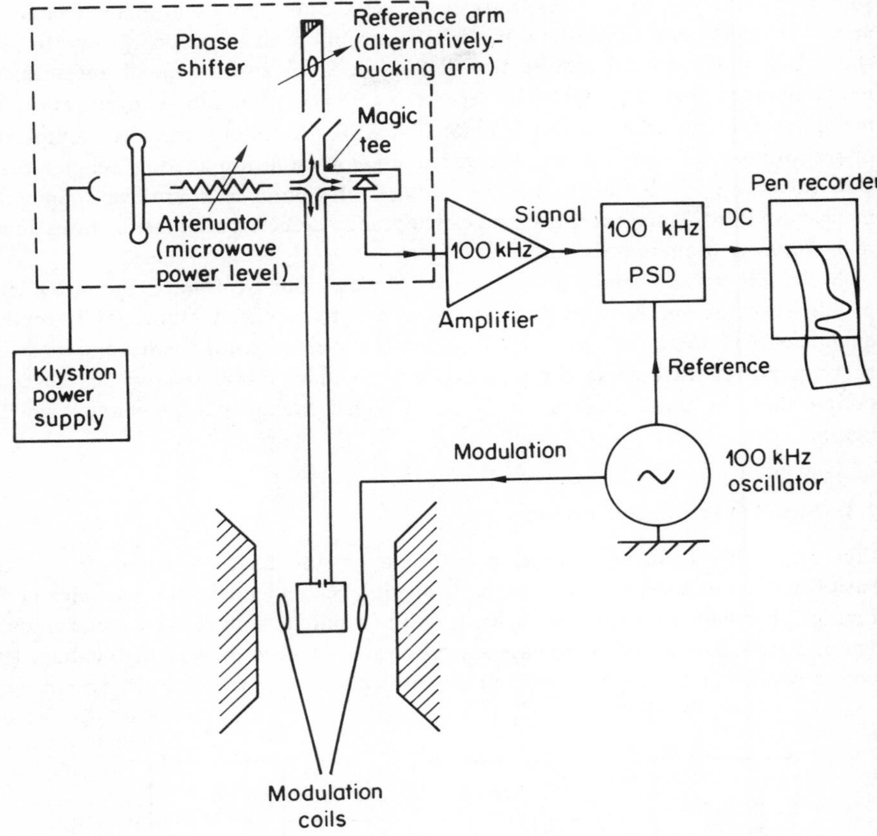

Figure 7.2 Basic layout of a practical ESR spectrometer

manually over larger ranges. The microwave radiation is transmitted via waveguide – copper tube of rectangular cross-section whose dimensions are of the order of the microwave wavelength (i.e. ~3 cm for X-band (9 GHz) spectrometers and ~8 mm for Q-band (35 GHz) spectrometers). The absorption cell is a microwave resonant cavity which serves to concentrate the microwave radiation at,the sample. At its simplest the microwave resonant cavity is a closed-off section of waveguide as indicated in Figure 7.1. The (tunable) length of the cavity is determined by the frequency of the radiation used and has coupling irises to allow the radiation to enter and leave the cavity. The coupling irises are simply small holes in the two cavity end walls as shown in the figure. The detection element is a simple diode, sensitive to microwave frequencies. The rectified current provided by this diode is determined by the intensity of the microwave radiation incident on it.

The ESR spectrometer differs from most other spectrometers in the manner used for scanning the absorption spectrum of the sample. Because of the difficulty of (manually) tuning the frequency source, and also the requirement that the microwave cavity be maintained in tune with this frequency, the magnetic field is scanned instead of the microwave frequency. This is an option which is available only in magnetic resonance spectroscopy.

Practical spectrometers differ from the simple system of Figure 7.1 in two basic ways. Firstly, a much more sensitive detection system is used than simply recording the detected DC current: magnetic field modulation which enables signal amplification and phase-sensitive detection is used. Secondly, a different waveguide geometry is used – a reflection cavity system instead of transmission cavity. This simplifies the insertion of the cavity between the pole pieces of the magnet and makes a much simpler arrangement for sample handling and/or magnetic field rotation. A schematic diagram of a practical spectrometer is given in Figure 7.2, and photographs of the layouts of various commercial 9 GHz (X-band) spectrometers are given in Figure 7.3–7.6. The various components are discussed in more detail below.

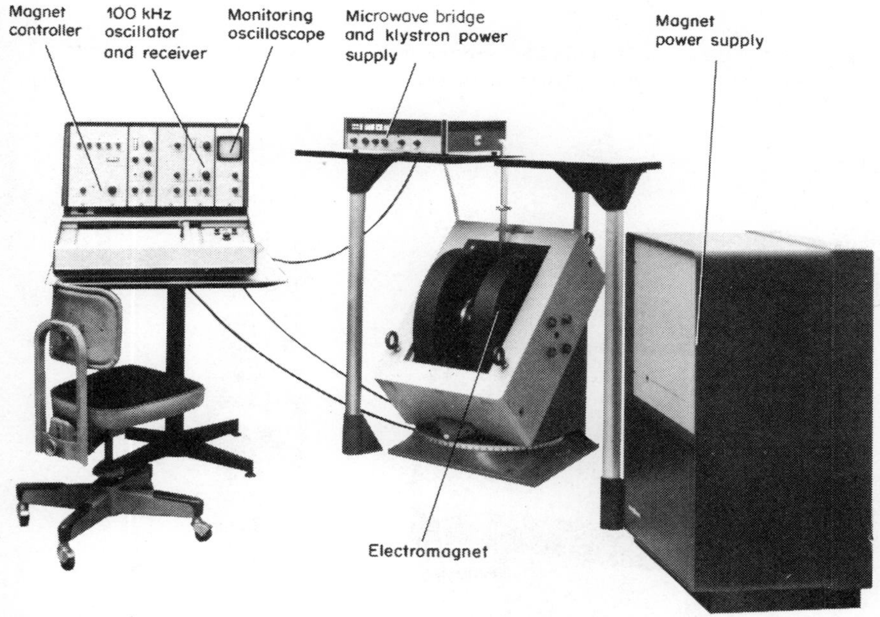

Figure 7.3 Varian E9 ESR spectrometer. This system also has facilities for low-frequency modulation. (Courtesy Varian Associates Ltd)

Magnet

A magnet is required which will produce magnetic fields in the region of 3 kG for 9 GHz spectrometers (X-band) and 13 kG for 35 GHz spectrometers (Q-band), and be able to sweep linearly over large magnetic field regions within this range. The fields produced must be both homogeneous and stable, but these requirements are by no means as stringent as for NMR, since both ESR linewidths and splittings are

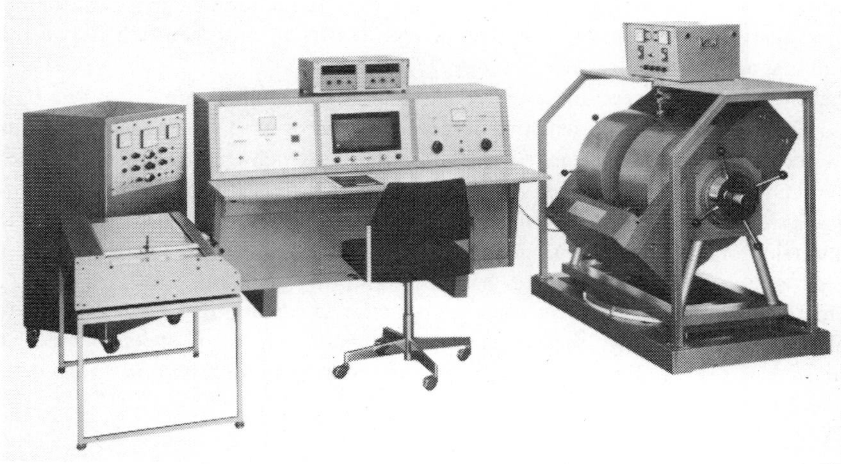

Figure 7.4 Bruker B-ER 418S ESR spectrometer, with proton NMR field measurement and digital microwave frequency measurement. (Courtesy Bruker Spectrospin Ltd)

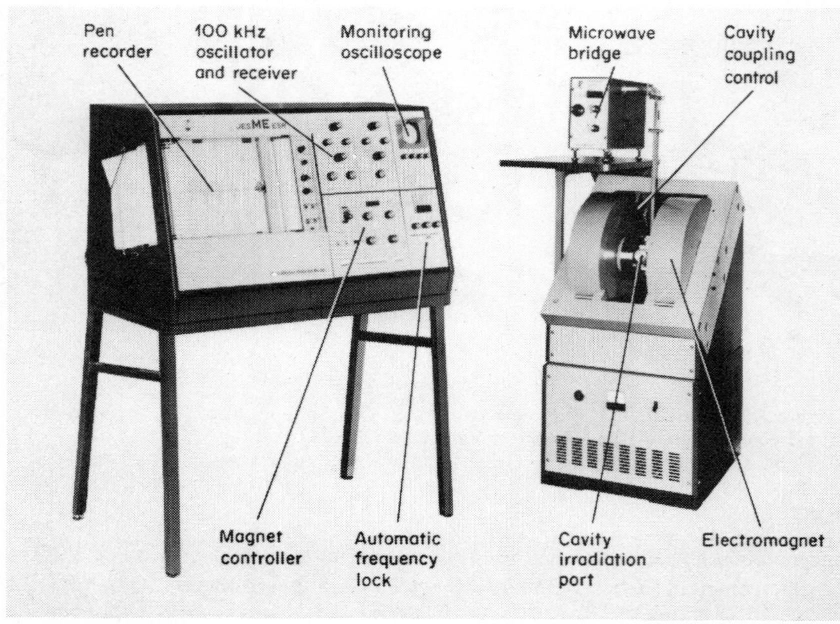

Figure 7.5 J.E.O.L. JES-ME ESR spectrometer. This system also has facilities for 80 Hz modulation. (Courtesy J.E.O.L. Co. Ltd)

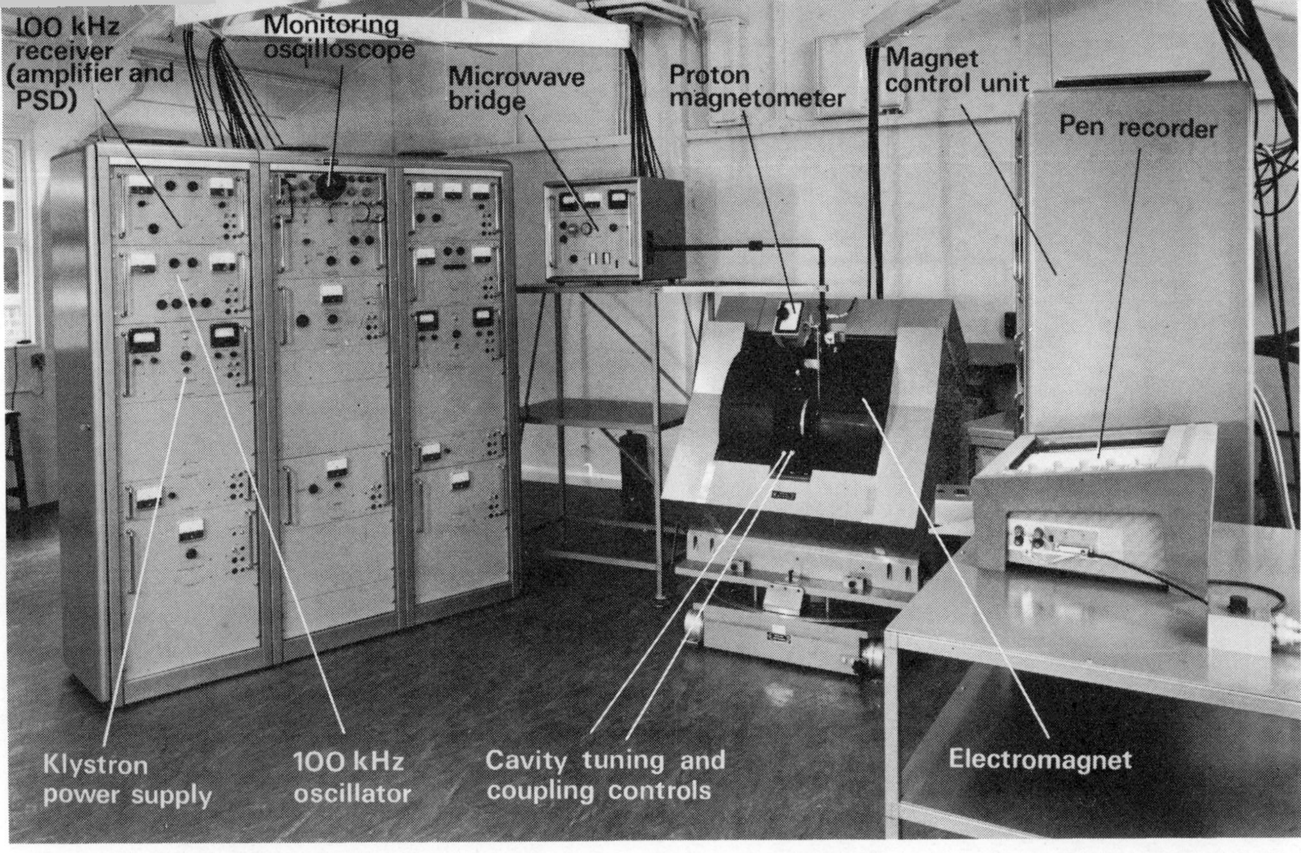

Figure 7.6 Decca X3 ESR spectrometer. The unmarked units are necessary for superheterodyne operation. (Courtesy Decca Radar Ltd)

considerably greater. In practice, water-cooled electromagnets are most often used High-quality electromagnets normally have adequate homogeneity and stability The field stability is often controlled by a Hall-probe magnetometer attached to a pole piece near the centre of the field. Care must be taken to ensure that the microwave cavity (and hence sample) is sitting in the most homogeneous part of the field. This can readily be done by moving the cavity about within the magnetic field to obtain a symmetrical ESR line on the oscilloscope.

Microwave Bridge

The microwave bridge is that part of the spectrometer enclosed by dotted lines in Figure 7.2. It is most usually contained in a separate unit mounted above the magnet. The unit normally contains controls for klystron tuning, klystron attenuation — which controls the amount of microwave power reaching the cavity — and also a switch and phase shifter for the reference (or bucking) arm.

In the system shown in Figure 7.2, the microwave power from the klystron is divided at the magic-tee junction between the reference arm and the arm containing the sample cavity. The power reflected from these arms is then directed, at the magic-tee, to the detector diode. If all the power incident on the resonant cavity were absorbed (critical coupling) and also none were reflected from the reference arm, then no net power would be directed at the detector. Under these conditions the detector is very sensitive to changes in the power absorption in the cavity, such as occur when the magnetic field is swept through the resonance of the sample in the cavity. Unfortunately the microwave diode does not detect very efficiently when the net current flowing through it is zero, and it is the function of the reference arm to leak a fixed amount of power to the diode, thereby enabling it to work at a favourable bias condition.

The magic tee is not the only way of providing this necessary bias current and several spectrometers employ either a microwave circulator or directional couplers in a so-called bucking arm. Whatever the source of the bias power it is essential that it be *in phase* with the power reflected from the cavity so as to avoid interference effects which grossly distort the lineshape. This adjustment is effected by the phase shifter in the reference arm. It is possible to dispense with the reference arm (with some loss in signal strength) by undercoupling the cavity so as to bias the crystal with power reflected from the cavity arm. This is discussed further in the next section.

Microwave Cavity

The requirements of the microwave cavity are basically that it shall be tuned to the klystron frequency, that the sample shall be situated in the region of maximum microwave *magnetic* field (perpendicular to the DC electromagnet field) and that there shall not be materials of strong microwave dielectric absorption in the regions of microwave electric field ('lossy' materials, e.g. water). Resonant cavities may be of rectangular or cylindrical cross-section, the former being more popular in commercial spectrometers. Typical cavities are shown in Figures 7.7 and 7.19.

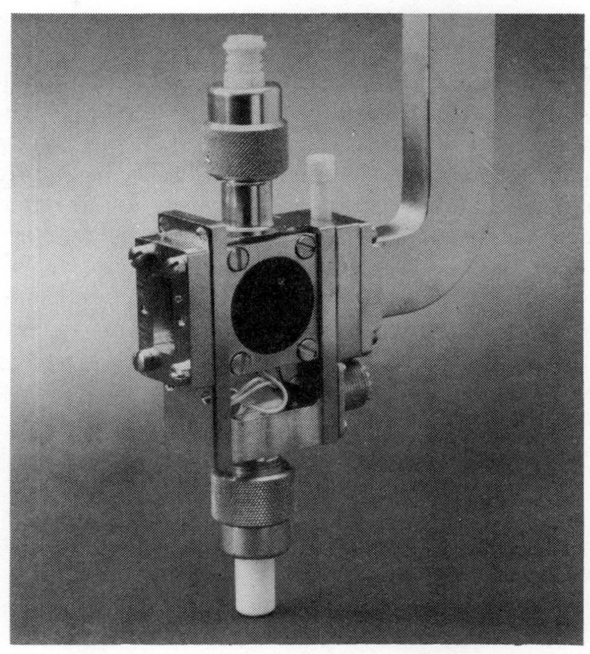

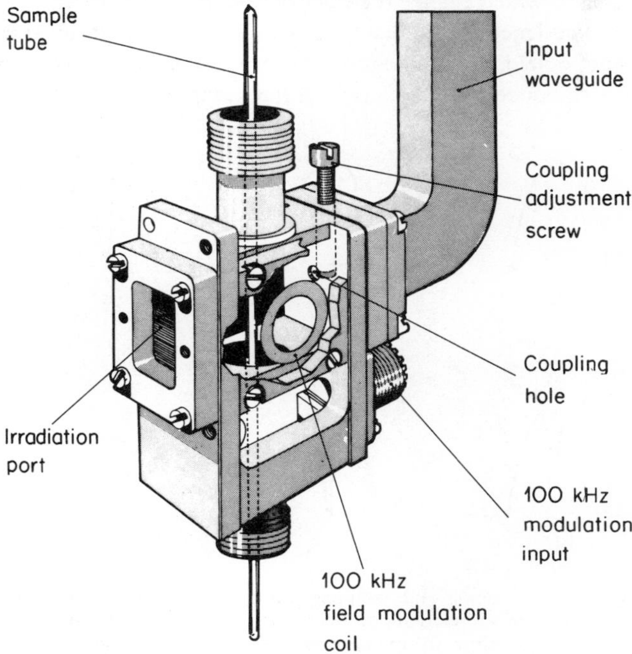

Figure 7.7 Rectangular ESR cavity. (Varian E-231). A detachable rod is keyed into the coupling control, allowing easy adjustment when the cavity is in the magnetic field. (Courtesy Varian Associates Ltd)

The microwave power from the klystron is coupled into the cavity via a hole in the wall and if the incoming microwaves are at the correct frequency, a resonant mode will be set up in the cavity. The resonant mode can be considered as being a kind of electrical and magnetic standing-wave pattern. The condition for a standing-wave pattern is that the length of the cavity shall be a whole number of half-wavelengths, thus the cavity may be tuned to the incoming microwaves by varying its length or the incoming microwaves tuned to the resonant cavity dimensions by tuning the klystron. Tuning is achieved by minimizing the power reflected to the detector diode (leakage current). Klystron tuning is employed in most spectrometers, but if cavity tuning is employed it is also possible to tune the cavity by altering its electrical wavepattern in a different way: by inserting a piece of dielectric into the cavity. (An important point worth remembering is that the sample itself causes an electrical perturbation in the cavity and thus retuning is required for samples of different materials or shapes. More crucially, the microwaves must be attenuated before removing a sample, since this immediately causes the cavity to go off-tune, resulting in a large reflection of power from the cavity which could easily burn out the detector diode.)

Since it is essential that klystron frequency and cavity remain in tune, most spectrometers have a cavity lock (automatic frequency control, AFC) system. This is a buffer system involving a feedback loop which changes the klystron frequency slightly in response to any small variations in the cavity operating conditions (e.g. temperature changes) which change the cavity frequency.

The cavity is designed such that the sample is situated in the maximum microwave magnetic field, giving maximum absorption on resonance. However, care must be taken with aqueous samples (which have extremely high dielectric loss) to

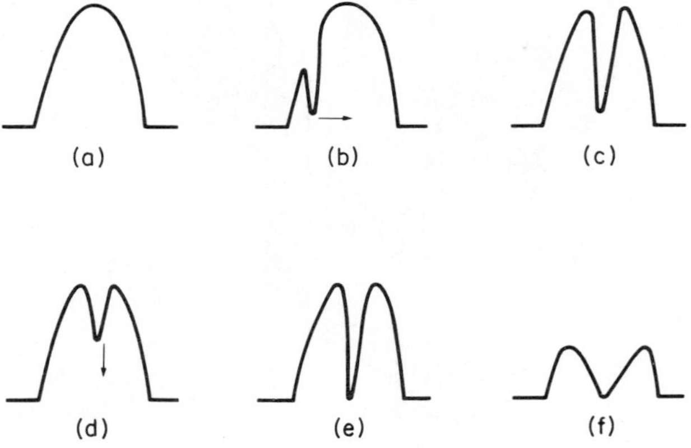

Figure 7.8 Tuning and coupling adjustment as indicated by displaying the klystron mode on the oscilloscope. (a) Klystron completely off-tune, (b) cavity absorption detected, but klystron not correctly tuned, (c) klystron on-tune, (d) cavity undercoupled, (e) cavity correctly coupled ('critically coupled'), (f) cavity overcoupled

ensure that they are kept out of high electric field regions of the cavity. This requirement restricts sample shape and is discussed in the section on sample handling. If such precautions are not taken, it is generally found impossible to tune the cavity with a lossy sample.

The amount of microwave power coupled into the cavity can be adjusted by a movable iris or reflecting stub as is indicated in Figure 7.7. If all the power incident on the cavity is absorbed by it, it is said to be critically coupled. Under these conditions maximum microwave power is reaching the sample. If the cavity is slightly undercoupled, a certain amount of power will be reflected back from the cavity, up the input waveguide. This reflected power will give a bias to the detector diode without the need for any phase shifter adjustment as was discussed above. The sequence of operations for tuning the cavity and adjusting the coupling, by displaying the klystron power output mode on the oscilloscope as a function of frequency, are indicated in Figure 7.8, (see also below in 'Operation' section).

Field Modulation and Phase-Sensitive Detection

The detection sensitivity is increased by modulating the magnetic field at the sample at a frequency of 100 kHz. This is achieved by modulation coils mounted rigidly on the outside cavity walls (see Figure 7.7). The magnetic field modulation system has two main advantages. Firstly, it filters out all noise which is not

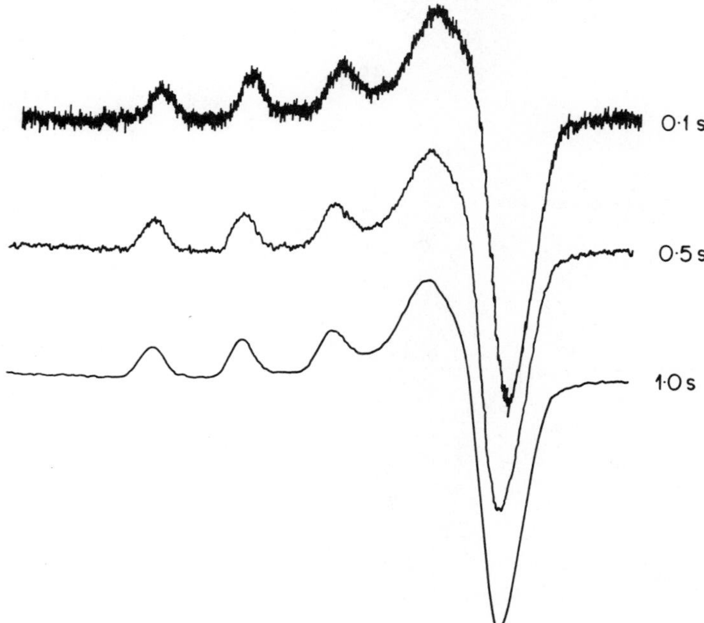

Figure 7.9 ESR spectrum of benzylamine oxidase recorded with various PSD time constants

modulated at 100 kHz, thus increasing the signal-to-noise ratio. Secondly, it produces an AC signal which is easier to amplify than a DC signal, thus giving improvement in signal strength.

The detector used to filter out all signals other than that modulated at 100 kHz is a phase-sensitive detector, PSD, (also called a lock-in amplifier or detector) which produces a DC output signal. The PSD operates by comparing the input signal with a 100 kHz reference signal derived from the oscillator which produces the original field modulation (see Figure 7.2).This reference channel of the 100 kHz oscillator is usually provided with a 'phase adjust' to bring the reference signal in

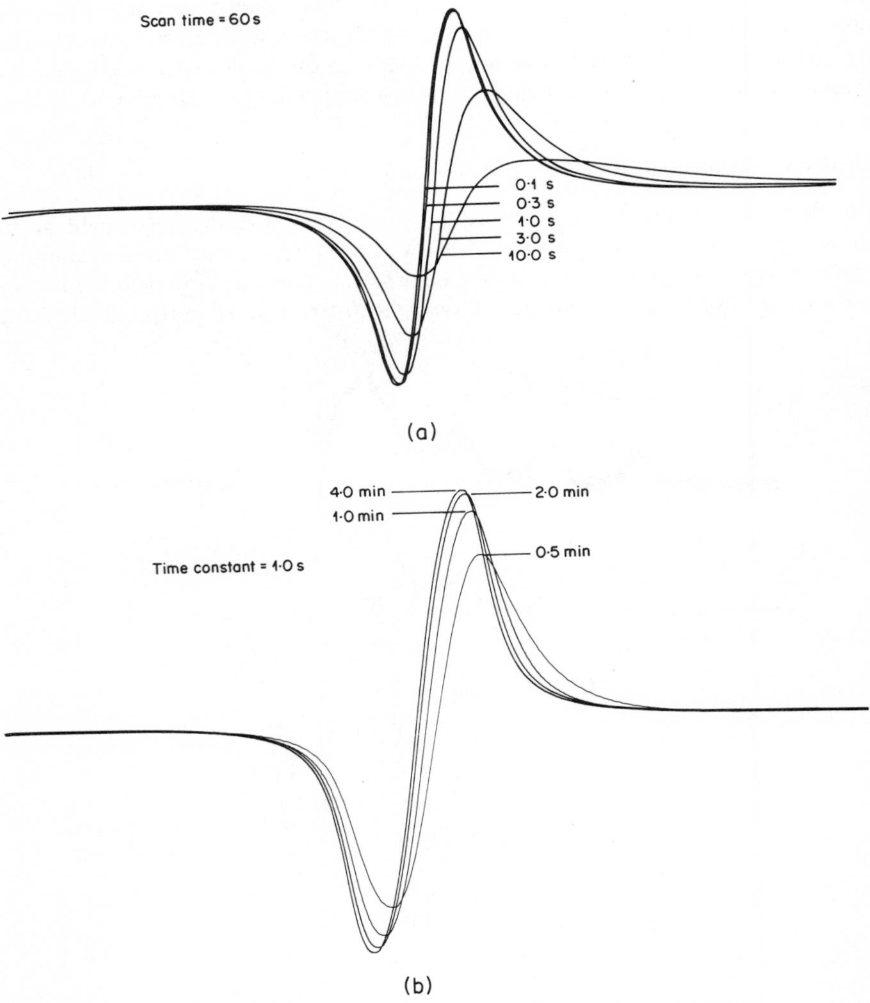

Figure 7.10 Effect of varying: (a) Time constant for fixed scan time. (b) Scan time for fixed time constant (Courtesy Varian Associates Ltd)

phase with that of the incoming signal. This can be done by simply maximizing the height of an ESR line observed on the monitoring oscilloscope. Like most filters, the PSD has a time constant (or response time) control, which can be used to filter out fast-varying noise. The time constant is a measure of the time taken by the PSD to respond to a change in signal level and thus can average out fast-varying noise. The potential increase in signal-to-noise is often very important in biological ESR, where frequently only small quantities of sample are available, e.g. highly purified enzymes. A typical use of long time constants to improve signal-to-noise is illustrated in Figure 7.9 using the copper-containing enzyme benzylamine oxidase. Care must be taken with the time constant setting, however, because if one sweeps too quickly through an ESR line, the limiting response of the time constant will cause distortions of the lineshape. This is illustrated in Figure 7.10 in which the time constant is varied for a fixed rate of scanning the magnetic field and also the magnetic field scanning rate is varied for a fixed PSD time constant. Clearly the two effects are complementary; to get an undistorted lineshape the time constant must

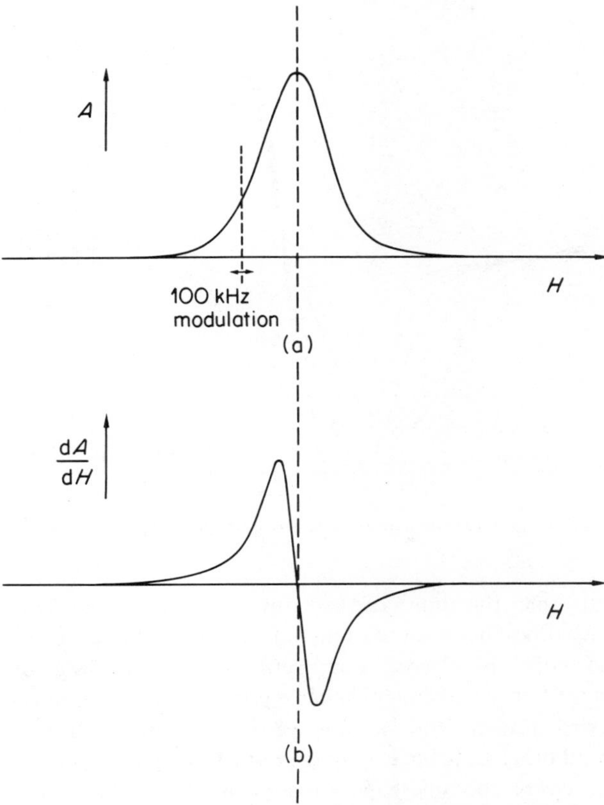

Figure 7.11 (a) Absorption lineshape indicating small field modulation. (b) First-derivative lineshape as produced by field modulation

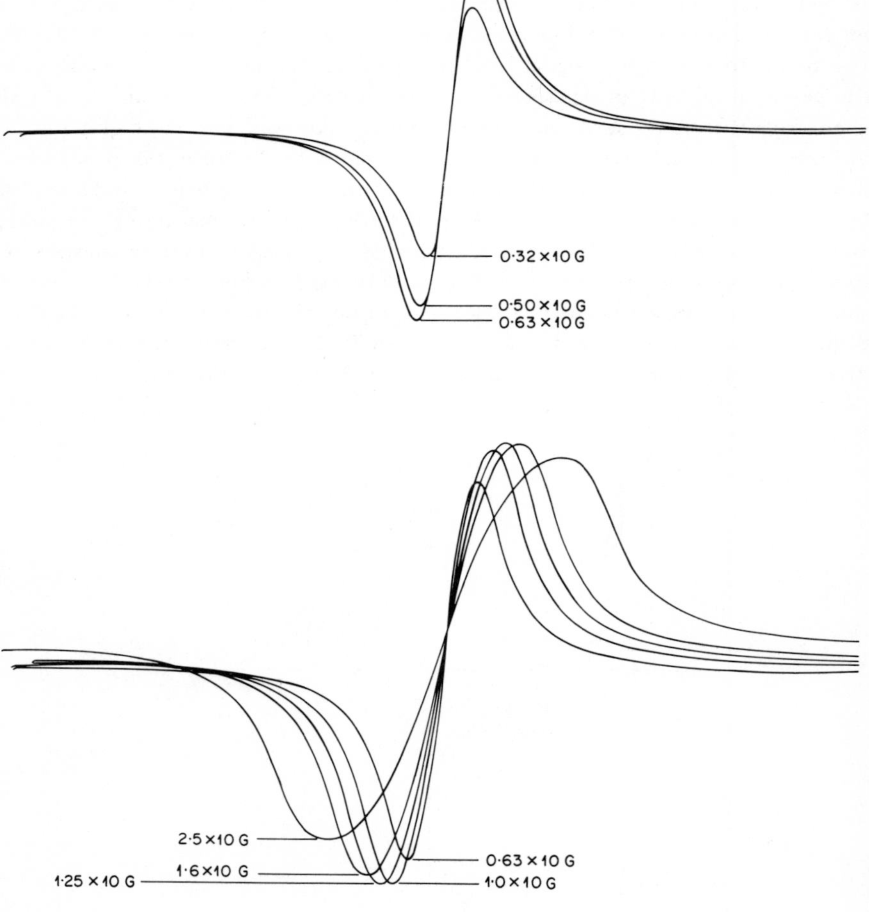

Figure 7.12 Effect of increasing modulation amplitude. (Courtesy Varian Associates Ltd)

be much shorter than the time taken to scan through the line. The settings chosen are thus a compromise between the time taken to scan the spectrum and the extent to which the noise is filtered out. Settings are optimized by varying time constants/scan time until no further change is produced in the lineshape.

An interesting feature will be noticed in the lineshapes of Figure 7.10; in common with all other ESR lines, they are not the simple absorption lineshape, but the first derivative of this lineshape – see Figure 7.11. This is a characteristic of phase sensitive detection: modulation of the magnetic field produces first-derivative detection. For the detection to be linear the magnetic field should be modulated through only a small part of the lineshape as it is swept through the ESR line. That is, the 100 kHz modulation amplitude must be small compared with the linewidth. If this is not so, distortion of the lineshape, 'modulation broadening', takes place as indicated in Figure 7.12. The modulation amplitude setting is thus optimized by decreasing until no further change is produced in lineshape. It is important to use the highest modulation amplitude consistent with no distortion since the signal strength increases with increasing modulation power as shown in the upper diagram of Figure 7.12.

Recording

The DC output from the PSD is normally fed to a pen recorder which traces out the spectrum as the magnetic field is swept. An x–y recorder is used and the x-deflection is driven directly from the magnetic field sweep unit, or frequently the field sweep is driven by the x-deflection of the recorder.

All spectrometers also have facilities for displaying ESR lines on an oscilloscope. This is extremely useful during setting-up procedures as indicated above. The oscilloscope display is achieved by sweep modulating the magnetic field through the ESR line at a low frequency, usually 50 Hz (mains frequency), by means of coils mounted either on the magnet pole faces or on the sides of the cavity and sweeping the oscilloscope x-deflection with this frequency also. A less common means of oscilloscope display is to sweep modulate the klystron reflector voltage. This is a considerably less sensitive detection mode than the steady field sweep with pen recording, but is useful for setting up a sample run, also the amplitude of the 50 Hz sweep is rather limited. Thus good detection is only obtained with strong signals and narrow lines. For this reason a strong standard sample with narrow lines such as DPPH (diphenyl picryl hydrazyl, a stable free radical) is sometimes used in tuning up a spectrometer. A speck of DPPH should be sufficient to produce a strong spectrum.

7.4 Operation – how to get a spectrum

To summarize the discussion of spectrometer function the sequence of operations necessary to obtain a spectrum is described below. The operational instructions have purposely been kept general.

A. *Cavity Tuning*

(1) Insert the sample rigidly in the cavity. In the case of a flat cell ensure that this has the correct (transverse) orientation in the cavity.

(2) Before switching on all units, ensure that the microwave power is set at zero (Klystron attenuator at infinity). (Klystron supply voltages are assumed to be set – these are not usually changed.)

(3) After the initial warm-up period increase the microwave power until the crystal detector current (leakage current) meter shows that the detector is receiving microwave power. This means the klystron is working and you are now in a position to tune the klystron to the cavity resonance.

(4) The microwave tuning is performed by the klystron tuning control (or less frequently by the cavity tuning rod). The cavity resonance is detected by modulating the klystron reflector voltage and displaying the klystron power output mode on the oscilloscope, or less easily by simply observing the detector crystal current

(a) For oscilloscope: switch on the mode sweep (reflector modulation), adjust the klystron/cavity tuner until the cavity absorption dip appears superimposed on the klystron mode. (This may require a systematic search.) Use the coupling adjustment to maximize the cavity dip and the tuning to position the dip in the middle of the oscilloscope sweep. The cavity is now on tune (see Figure 7.8).

or

(b) For detector meter (leakage-current meter): search through the tuning range to find the dip in the detector current level. Having found the dip, minimize the detector current by alternate adjustment of first the tuning and then the coupling. When the detector current is reduced to zero (at the bottom of the dip), the cavity is on tune.

B. *Cavity Lock, Power Level and Detector Biasing*

(1) Now switch from mode sweep to cavity lock/AFC ('operate') (AFC modulation level, gain and response are assumed set – these are not usually changed). If possible, check that the AFC is working by slightly changing the klystron reflector voltage and verifying that the AFC meter follows this change.

(2) The microwave power can now be turned up to the desired level. This will probably require some readjustment of the cavity coupling, depending on the detector biasing, to keep the detector current zero as in part A. (4) (b) above. (Do not alter the klystron frequency tuning at this stage.)

(3) There are two possible methods of detector biasing:

(a) With the reference arm (phase tuning): switch in the reference power, adjust the phase tuning to give maximum detector current. If the reference arm has a variable amplitude level, use this to set the detector current to the manufacturer's recommended level, in conjunction with maximizing the phase.

or

(b) Simply undercoupling the cavity: off-set the coupling adjustment from critical coupling (zero detector current) until the necessary bias level is indicated on the detector meter. (This reflected power is sometimes achieved by means of a slotted line in the cavity arm – such a system also requires phase adjustment similar to (a).)

Note that in some cases, depending in the sample, it may be found impossible to critically couple the cavity. It will then be found that as the microwave power is increased, the detector current will quickly rise above the recommended value and be in danger of burning out the detector diode. Thus one is restricted to low power operation, or in the case of reference arms with variable amplitude levels it is possible to off-set this high detector current. This is done by tuning the phase to a *minimum* detector current rather than a maximum, and using the amplitude level to set the detector current to the required level at the desired microwave power.

C. *Search for Spectrum*

(1) The magnet (and possibly the klystron) requires cooling water, these should have been switched on and allowed to stabilize for some time. N.B. do not switch the magnet on or off in steps of greater than 1kG.

(2) Switch to oscilloscope display.

(3) Manually scan the magnetic field using the field control unit, or the deflection of the recorder, while watching the oscilloscope for a line to appear. Normal ($g = 2$) lines will appear at around 3 kG for X-band spectrometers and at around 13 kG for Q-band spectrometers.

D. *Optimizing Detection*

(1) Choose a strong, narrow line on which to tune up and optimize signal strength.

(2) Adjust the reference phase of the 100 kHz oscillator until the signal viewed on the oscilloscope is maximized.

(3) Adjust the 100 kHz oscillator power to maximize the signal *without* broadening.

(4) Adjust the microwave power to give maximum signal before the onset of saturation.

(5) The oscilloscope modulation sweep can now be switched off and the pen recorder used.

E. *Recording a Spectrum*

(1) Record a spectrum on the pen recorder by automatically sweeping the magnetic field over the region of spectral interest. The magnetic field sweep and 100 kHz receiver gain setting required to keep the spectrum on scale are best found by trial and error.

(2) Choose the optimum PSD time constant (response time) for a given scan time by repeatedly running pen-recorder charts with decreasing time constant until no further decrease in lineshape distortion is detected.

(3) A spectrum can now be recorded under optimum conditions.

If the sample has a strong spectrum the optimization and time constant adjustments are unnecessary and one need only check that settings are not so high as to cause lineshape distortions. For a series of similar samples these settings can safely be left unchanged, and for similar sample configurations and sizes the tuning is unlikely to change very much either.

Some spectrometers (e.g. the Varian E-line systems) have multifunctional switches which simplify operation by performing several of the above steps simultaneously.

7.5 Measurement

The most important measurable features of an ESR spectrum are the point about which the spectrum is centred, indicated by the *g*-value, and the splittings in the spectrum, most usually hyperfine splittings determined by the *A*-value. The *g*-value is related to the field, H, about which the spectrum is centred by

$$h\nu = g\beta H \tag{7.1}$$

A measurement of *g* thus requires measurement of both *H* and the microwave frequency, v. A useful relation obtained from the numerical constants *h* and β is

★ $$g = \frac{h}{\beta} \cdot \frac{\nu}{H} = 0.71444 \times \frac{\nu(\text{GHz})}{H(\text{kG})} \tag{7.2}$$

The microwave frequency is normally measured by means of a cavity wavemeter, a resonant cavity which is tuned to the microwave frequency by a micrometer screw. The resonance position is detected by a sharp dip in the leakage current to a diode detector.

The magnetic field values can often be obtained directly from the field control unit. These can be quite accurate for field sweeps or differences (such as are required in measuring hyperfine constants) but less so for absolute values of field positions as required for *g*-value measurements. In this case a standard of well-known *g*-value and narrow linewidth may be used as a *g*-marker to calibrate absolute field position. DPPH (diphenyl picryl hydrazyl) is a convenient *g*-marker, its *g-value is*

$$g(\text{DPPH}) = 2.0036 \tag{7.3}$$

and the field at which it occurs is

$$H_{\text{DPPH}}(\text{kG}) = 0.35658 \times \nu(\text{GHz}) \tag{7.4}$$

To less accuracy, *g*-values may be measured without measuring the microwave frequency and with an approximate value of the absolute field, if a standard of similar *g*-value, g_0, is used. The unknown *g*-value is then given approximately by

★ $$g \cong g_0 \left(1 + \frac{\Delta H}{H_0}\right) \tag{7.5}$$

where H_0 is the field position of the standard and $\Delta H = H_0 - H$ is the difference in field position between standard and unknown, respectively. Since ΔH is much smaller than H_0, the latter need not be determined very accurately, and all measurements can be made from the field controller.

Accurate absolute values of magnetic field can be measured using a proton magnetometer (see Figure 7.6) which is tuned to give the nuclear magnetic resonance frequency of protons in the magnetic field. The magnetic field is then related to the proton NMR frequency by

★ $$H(\text{kG}) = 0.23487 \times \nu_{\hat{p}}(\text{MHz}) \tag{7.6}$$

To measure hyperfine constants it is only necessary to measure field splittings since they are frequently quoted in gauss. However, the rather more exact energy units are sometimes used. The appropriate relationship is

$$A\ (\text{energy}) = A(\text{G}) \times g\beta \tag{7.7}$$

Hence values in energy units depend on the g-value. In the common energy units

$$\beta = 1.39969\ \text{MHz/G} = 0.46686 \times 10^{-4}\ \text{cm}^{-1}/\text{G} \tag{7.8}$$

Taking $g = 2.0036$, one gets for these energy units

Frequency units:

$$A(\text{MHz}) = 2.80442 \times A(\text{G}) \tag{7.9}$$

Wavenumbers:

$$A(\text{cm}^{-1}) = 0.93540 \times 10^{-4} \times A(\text{G}) \tag{7.10}$$

A simple example. The experimental spectrum of an aqueous solution of the spin label TEMPO is given in Figure 7.13 with proton resonance markers at 0.02 MHz intervals calibrating the sweep. The wavemeter micrometer reading was

0.2740 ins $\equiv$ 9.276 GHz (deduced from wavemeter calibration)

The central line of the spectrum specifies the TEMPO g-value. Interpolation between proton resonance markers shows it to occur at

$$14.040 + 0.02\left(\frac{5.0}{5.8}\right) = 14.0572\ \text{MHz}$$

$$\equiv 0.23487 \times 14.0572 = 3.3016\ \text{kG}.$$

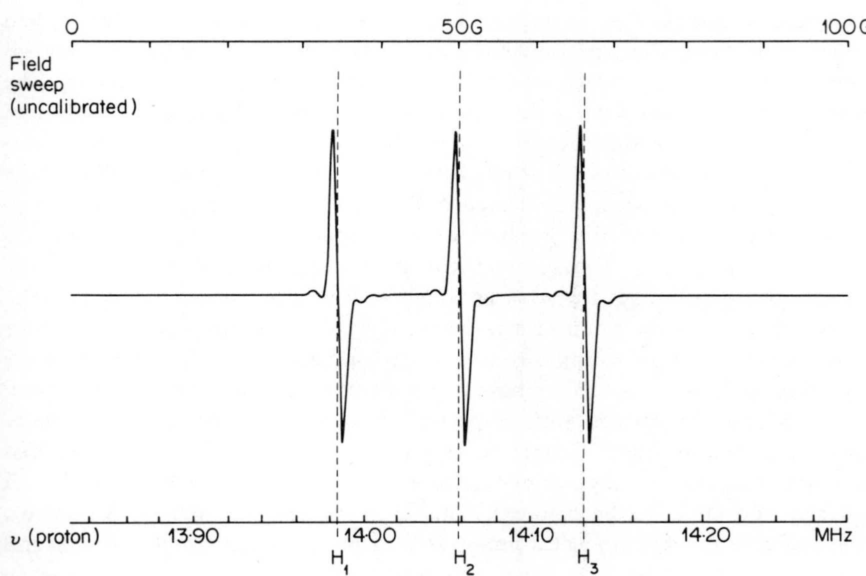

Figure 7.13 Experimentally recorded spectrum of TEMPO spin label with manual proton resonance field calibration

Hence

$$g = 0.71444 \times \frac{9.276}{3.3016} = 2.007$$

The positions of the two outer lines (given by interpolation) are

$$H_1 = 0.23487 \left[13.980 + 0.02 \left(\frac{1.2}{5.8} \right) \right] = 3.2845 \text{ kG}$$

and

$$H_3 = 0.23487 \left[14.120 + 0.02 \left(\frac{3.5}{5.8} \right) \right] = 3.3192 \text{ kG}$$

giving hyperfine separations of

$$A = 17.1 \text{ G}$$

or

$$A = 17.6 \text{ G}$$

which is to be compared with the value of 17 G deduced directly from the field sweep scale (from the electromagnet controller) given in Figure 7.13. Expressed in energy units, the hyperfine splitting is

$$A = 17.4 \times 2.007 \times 1.3997 = 48.9 \text{ MHz}$$

or

$$A = 17.4 \times 2.007 \times 0.46686 \times 10^{-4} = 16.3 \times 10^{-4} \text{ cm}^{-1}$$

It is very simple to determine the centres of lines which have symmetrical lineshapes such as those from single crystals or molecules rotating rapidly in solution as in the example. The centre is just the point of maximum slope at which the line crosses the baseline as indicated in Figure 7.11. However, for the so-called powder or polycrystalline spectra which arise from such systems as frozen solutions of metalloproteins, particularly enzymes, the situation is much less clearcut. The powder spectrum arises from a random distribution of rigidly oriented molecules and thus consists of a superposition of absorption lines corresponding to orientation in all possible directions. The observed spectrum is the first differential of the resulting absorption envelope, indicated in Figure 7.14. This illustrates the ambiguity involved in determining g-values from powder spectra. For derivative-like pseudo-lines which cross the baseline, the g-value can be determined from the baseline crossing point, but for other pseudo-lines it is not clear whether to take the peak of the curve or the point of maximum slope following the peak. In such cases it is necessary either to adopt a consistent empirical rule which can be used for comparison purposes, or to computer simulate the entire powder spectrum. Powder spectra for species with hyperfine structure are generally even more complicated, but relatively simple spectra often arise from systems with axial symmetry, because the hyperfine splitting in the perpendicular direction is frequently too small to be resolved. This is illustrated in Figure 7.15 for two systems of considerable biological importance: a paramagnetic metallo-protein and a nitroxide lipid spin label. In these cases g-values and hyperfine splittings can be measured from clearly defined features in the spectra as indicated in the figure, and as explained previously in Chapter 6.

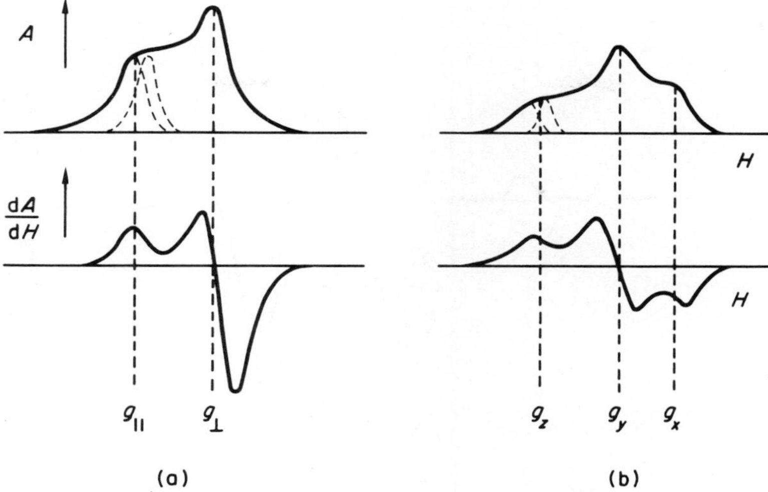

Figure 7.14 Absorption envelopes and first-derivative spectra for polycrystalline powder samples of the type found with non-haem iron proteins. (a) Spectrum with axial symmetry (e.g. reduced adrenodoxin), (b) spectrum with rhombic symmetry (e.g. reduced spinach ferredoxin). The individual component lines of the absorption envelope are indicated by the dotted lines

The total area under the ESR absorption curve is proportional to the amount of paramagnetic species in the sample and can thus be used as a quantitative assay. A calibration standard is required: Cu EDTA (1mM Cu in 10mM EDTA) may be used for paramagnetic ions and DPPH in organic solvent (whose concentration can be determined from its molar absorption: A_m [525 nm] = 11.9×10^3) for free radicals. (DPPH in organic solvent gives a typical free radical spectrum, unlike the extremely narrow single line used in spectrometer tuning obtained from solid DPPH). Such estimations are normally not very accurate because of differences in tuning and instrumental settings and also differences in line shapes between sample and standard. Variations in instrumental settings can be to some extent offset by normalization using an encapsulated small speck of DPPH in both sample and standard runs.

7.6 Sample Handling

Aqueous Samples

Since the samples normally encountered in biochemical applications are aqueous, we consider these first. Unfortunately, water is extremely lossy at microwave frequencies and this causes trouble in tuning the cavity, making it impossible to tune in bad cases. The large dielectric absorption must be cut down by reducing the amount of sample in the microwave electric field of the cavity. This inevitably

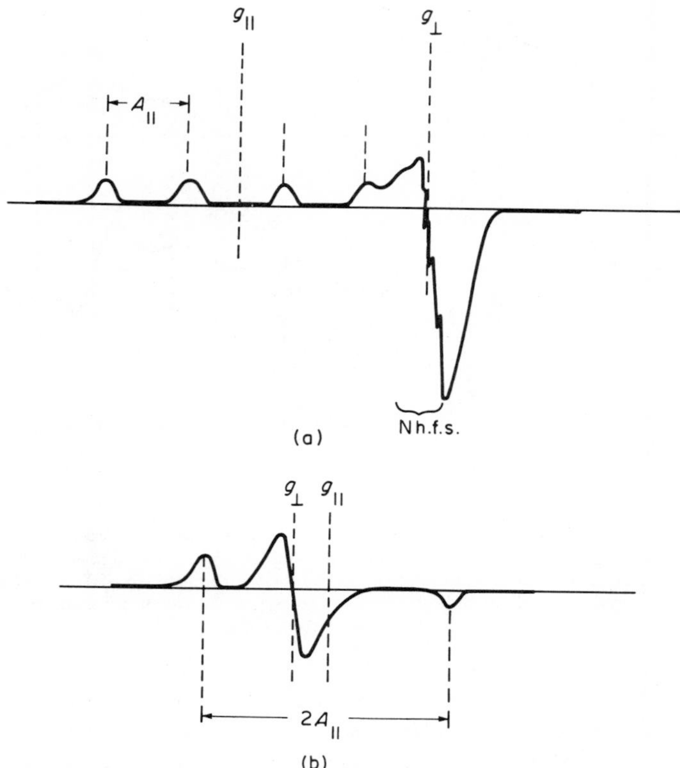

Figure 7.15 Polycrystalline powder spectra of frozen solutions, indicating the method of measuring the parameters. (a) A typical copper protein (e.g. copper conalbumin). (b) A spin label

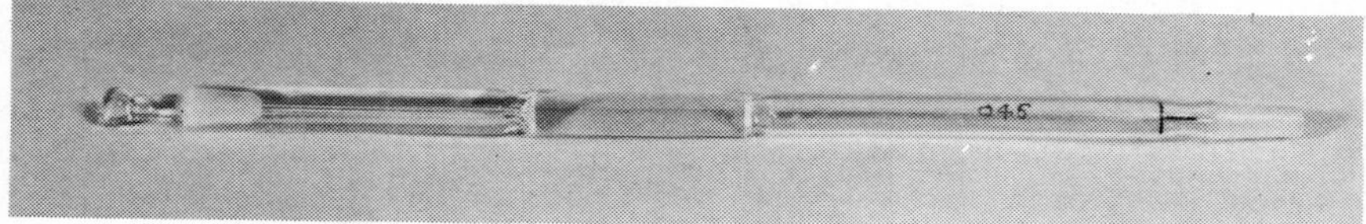

Figure 7.16 Flat, quartz, aqueous sample cell

means a reduction in the quantity of sample which can be used, but the optimum filling factor is achieved by using a flat cell as shown in Figure 7.16. The plane of the cell is placed transverse to the length of the cavity so as to locate the whole of the sample in a region of minimum electric field and maximum magnetic field, thus minimizing dielectric absorption and maximizing magnetic absorption. A simpler solution, if signal strength is not critical, is to cut down the quantity of sample by using a thin-walled glass capillary tube which can be placed concentrically inside a conventional sample tube. Such tubes are easily made from sealed-off dropping pipettes.

If only a limited quantity of material is available it is helpful if the flat cell is designed such that the dead volume of the cell is kept to a minimum. This can be conveniently done if the lower limb of the cell, below the flat region, has a capillary bore and is terminated in a small, male ground joint. In this way the cell can be used like a pipette and it is possible to perform a complete titration with a sample volume of 0.2 ml. When performing titrations it is also useful to attach a small syringe to the lower limb of the cell. Small quantities of a concentrated solution of the added reagent can then be introduced at the top of the cell and mixing performed by drawing the sample into the syringe and forcing it back and forth into the cell. Using this method small quantities of material (of the order of 0.4 ml) may be titrated without disturbing the position of the cell in the cavity, thus avoiding resetting errors by ensuring that all samples are run under identical conditions.

Sample size is quite important since signal strength cannot be improved indefinitely by increasing sample concentration. At high concentrations one begins to see the effects of magnetic interaction between the paramagnetic centres. This 'interaction broadening' is illustrated in Figure 7.17 for the small spin label,

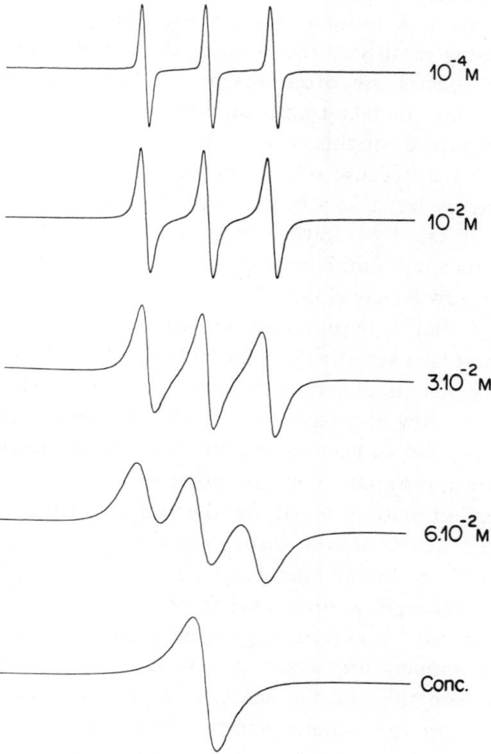

Figure 7.17 Interaction broadening of nitroxide spin label spectrum as a result of increasing concentration

TEMPO, in aqueous solution. Clearly at high concentrations all the structure of the spectrum is swamped by a single broad line. To eliminate interaction broadening in small molecules it is necessary to use concentrations $\leqslant 10^{-3}$ M. Macromolecules, e.g. proteins, are by their very nature magnetically dilute since they contain a very large number of diamagnetic atoms in proportion to their paramagnetic centre. However, there are handling problems with macromolecules at high concentration because of viscosity effects, denaturation, aggregation, etc. Another source of interaction broadening can come from atmospheric molecular oxygen which is paramagnetic. An improvement in resolution of narrow lines in solution spectra can often be obtained on de-oxygenating the sample either by freeze–thaw or bubbling nitrogen through the solution.

Temperature Variation

Variable temperature facilities are necessary for determining activation energies and associated thermodynamic parameters. However, perhaps the practically most significant application is the use of low temperatures in the studies of metalloproteins. Low temperatures provide three basic sources of increased sensitivity. Firstly, freezing aqueous solutions removes the dielectric losses associated with liquid water, increasing sensitivity and allowing the use of larger samples. Secondly, transition-metal-ion spectra are often sharper at lower temperatures because of longer relaxation times. (In fact transition-metal-ion spectra are often not observable at room temperature for this very reason.) Finally, a lower temperature gives increased signal strength because of the increased population difference between upper and lower energy levels as a result of the Boltzman distribution. Freezing a solution of a small, rapidly rotating molecule (e.g. lipid spin label) produces dramatic effects in its spectrum, changing it from sharp, motionally narrowed lines to a polycrystalline powder envelope. For a macromolecular solution the effective viscosity is so high that a pseudo-powder spectrum is obtained even at room temperature and increased sensitivity is the only spectral change on going to lower temperatures. This is not, however, necessarily the case for spin labels attached to macromolecules, since they may have,considerable motional freedom relative to the macromolecule, giving rise to narrow lines at room temperature. Low-temperature operation is thus only appropriate to metalloproteins.

The most convenient method of varying the sample temperature is by containing it in an open-ended quartz dewar through which chilled/heated nitrogen gas is passed – see Figure 7.18. For temperatures below room temperature the nitrogen gas is first passed through a heat exchanger immersed in liquid nitrogen (or alternatively is produced by evaporating liquid nitrogen) before passing over the heater. There is a temperature sensor at the inlet to the sample dewar and a feedback loop between this and the heater maintains a steady temperature at the sample. Such a system can achieve sample temperatures in the range -180°C to $+300^\circ$C. If a single low temperature is required, a dewar containing liquid nitrogen can be inserted in the cavity. Although this is capable of a slightly lower temperature than the gas-flow system, it is more troublesome because boiling of the

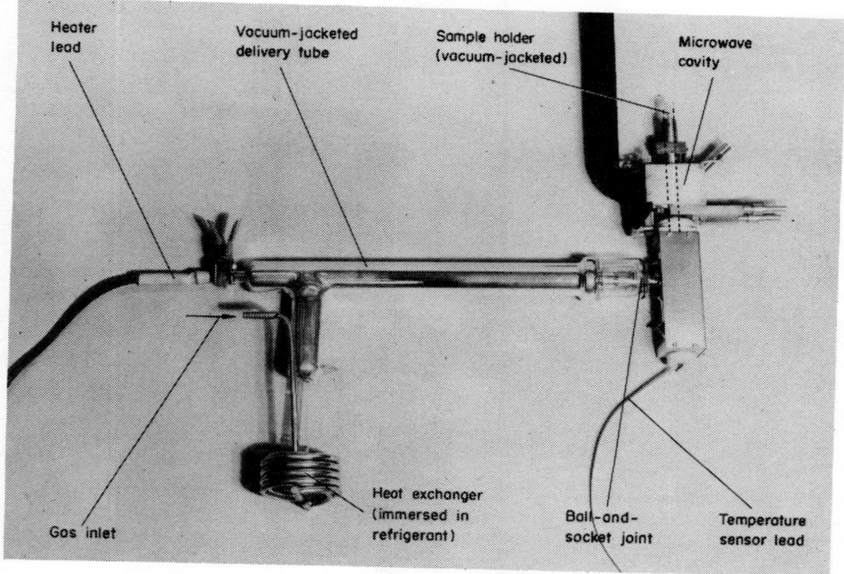

Figure 7.18 Nitrogen gas-flow variable temperature system. The cavity assembly fits within the magnet pole pieces

liquid nitrogen in the cavity causes considerable noise and frequently overpowers the cavity lock (automatic frequency control) system.

Non-Aqueous Solutions and Dry Powders

Solutions in non-lossy solvent (not water!) can be contained simply in cylindrical quartz tubes as indicated in Figure 7.7. The quartz used for the sample tube must be of a quality which is free from paramagnetic impurities. Various tube diameters may be used with the appropriate size of retaining collars, depending on the quantity of sample available.

Standard sample tubes can also be used for powdered solids provided they are magnetically dilute and contain no water, e.g. lyophilized tissue.

Single Crystals

As indicated in the previous chapter, the maximum amount of information can be obtained, at high resolution, from single-crystal ESR spectra. Unfortunately, for biological samples this method is limited by the small number of molecules which can be obtained as single crystals of sufficient size. For those single crystals which are available it is necessary to be able to perform angular variations of the magnetic field direction with respect to given axes of the crystal. This is easily accomplished by means of a goniometer sample mount such as the one illustrated in Figure 7.19. The crystal is rigidly mounted on a quartz rod which can be rotated about a vertical

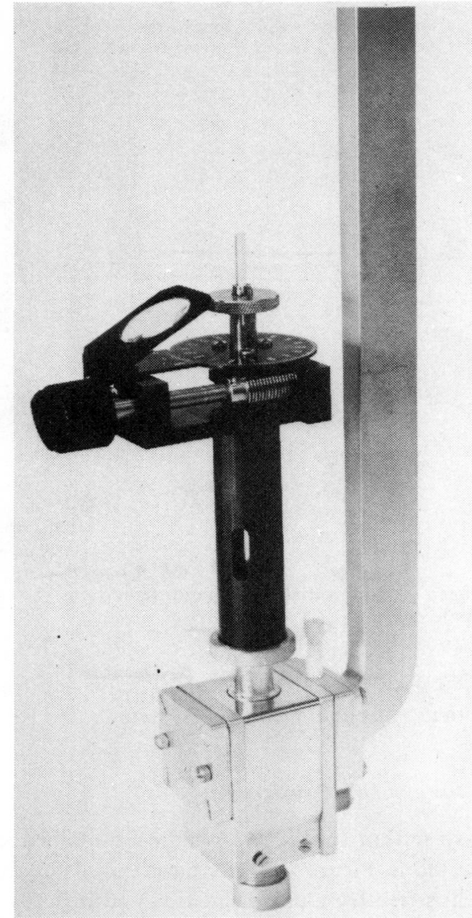

Figure 7.19 Rectangular cavity with goniometer sample mount for single-crystal rotation studies. (Courtesy Varian Associates Ltd)

axis. An alternative method is to have the sample statically mounted in the cavity and to rotate the magnet. However, for several common cavity configurations (such as those indicated in Figures 7.7 and 7.19) it is impossible to rotate the magnet.

Biological Tissues

Biological tissues, as opposed to biological molecules, may be studied *in vitro* by ESR as long as their geometry is restricted to limit the amount of water introduced into the microwave electric field. A simple biological tissue cell, similar to the flat

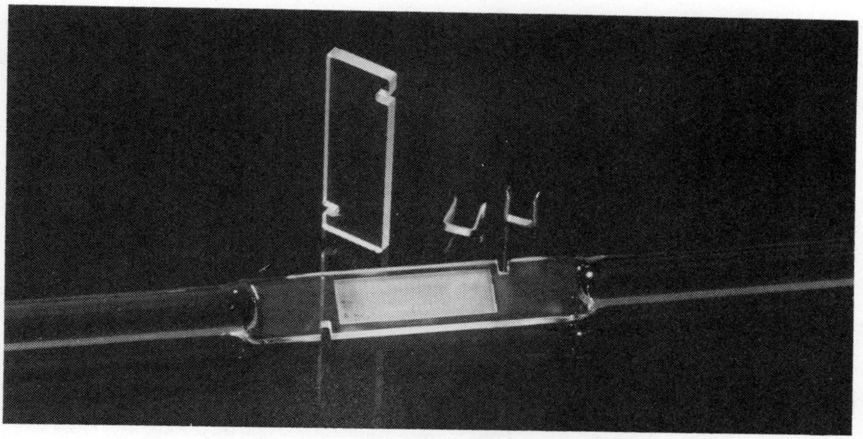

Figure 7.20 Biological tissue cell. (Courtesy Varian Associates Ltd)

aqueous sample cell, is illustrated in Figure 7.20. Such a cell is particularly useful for studying oriented tissues and permits the introduction of a small quantity of aqueous bathing phase. More complicated cells have been constructed, e.g. for exciting nerve tissue whilst in the cavity, and blood cells have been partially oriented by flowing them through a flat aqueous sample cell.

7.7 Other Special Techniques for Biological Work

Irradiation

There has been considerable interest in radiation biology during the past twenty-five years; since irradiation of biological material often leads to the production of radicals, facilities are needed for simultaneously irradiating and observing the ESR spectrum of a sample. The sample can be either a single crystal (often mounted on a goniometer rod) a tissue homogenate contained in a thin cell or a frozen solution. Irradiation is effected through a window in the cavity (Figure 7.7).

A sample holder capable of irradiating solid particulate samples (actually used for bacterial spores) at high dose rates outside the cavity is shown in Figure 7.21. The material is irradiated in the exposure chamber A which has a beryllium window and is immersed in liquid nitrogen. During irradiation the quartz tip B of the ESR tube is protected from stray X-rays by wrapping it in lead. After irradiation the quartz tip is precooled with liquid nitrogen and the sample then dumped quickly into the tip from the large exposure chamber. The sample can now be stored in the quartz tip immersed in liquid nitrogen and transferred to the ESR cavity at liquid nitrogen temperature. This procedure, by constantly maintaining the sample at liquid nitrogen temperature, freezes in the irradiation-induced free radicals.

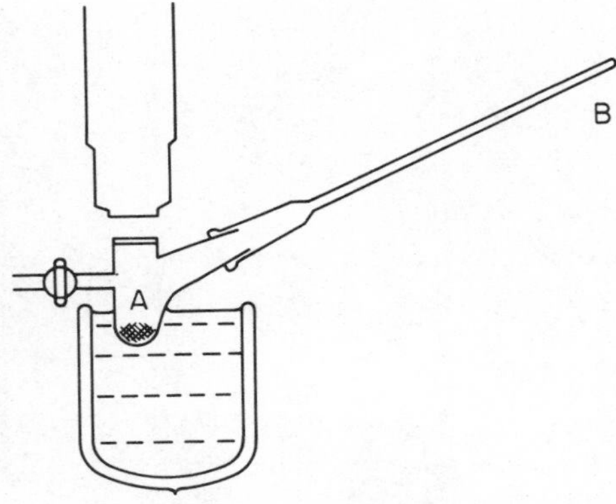

Figure 7.21 Low-temperature X-ray irradiation apparatus. (After a design by Dr B. Smaller)

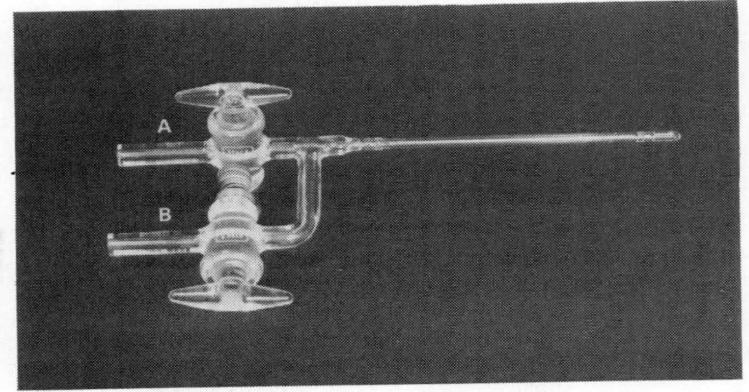

Figure 7.22 ESR sample tube for anaerobic studies

Anaerobic Studies

ESR studies on oxidative enzymes frequently require working under anaerobic conditions. An ESR tube adapted for anaerobic work is shown in Figure 7.22. Oxygen-free enzyme would be introduced from a syringe to the tube via tap A whilst a stream of oxygen-free argon is maintained through tap B. The enzyme reaction would be initiated by adding reducing substrate, again with an argon stream through B; after a suitable reaction time the sample would be frozen by immersion in liquid nitrogen and ESR studies made at low temperatures.

Biological Tissue Techniques

The types of sample holders suitable for biological tissue have already been discussed. This section deals with techniques of sample preparation. The three basic methods used are the freeze-drying technique, the surviving-tissue technique and the rapid-freeze technique.

In the freeze-dry technique, water is removed from the tissue by lyophilization and the sample then examined in a standard ESR tube. This method provides good sensitivity, but it is uncertain what proportion of the *in vivo* free radicals survive the freeze-drying process. It is also possible that artefactual free radicals are generated by the freeze-drying. For these reasons, the freeze-dry technique is not now commonly used in serious quantitive work.

The surviving-tissue technique approaches most closely to the *in vivo* situation. The organs to be studied are removed as quickly as possible from the animal and stored on ice. Tissue slices are cut as required (~0.5 mm thick) and examined in a tissue cell, or in aqueous suspension in a flat aqueous sample cell. The disadvantage of this method is the low sensitivity because the high water content necessitates small samples.

The rapid-freeze technique overcomes the difficulty of high water content by using frozen samples. In this method the freshly obtained tissue is rapidly frozen in liquid nitrogen. The samples are then examined in the spectrometer at this temperature. The procedure is thus analogous to the rapid freeze flow technique discussed in Chapter 9. Sensitivity enhancements are obtained as in the low-temperature observation of metalloproteins. Indeed, the rapid-freeze technique is essential for observing paramagnetic ions in tissue.

The CAT

Although ESR is an inherently sensitive technique, in biological problems one is often dealing with small quantities of sample or, more acutely, extremely dilute samples such as surviving tissue or spin labels biosynthetically incorporated into natural tissue. In such cases the CAT produces an extremely useful source of signal enhancement. As already discussed in the NMR section, the CAT stores and adds repeated sweeps through the weak spectrum, the randomly fluctuating noise thus tending to cancel out whilst the ESR signal itself accumulates. The statistics of random noise show that the noise is reduced in proportion to the square root of the number of accumulations. Thus it only takes 4 scans to improve the signal-to-noise by a factor of two, but 16 scans for a further factor of two improvement, etc. An example of the improved signal-to-noise obtained by this signal averaging technique is given in Chapter 3, for an NMR sample. The principles are exactly the same for an ESR sample.

7.8 Summary

(1) The ESR spectrometer is an absorption spectrometer in which the magnetic field is scanned instead of frequency.

(2) The sample is placed in a resonant cavity which must be tuned to the microwave frequency. This is normally done by tuning the klystron frequency.

After tuning, the klystron is locked to the cavity frequency using an automatic frequency control.

(3) The microwave detection is via a bridge, and the required diode detector bias is achieved by slightly undercoupling the cavity, or by means of the reference (or bucking) arm which requires phase adjustment. Signal strength can be increased by increasing the microwave power if the sample is below saturation.

(4) Magnetic field modulation with phase sensitive detection is used. This requires phase adjustments in the reference channel of the 100 kHz oscillator. Improved signal strength is obtained by increasing the gain of the 100 kHz amplifier (though this increases the noise proportionately) or by increasing the modulation power (though over modulation can broaden the spectra). Improved signal-to-noise can be obtained by using a longer PSD time constant, though a compromise is necessary with magnetic field scan time to avoid lineshape distortion.

(5) Oscilloscope display by field or frequency modulation is used in tuning up the spectrometer and searching for spectra. Spectra are recorded for measurement on the pen recorder.

(6) DPPH is a useful sample for tuning up the spectrometer, and also as a standard *g*-marker.

(7) Measurement of *g*-values requires both frequency and absolute field. Measurement of splitting, e.g. hyperfine constants, requires only field sweep.

(8) Aqueous samples are lossy and require special care. Low temperatures – freezing – are recommended for metalloproteins to overcome this and also improve sensitivity.

Chapter 8
ESR Applied to Biomolecules

8.1 Small biomolecules

In principle, all biological oxidations or reductions could take place in one-electron steps. The radical intermediates might be expected to be reactive and detection by ESR would only be feasible in special cases, for example when the unpaired electron is delocalized. Flavin and quinone radicals are the best characterized examples in this category. Unstable radicals, for example from enzyme substrates, may be detected by rapid reaction techniques. The study of radicals generated by metabolic processes has in many cases been aided by similar studies on radicals produced from model compounds by chemical oxidation.

Flavin radicals

Protein having flavin mononucleotide and flavin adenine dinucleotide as coenzymes participate in a wide variety of biological oxidative processes. Reduction of the flavin ring is the key reaction involved in all flavoproteins; the overall two-electron reduction can proceed in one-electron steps. Detailed characterization of radical intermediates has come from ESR studies on simple riboflavin derivatives particularly lumiflavin (see Figure 8.1). Limited reduction under anaerobic conditions yields several semiquinone radical species. By choosing an appropriate pH, the cationic, neutral or anionic species can be studied selectively. Alternatively the chelate formed between the radical and a diamagnetic metal ion (for example Zn^{2+} or Cd^{2+}) both increases the radical signal intensity by driving the equilibrium

$$\text{flavin}_{ox} + \text{flavin}_{red} \rightleftharpoons 2 \text{ semiquinone}$$

to the right and simplifies the spectrum since the chelate is formed only with the anionic radical species.

The ESR spectra of anion radicals formed from two lumiflavin derivatives are shown in Figure 8.2. The extensive hyperfine structure is due to interaction between the unpaired electron and various nitrogen and hydrogen nuclei around the ring system. It can be seen that replacement of the hydrogen at position 3 by an alkyl grouping has little effect on the spectrum. This indicates that the unpaired electron density at position 3 is low. Similarly isotopic replacement of the nitrogens in positions 1, 3, 5 and 10 or the proton at position 9 has allowed complete spectral

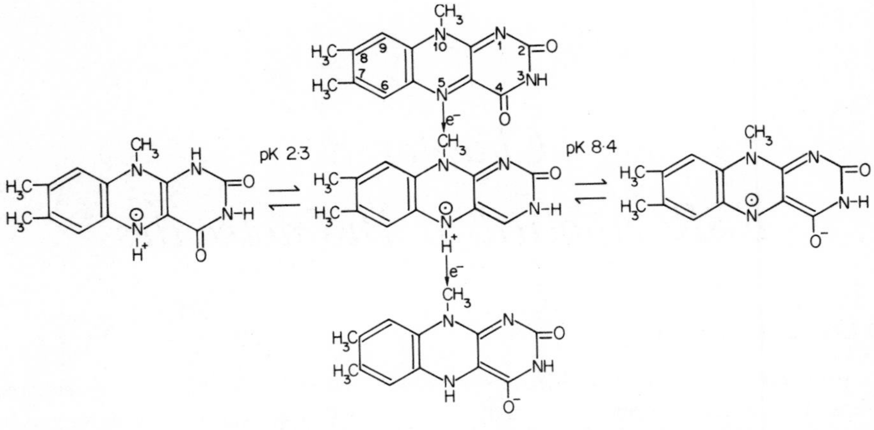

Figure 8.1 Structures of lumiflavin and its reduction products at different states of protonation

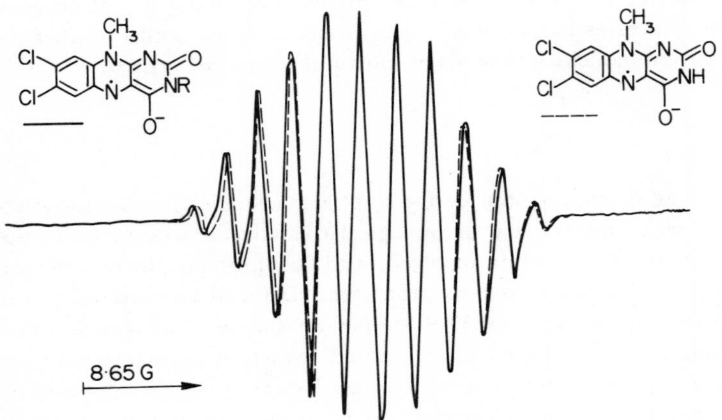

Figure 8.2 ESR spectra of 7,8 dichloro-10-methyl isoalloxazine radicals prepared by partial reduction of the flavin dissolved in dimethyl formamide at alkaline pH. (From Ehrenberg, Müller and Hemmerich, 1967). R = $-CH_2CO_2H$

assignment (Ehrenberg, Müller and Hemmerich, 1967; Müller, Erriksson and Ehrenberg, 1970); however, accurate measurement of the various hyperfine splittings has only been possible since the advent of ENDOR (see Chapter 9). The hyperfine splittings have been used to calculate spin densities (see Chapter 6) and the results compared with those derived from molecular orbital theory (Song, 1969) are shown in Table 8.1.

From this table, it can be concluded that the electron is not delocalized onto the pyrimidine ring and thus this ring is unlikely to participate in electron transfer

Table 8.1
Spin densities at various positions on flavin semiquinone anion calculated from ESR hyperfine splittings and from molecular orbital theory

Position	Atom	Spin density	
		calculated from hyperfine splittings	calculated from molecular orbital theory
1	N	–	−0.002
3	N	–	−0.036
5	N	0.256–0.394	0.361
6	C	0.129–0.167	0.201
7	C	–	−0.117
8	C	0.148–0.190	0.140
9	C	0.033–0.048	−0.060
10	N	0.112–0.173	0.164

processes. High electron densities are found on N5, N10, C6 and C8 suggesting that these atoms probably participate in electron transfer.

At the mid-point for reduction, a large proportion of the total flavin present in metal-free flavoproteins can be accounted for as semiquinone radical. For flavoproteins containing redox-active metals, the levels of semiquinone radical are sometimes much reduced due to greater delocalization of the electron over other redox components, and also the ESR signal height is decreased due to spin–spin broadening between the different paramagnetic species. Kinetic studies have shown that the flavin radical is produced in times less than the time for the catalytic cycle which is consistent with the radical being a participant in catalysis.

Substrate radicals generated by peroxidase

Early stopped-flow studies by Chance (1952) pointed to the existence of two, coloured enzyme substrate intermediates produced by the action of peroxidase. The kinetics of appearance and disappearance of these intermediates were determined and an overall catalytic pathway proposed (Figure 8.3). Oxidation of the enzyme by hydrogen peroxide yields compound I (green) which is reduced by the electron donor molecule AH_2 to compound II (red). Conversion of compound I to compound II and subsequent reduction by a second molecule of donor substrate both produce substrate radicals which disappear by non-enzymic dismutation.

It can be readily shown that the steady-state concentration of AH• will be given by:

$$[AH^{\bullet}] = \left\{ \frac{k_3 [E] [AH_2]}{kd} \right\}^{1/2} \tag{8.1}$$

where k_d is the rate constant for the dismutation reaction and all other terms are as indicated in Figure 8.3.

Continuous-flow ESR experiments by Yamazaki, Mason and Piette (1959, 1960)

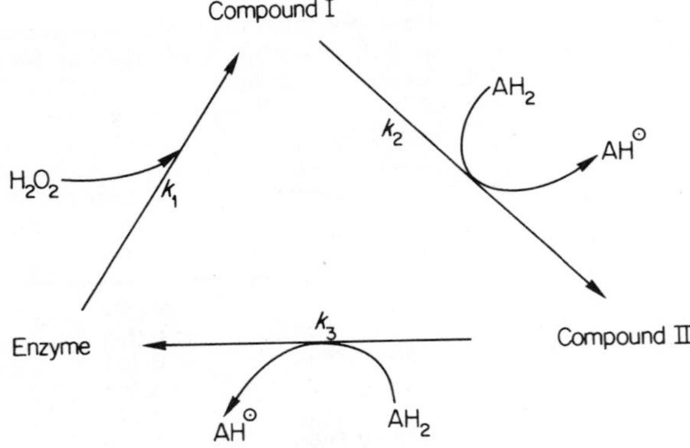

Figure 8.3 Catalytic pathway for the enzyme peroxidase. The rate constants for the various reactions are k_1, k_2 and k_3

not only showed the identity of the substrate radical but also gave values for the steady-state concentration of $AH^{\odot}$ in accordance with equation (8.1). The oxidation reaction with ascorbate as reducing substrate would be

CH_2OH | HO—CH, H, O, =O, HO, OH $\xrightarrow{H^{\odot}}$ CH_2OH | HO—CH, H, O, =O, $O^{\odot}$, OH

where the unpaired electron could be delocalized onto the ring. Interaction with the C–H proton would yield a doublet with a splitting of about 2 gauss and this is clearly seen in Figure 8.4.

The concentrations of ascorbate radical at various concentrations of enzyme, H_2O_2 and ascorbate are shown in Table 8.2.

From experiments 1 and 2, it can be seen that when the enzyme concentration changes by a factor of 4, the radical concentration changes by a factor of 2. In other words $[AH^{\odot}] \propto [\text{enzyme}]^{1/2}$.

From experiments 2 and 3, it can be seen that when the H_2O_2 concentration changes by a factor of 4, the radical concentration is scarcely affected. Both sets of results are consistent with equation (8.1). Also, since the free radical levels exceed by an order of magnitude the concentration of enzyme, they must exist free in solution, and cannot arise from compounds I or II.

The decay curve for the radical produced from hydroquinone by alkaline oxidation can be monitored either by ESR or by optical density at 424 nm. As shown in Figure 8.5, the two decay curves are identical. They are also identical to the decay curve from the radical produced by action of peroxidase on hydroquinone which is further evidence for its identity, in this case.

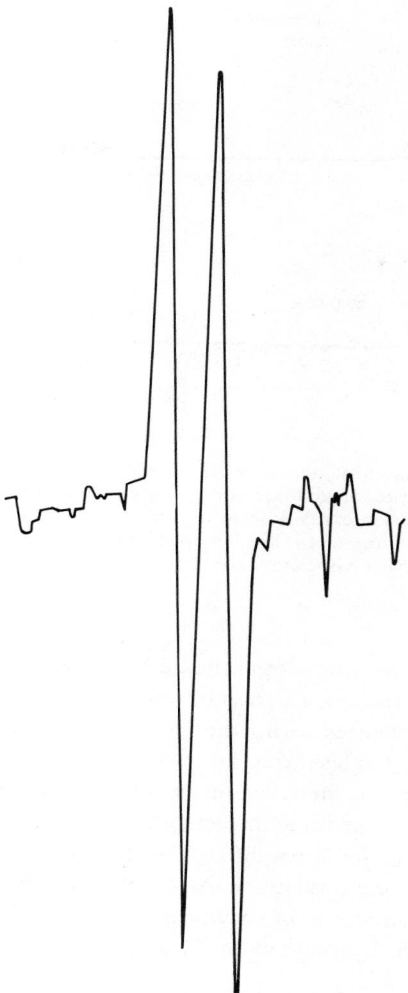

Figure 8.4 The ESR spectrum of ascorbate free radical produced enzymically by turnip peroxidase using the continuous-flow technique. (From Yamazaki and Piette, 1961. Reproduced by permission of Elsevier Scientific Publishing Company)

Table 8.2

Experiment number	Peroxidase	H_2O_2	Ascorbate	Ascorbate radical
1	1×10^{-8} M	2×10^{-2} M	2×10^{-2} M	2.1×10^{-7} M
2	4×10^{-8} M	2×10^{-2} M	2×10^{-2} M	4.5×10^{-7} M
3	4×10^{-8} M	5×10^{-3} M	2×10^{-2} M	3.8×10^{-7} M

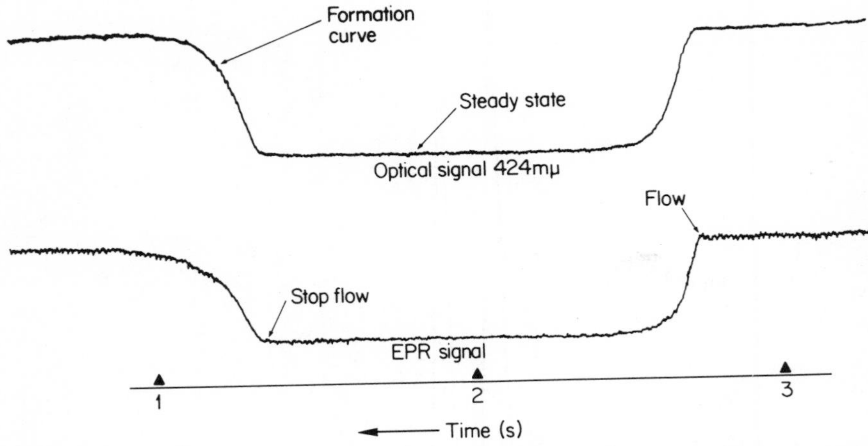

Figure 8.5 Simultaneous ESR and optical absorption measurements on the radical produced by aerial oxidation of hydroquinone using continuous flow in conjunction with a VARIAN optical transmission cavity accessory. During flow, no signal is observed since the flow is faster than the reaction; when flow is stopped, the formation of a free radical occurs. (Figure by courtesy of Varian Associates Ltd)

8.2 Metalloproteins

In order to understand the diverse roles played by proteins, we need to know (i) the three-dimensional structure of a particular protein down to the atomic level and (ii) how this structure changes during the functional process. Over the past twenty years, X-ray diffraction has been very successfully applied to solve the structures of several proteins. There are, however, many proteins which will be difficult to crystallize, for example those found in membranes and others whose high molecular weight presents problems for X-ray diffraction studies. Again X-ray crystallography requires a fixed protein conformation; any conclusions about enzyme mechanisms derived from even the structures of enzyme inhibitor complexes fall into the realms of plausible speculation. Dynamic methods are needed to establish the speculations as facts.

Both NMR and ESR are capable of giving dynamic as well as structural information down to the atomic level. The particular merit of ESR is its specificity. Paramagnetic centres in metalloproteins are associated with some or all of their functions. Thus changes occurring at the active sites of such metalloenzymes can be monitored specifically by ESR, without the diamagnetic remainder of the protein confusing the spectrum. The application of ESR to the study of metalloproteins will be illustrated by the examples of myoglobin, an iron-containing protein and the enzyme laccase which contains copper.

Myoglobin

Proteins containing the haem ring system are involved in both electron transfer and oxygen carrier functions. A most important group of haem proteins, the cytochromes, transfer electrons sequentially from flavoproteins to molecular oxygen; the cytochromes undergo reversible Fe^{2+}–Fe^{3+} valence changes during their catalytic cycle. Although many cytochromes have been purified, they are usually bound to membranes and therefore difficult to obtain in the homogeneous form needed for biophysical studies. The exception to this is cytochrome-*c* which has been crystallized and its structure determined by X-ray diffraction analysis (Dickerson *et al.* 1971). By contrast, the two proteins responsible for oxygen transport to the muscles (haemoglobin and myoglobin) are readily purified to homogeneity and have consequently been studied by a variety of biophysical methods. In respect of both structure and function, myoglobin is simpler than haemoglobin; thus myoglobin resembles one of the four haemoglobin subunits and shows no cooperativity in oxygen binding.

Mention has been made in Chapter 1 that oxygen binds to the haem iron centre of myoglobin. Five of the coordination positions to the iron are provided by nitrogens (from the porphyrin ring and a polypeptide chain histidine). The sixth coordination position in myoglobin can be occupied by water, oxygen or other small molecules (see Table 8.3).

Table 8.3
The valence of iron centre in myoglobin according to the ligand coordinated at the sixth position

Name	6th Coordinating group	Valence of the iron
Deoxymyoglobin	–	Fe^{2+}
Oxymyoglobin	O_2	Fe^{2+}
Acid met myoglobin	H_2O	Fe^{3+}
Cyano met myoglobin	CN^-	Fe^{3+}
Myoglobin fluoride	F^-	Fe^{3+}
Myoglobin azide	N_3^-	Fe^{3+}

ESR studies on myoglobin were initiated to provide information on co-ordination to the sixth position of the haem. During the course of these studies, it became apparent that in addition information could be derived concerning the orientation of the haem planes with respect to the rest of the protein (Bennett *et al.*, 1957).

The ferrous centre in native myoglobin is unsuitable for ESR studies since in the low-spin form it is diamagnetic whilst the zero field splitting in the high-spin form (see Chapter 6) does not allow ESR transitions to be observed. Thus ESR studies have in general been made on metmyoglobin in which the iron is present as high-spin Fe^{3+}. Even for metmyoglobin it is not easy to observe an ESR signal since the electron spin–lattice relaxation time of high-spin Fe^{3+} is short; all the measurements have normally to be made at liquid-nitrogen temperatures or below. The *g*-value anisotropy in metmyoglobin is large; *g*-values of 6 and 2 are observed when the magnetic field is applied in or perpendicular to the haem plane respectively. It is the *g*-value anisotropy which gives a very sensitive method for determining the orientation of the haem planes with respect to the crystallographic axes.

In principle, all that is required is to mount a crystal of metmyoglobin in the ESR cavity and rotate it about all possible axes until a g-value of 2.0 is obtained. It is then known that the magnetic field is being applied along the direction perpendicular to the haem plane. In practice, rotation about all axes is difficult and the approach has therefore been to mount the crystal in different crystallographic planes in turn and to plot the g-value variation for this plane. There is yet another practical difficulty; each unit cell of the crystal structure contains two molecules of myoglobin. Thus there will be two differently oriented sets of haem planes in the crystal and hence two sets of g-value variations as the crystal is rotated. The results for rotation around the *ab* plane are shown in Figure 8.6.

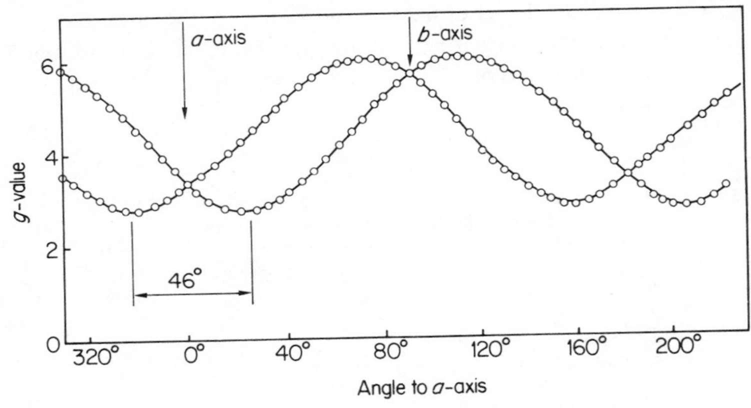

Figure 8.6 The g-value variations for acid met myoglobin during rotation of the magnetic field around the *ab* plane. Two curves are obtained from the two molecules per unit cell. (From Ingram, 1969. Reproduced by permission of Adam Hilger Ltd)

The minimum g-value (not exactly 2.0 since neither normal to the haem plane lies in the *ab* crystallographic plane) lies at an angle of 23° to the a-axis and has a value of 2.64. Substitution of this g_θ value into the version of equation (6.5) appropriate for metmyoglobin

$$g_\theta^2 = 4(1 + 8 \sin_\theta^2) \tag{8.2}$$

gives a value of θ equal to 17.5° which is the angle between the *ab* plane and the haem normal. The angle can be checked by similar measurements in other crystallographic planes.

This success with myoglobin gave Ingram and his colleagues confidence in applying a similar approach to haemoglobin. In this case, the crystallographic unit cell contains a single molecule of the haemoglobin tetramer. Single-crystal ESR studies showed immediately that the haem planes were not parallel to each other as had previously been assumed. The results from the detailed ESR analysis of haemoglobin are given in Bennet *et al.* (1957).

All the above studies were made on single crystals. It is the exception rather than the rule that large single crystals of metalloproteins are available. What information therefore can be derived from ESR studies on frozen solutions of haem proteins?

Values for g_x, g_y and g_z can be measured with accuracy from polycrystalline spectra. Thus myoglobin azide, which has iron present as low-spin rather than high-spin ferric, has g-values in the region of $g = 2$ as shown in Figure 8.7.

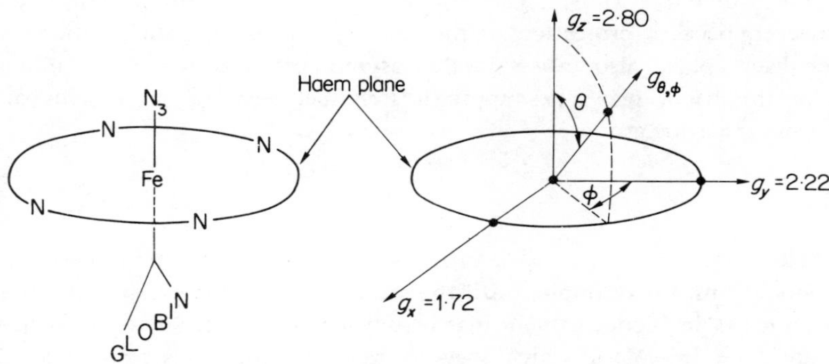

Figure 8.7 Principal g-values for myoglobin azide. (From Ingram, 1969. Reproduced by permission of Adam Hilger Ltd)

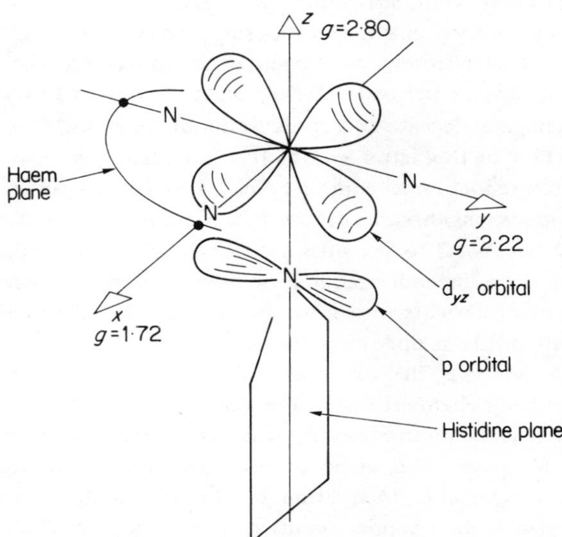

Figure 8.8 Interaction of the p orbital from the co-ordinating histidine nitrogen with the d_{yz} orbital on the iron atom of myoglobin azide. (From Ingram, 1969. Reproduced by permission of Adam Hilger Ltd)

Since the haem plane is symmetrical, one might have guessed that there would be axial symmetry, i.e. $g_x = g_y$. This is in fact true for haem itself so either the histidine at position 5 or the azide at position 6 must have affected the g-values. Qualitative application of ligand field theory shows that if the maximum g-value in the haem plane ($g = 2.22$) is associated with the y-direction, then the d_{yz} orbital will have highest energy and the p orbital on an imidazole ring nitrogen from the histidine coordinated at position 5 will also be parallel to the y-axis (see Figure 8.8). It can be seen that the orientation of the histidine with respect to the haem plane is therefore known. The situation is somewhat more complicated than this, however, because projection of the azide group, in the 6th position, down onto the haem plane also causes g-value asymmetry, and in fact the minimum g-value in the haem plane lies approximately between the projections of the histidine and the azide groups.

Laccase

Copper, like iron, is found in a wide variety of oxygen-carrying and redox proteins. The haemocyanins, for example, fulfil the same role in molluscs and arthropods as haemoglobin has in blood, namely that of oxygen transport. Solutions of haemocyanin are blue in colour which suggests that the copper is present as Cu^{2+}. However, no ESR signal can be detected, even at low temperatures, which indicates that the copper sites are diamagnetic. This conclusion is supported by magnetic susceptibility measurements. Obviously studies on the copper sites in haemocyanin will require techniques other than ESR.

There are many copper enzymes catalysing redox reactions, in most cases involving electron transfer from a reducing substrate to oxygen. The oxygen can be reduced either to hydrogen peroxide (2-electron reduction) or to water (4-electron reduction). The enzymes laccase and cytochrome oxidase (see Section 8.5(ii)) are examples of enzymes in this latter group. It is interesting to note that enzymes catalysing 4-electron reduction all contain at least 4 metal ions per mole of enzyme. Thus laccase (4 copper ions) has this property in common with cytochrome oxidase (2 copper ions, 2 haems). This provides a rationalization for detailed biophysical studies on laccase since an understanding of how oxygen is reduced to water by laccase should provide insights into how the complex membrane-bound enzyme cytochrome oxidase fulfils its important functions.

Laccase, which catalyses the oxidation of hydroquinones, contains 4 copper atoms as determined by chemical assay. The ESR spectrum of a frozen solution of laccase run at 9 GHz is shown in Figure 8.9 and indicates that some of the copper is present as Cu^{2+}. Moreover, the shape of the spectrum is consistent with axial symmetry at the copper site. Integration of the area under the spectrum and comparison with that from a copper standard shows that only 2 of the 4 coppers contribute to the signal. Obviously ESR can only provide information about these two copper sites.

Attention is drawn to a 'bump' (indicated by the arrow in Figure 8.9) at low field and to the difference in linewidths of the hyperfine lines. Both these features

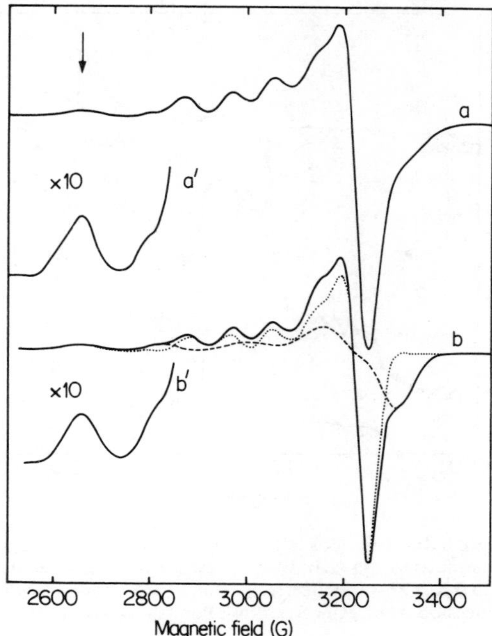

Figure 8.9 (a) Experimental, and (b) simulated, 9 GHz ESR spectrum of laccase recorded at 77 K. Part of the spectrum (a′ and b′) is shown with 10 times higher gain. The dotted and dashed lines in (b) are the separated contributions from the two Cu^{2+} centres. (From Malmström *et al.*, 1968. Reproduced by permission of Elsevier Scientific Publishing Company)

suggest that in fact the spectrum is composed of two overlapping signals. This was verified by ESR studies at 35 GHz which gives enhanced resolution of the spectrum (Figure 8.10). Computer simulation also allows the contributions from the two Cu^{2+} centres (designated type 1 and type 2) with different ESR parameters to be separated; spectra simulated in this way for 9 GHz are shown in Figure 8.9.

The properties of types 1 and 2 Cu^{2+} centres in laccase are clearly distinct.

Type 1 copper is characterized by a narrow hyperfine splitting (A_{11}) of 250 MHz; this value should be compared with that of 470 MHz for simple copper complexes like copper–EDTA. Narrow hyperfine splitting indicates extensive delocalization of the electron density from the copper and suggests that type 1 copper has a redox function. Reduction of laccase with the substrate hydroquinone leads to loss of the type 1 ESR signal which supports a redox role for type 1 Cu^{2+} centres.

Type 2 copper by contrast has A_{11} = 475 MHz which is close to that of simple copper complexes; type 2 copper, unlike type 1, is not reduced by hydroquinone,

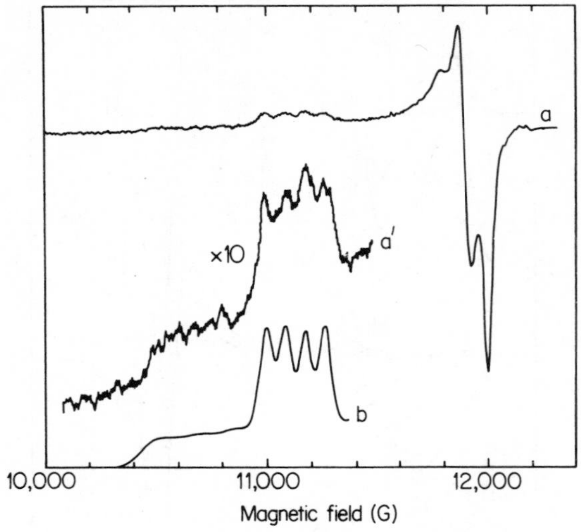

Figure 8.10 (a and a′) Experimental, and (b) part of the simulated, 35 GHz ESR spectrum of laccase recorded at 110 K. (From Malmström *et al.*, 1968. Reproduced by permission of Elsevier Scientific Publishing Company)

so its function in the enzyme is not obvious. It has been found that inhibitors like cyanide and fluoride bind specifically to type 2 copper. Unambiguous evidence for this has come from experiments with $K^{13}CN$ and $Na^{19}F$ when only the type 2 copper ESR signal shows hyperfine splitting due to interaction with the $I = ½$ nuclei of ^{13}C or ^{19}F. The experiments with fluoride are shown in Figure 8.11; with equimolar fluoride the type 2 copper hyperfine peaks are split into doublets while at high fluoride concentrations, they are split into triplets with an intensity distribution 1:2:1. These results can be explained by interactions of the type 2 Cu^{2+} with one or two ^{19}F nuclei. Thus it seems plausible to suggest that type 2 copper might function as a site in the enzyme for binding effectors, which regulate enzymic activity, or alternatively as a site for stabilizing intermediates produced by the catalytic process (Bränden,*et al.*, 1971).

The function of the remaining two diamagnetic coppers is suggested from the results of anaerobic titration experiments with ascorbate (Reinhammar and Vänngård, 1971) which show that the enzyme is capable of accepting four electrons. Ascorbate, unlike the true substrate hydroquinone, reduces both type 1 *and* type 2 coppers; this accounts for two of the electrons. Since there are no other known redox sites on the enzyme, it follows that the remaining two electrons would reduce the two diamagnetic coppers. Thus these diamagnetic coppers in laccase would need to be spin-paired Cu^{2+} rather than simply Cu^{+} as we might have originally suspected.

Kinetic studies using both ESR and spectrophotometric detection have shown that all electrons from reducing substrate enter the enzyme molecule through type

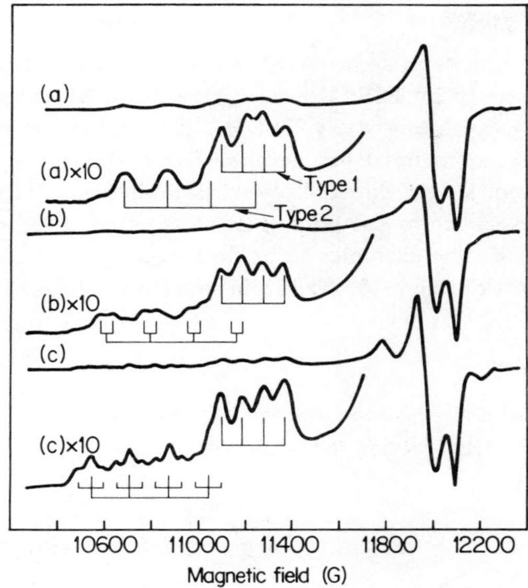

Figure 8.11 35 GHz ESR spectra from native and fluoride-treated laccase. (a) No fluoride; (b) equimolar fluoride; (c) 20-fold excess fluoride. (From Malkin *et al.*, 1968)

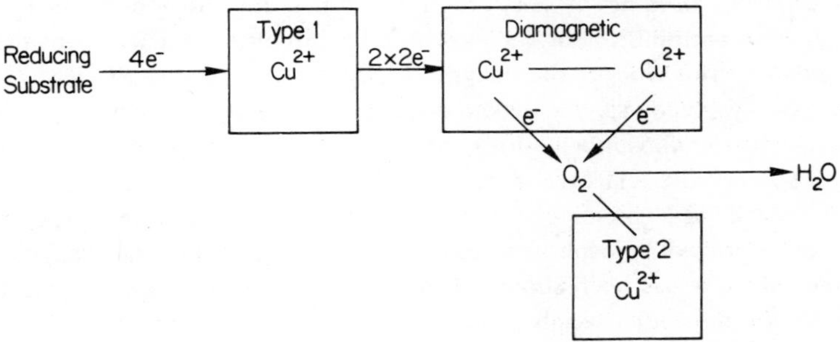

Figure 8.12 Schematic representation of how the different copper sites function in laccase

1 copper. Intra-molecular electron transfer to the diamagnetic pair, which have been activated by the binding of oxygen, then probably takes place. Intermediate species in the four-electron reduction of oxygen to water have not been detected, which suggests that they might remain bound to the diamagnetic pair and to the type 2 copper. A schematic representation of how the copper sites function in laccase is shown in Figure 8.12. It can be seen from this example that ESR in conjunction with other biophysical techniques can provide considerable information about metal-containing redox enzymes.

8.3 Spin-labelled proteins

The vast majority of proteins do not have an inherent paramagnetic centre and thus are unsuitable for study by ESR. However, the advent of spin labelling makes all proteins potentially capable of study by ESR. The application of spin labelling to the study of biological material has developed over the last decade. Many of the early qualitative studies were directed towards monitoring conformational changes in the protein subsequent to the binding of some effector molecule, for example substrate or inhibitor. The examples to be discussed in this section illustrate what quantitative information can be derived from spin-label studies of proteins.

Phosphofructokinase

This enzyme catalyses the conversion of fructose-6-phosphate to fructose-1,6-diphosphate, an early reaction in the glycolytic pathway.

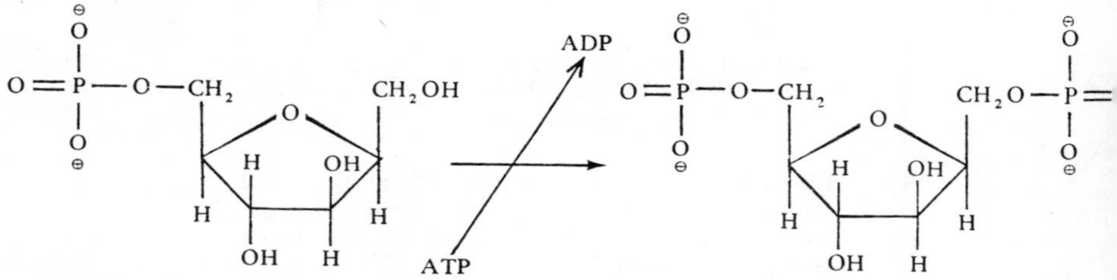

$O{=}P(O^{\ominus})_2{-}O{-}CH_2$ … CH_2OH (furanose ring: O; H, OH; H, H; OH, H) $\xrightarrow[\text{ATP}]{\text{ADP}}$ $O{=}P(O^{\ominus})_2{-}O{-}CH_2$ … $CH_2O{-}P(O^{\ominus})_2{=}$ (furanose ring: O; H, OH; H, H; OH, H)

Mg^{2+} is also essential for this reaction; probably formation of an Mg–ATP complex facilitates binding of ATP to the enzyme. In addition to its role as a substrate, ATP is an inhibitor of the enzyme; this inhibition in part forms the basis for the regulatory function of the enzyme in glycolysis – when sufficient ATP has been produced by glycolysis and linked oxidative processes (the tricarboxylic acid cycle and oxidative phosphorylation), phosphofructokinase is partially inhibited and remains so until the ATP level decreases.

It is of considerable biochemical importance to understand the catalytic and regulatory properties of phosphofructokinase in terms of structural changes within the enzyme. Since it has been shown (Jones *et al.*, 1972) that a single sulphydryl group per 90,000 molecular weight protomer can be spin-labelled, by the reagent

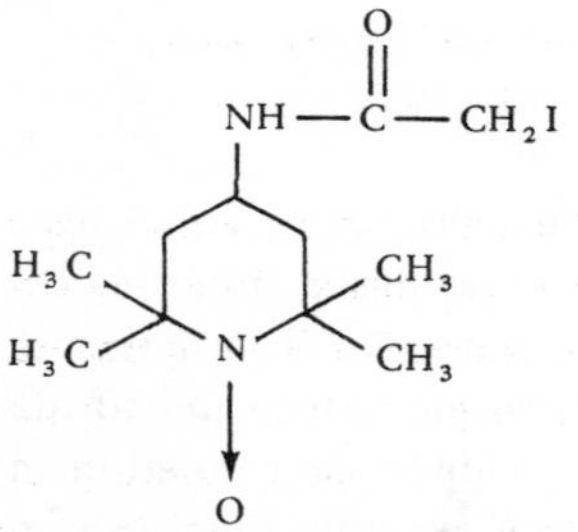

$NH{-}C({=}O){-}CH_2I$ on a piperidine ring bearing H_3C, H_3C, CH_3, CH_3 and $N \rightarrow O$

4-(2 iodoacetamido)-2,2,6,6,tetramethylpiperidino-oxyl, ESR can be used to study the enzyme. Under these conditions the spin-labelled enzyme is fully active

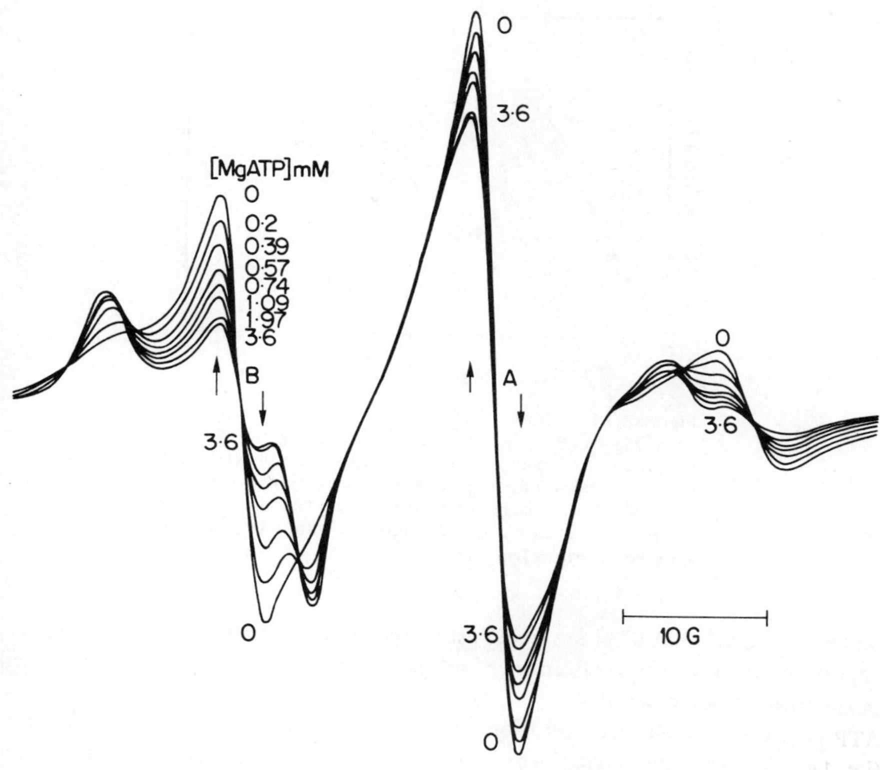

Figure 8.13 ESR spectra of spin-labelled phosphofructokinase titrated with Mg—ATP. (From Jones *et al.*, 1972)

and retains its allosteric kinetics. The spectral changes resulting from titration with Mg—ATP are shown in Figure 8.13. Sharp isosbestic points can be clearly seen suggesting that the spin label is located in two environments, which can be interconverted through a conformational change. Qualitatively we can see from Figure 8.13 that Mg—ATP binding causes immobilization of the spin label (c.f. Figure 6.18). The bindings curve for Mg—ATP at pH 7.5, as obtained from the spin-label-detected conformational change in the enzyme, is sigmoidal (see Figure 8.14) which suggests that positive cooperativity between Mg—ATP sites occurs.

Since the spectra in Figure 8.13 are all overlaps of two components, it is not possible accurately to assign rotational correlation times to these components through application of equation (6.19). However, the spectrum obtained in the absence of Mg—ATP is partially immobilized and corresponds to a correlation time (from equation 6.19) of approximately 4×10^{-9} S. This value clearly shows that the spin label has mobility separate from that of the whole protein molecule for which a value of 10^{-7} S/can be calculated from equation (6.18) and indicates that caution must be exercised when distances of substrate protons or paramagnetic

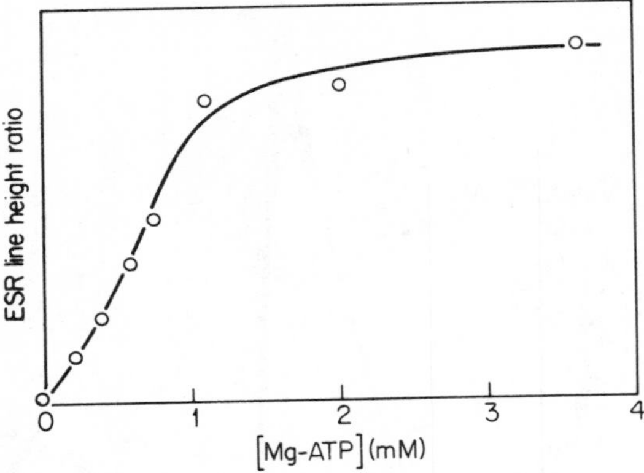

Figure 8.14 Binding curve for phosphofructokinase with Mg–ATP at pH 7.5. The ordinate is the line-height ratio of peak A to peak B, in the ESR spectrum of Figure 8.13, which is inversely proportional to the fraction of the enzyme which is in the conformation corresponding to the higher mobility state (B) of the spin label. (From Jones *et al.*, 1972)

centres from the spin label are being estimated. Distance measurements are a very important quantitative application of protein spin labelling and consequently will be discussed in some detail.

In order to obtain distance information, magnetic dipole interaction effects of the spin label on the NMR linebroadening behaviour of individual ATP protons must be determined. Measurement of the spin–lattice ($T_{1\mathrm{M}}$) and spin–spin ($T_{2\mathrm{M}}$) relaxation times for various protons on ATP bound to spin-labelled enzyme allows an accurate calculation to be made of the dipolar correlation times (τ_c) for the spin-label–proton interactions; correlation times for the different motions affecting nuclear relaxation have been discussed in Chapter 2. The distances (r) of different ATP protons from the nitroxide may be calculated from the NMR linebroadenings (i.e. $1/T_{2\mathrm{M}}$ values) and the corresponding correlation times, using the equation

$$\frac{1}{T_2\mathrm{M}} = \frac{4\tau_c}{15} \cdot \frac{\gamma_I{}^2 g^2 S^2 (S+1)\beta^2}{r^6} \tag{8.3}$$

Further details of this calculation can be found in Jones *et al.* (1973). Table 8.4 gives the values of τ_c and r determined in this way.

From these data we can start to map the orientation of the ATP with respect to the spin label. However, in view of what has been said earlier in this section about the mobility of the spin label, this distance information could be in error. Fortunately we can obtain a check on the distance since the paramagnetic Mn^{2+} ion substitutes for Mg^{2+}.

The ESR spectrum of spin-labelled enzyme titrated with Mn–ATP is shown in Figure 8.15. Comparison of this spectrum with that from Mg–ATP/ binding (Figure 8.13) reveals a marked decrease in the central peak. This quenching effect is

Table 8.4
Distances of various ATP protons from the nitroxide in spin-labelled phosphofructokinase, calculated from the NMR line broadenings and the corresponding correlation times. The positions of the protons are given in Figure 8.16

Position of proton	$\tau_c \times 10^9$ s	r Å
H-2	13	7.2
H-8	6	7.5
H-1′	10	7.0

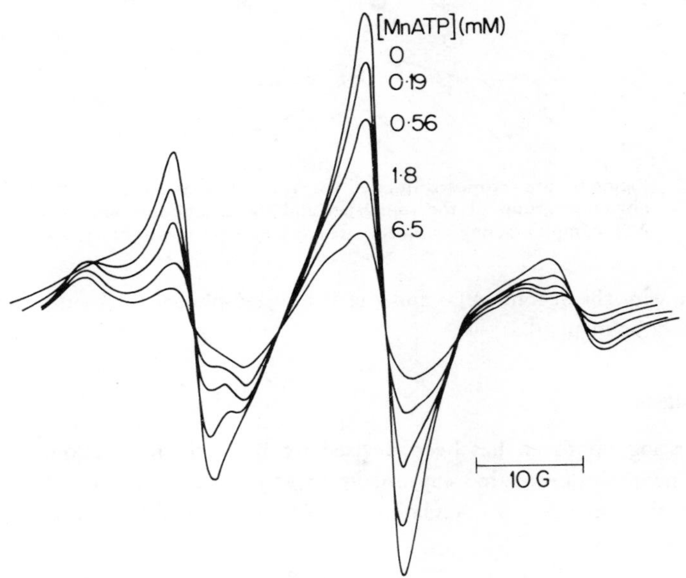

Figure 8.15 ESR spectra of spin-labelled phosphofructokinase titrated with Mn–ATP, showing the dipolar quenching effect. (From Jones *et al.*, 1973)

due to dipolar interactions between the paramagnetic Mn^{2+} and the spin label. The distance of separation of these dipoles (12 Å) can be calculated from the titration data (see Jones *et al.*, 1973) and is self-consistent with the distances of ATP protons from the spin label. A speculative model for the Mn–ATP binding site on the enzyme is shown in Figure 8.16. Whilst this is an advance in our knowledge of phosphofructokinase it should be pointed out that these results do not show whether ATP binding is occurring at the active and/or the inhibitor site nor how this cooperativity is related to the sigmoid kinetics with respect to fructose-6-phosphate concentration which are only observed below pH 7.0. If other selective binding sites for protein spin labels to phosphofructokinase can be found, there is

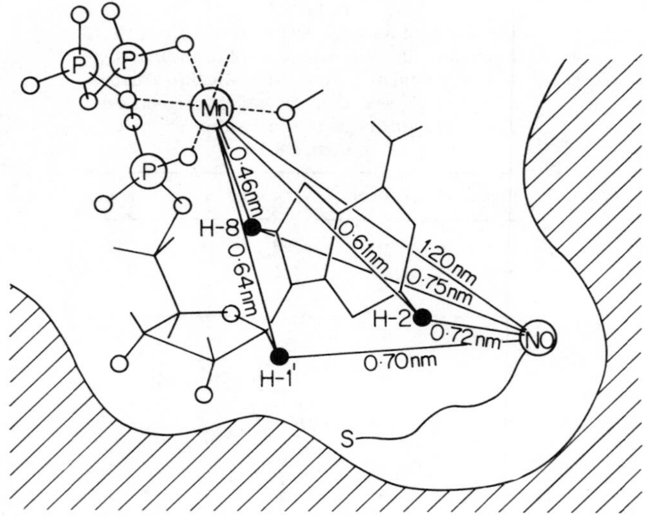

Figure 8.16 Proposed model for the relationship between the nitroxide group of the spin label and the neighbourhood metal–ATP complex bound to phosphofructokinase. (Jones *et al.*, 1973)

no reason why the second ATP and the fructose-6-phosphate binding sites should not similarly be mapped.

Chymotrypsin

An interesting approach has been devised by Berliner and McConnell (1966) to label the proteolytic enzyme chymotrypsin at its active site. In the hydrolysis of esters by this enzyme, an acylated enzyme intermediate is formed and later hydrolysed.

$$R-\overset{\displaystyle O}{\overset{\|}{C}}-OR' \xrightarrow[\text{HOR}']{\text{Enzyme}} R-\overset{\displaystyle O}{\overset{\|}{C}}-\text{Enzyme} \xrightarrow{H_2O} R-\overset{\displaystyle O}{\overset{\|}{C}}-OH + \text{Enzyme}$$

The substrate

H_3C, H_3C, CH_3, CH_3, N→O, C(=O)–O–C_6H_4–NO_2

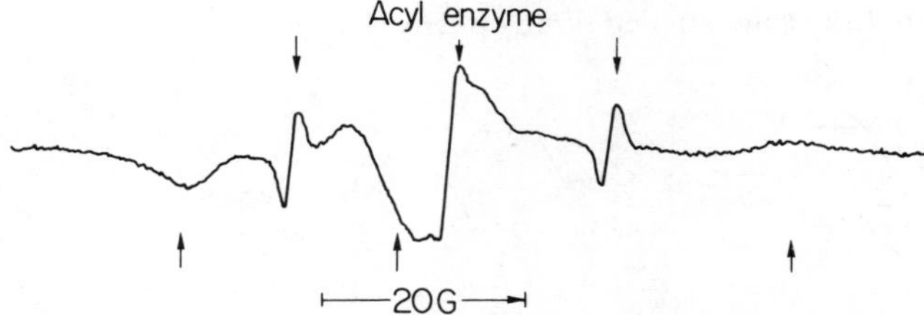

Figure 8.17 Resonance spectrum of spin labelled acyl chymotrypsin at pH 3.5. Broad resonance lines indicated by 'up arrows' (↑) are due to the acyl group immobilized at the active site. The three narrow 'down arrows' (↓) arise from free nitroxide in solution due to slow deacylation at this pH. (From Berliner and McConnell, 1966)

thus leads to binding of the spin label and release of nitrophenol in the first step. The kinetics of nitrophenyl release can be monitored by visible spectroscopy whilst the kinetics of the second step (release of spin-labelled acid) can be monitored by ESR. At low pH, the second step is slow and the ESR spectrum of the acyl enzyme can be observed. The spectrum (Figure 8.17) is characteristic of a strongly immobilized spin label indicating that the active centre must be sufficiently flexible to admit the substrate but sufficiently rigid thereafter to immobilize the acyl grouping.

Other studies have been made of spin-labelled inhibitor binding to chymotrypsin. These inhibitors are derivatives of sulphonyl fluoride which bind to the active site serine. It was found that the derivative

SO_2F

O=C

O

H_3C CH_3

H_3C N CH_3

O

was only weakly immobilized which suggests that the active site 'cleft' is only large enough to accomodate the aromatic ring of the inhibitor or acyl portion of the substrate.

Antibody–hapten interactions

A further example of the use of spin labels to probe the depth of active site clefts is the important one of antibody–hapten interactions. Stryer and Griffith (1965) have prepared the spin-labelled dinitrophenyl hapten

H_3C CH_3

$O \leftarrow N$ $=N—NH—$ NO_2

H_3C CH_3 O_2N

and used it to study binding to rabbit antidinitrophenyl antibody. The free radical was strongly immobilized when bound to the antibody with a correlation time, τ_c, of 4×10^{-8} S (Figure 8.18). It is further possible to titrate antibody *vs* spin-labelled hapten, the end-point being when the highly mobile free nitroxide signal appears superimposed on the immobilized signal (see Figure 8.18). In this way, the number of binding sites has been determined as two per antibody.

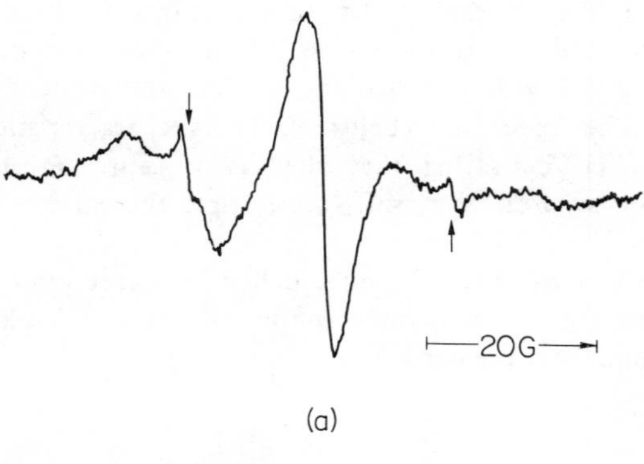

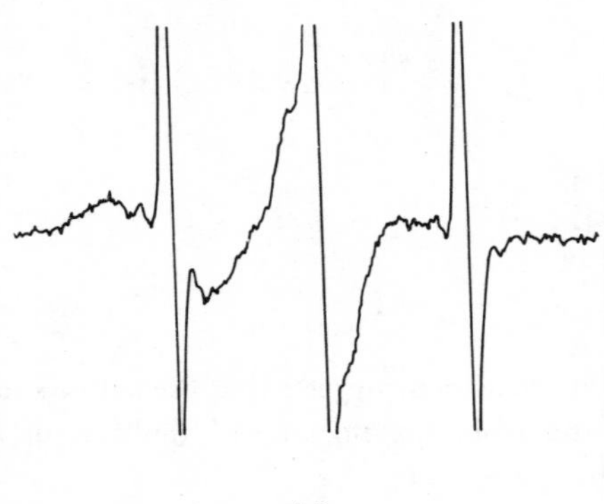

Figure 8.18 ESR titration of the binding of dinitrophenyl nitroxide hapten to antibody. The hapten/antibody ratio is 1.8 in (a) and 2.3 in (b). (From Stryer and Griffith, 1965)

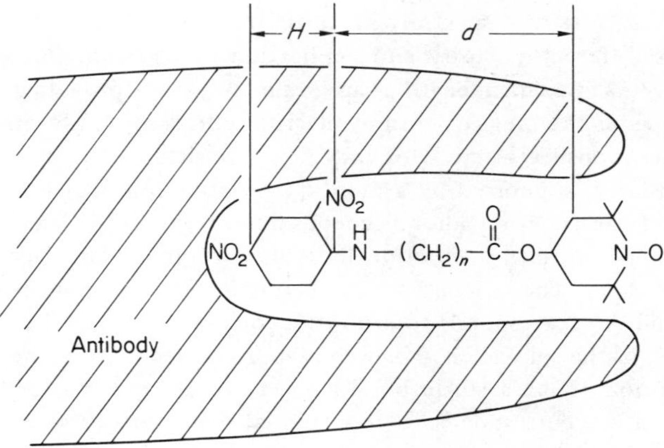

Figure 8.19 Schematic representation of the antibody binding site and the spin-labelled hapten used by Hs ia and Piette (1969)

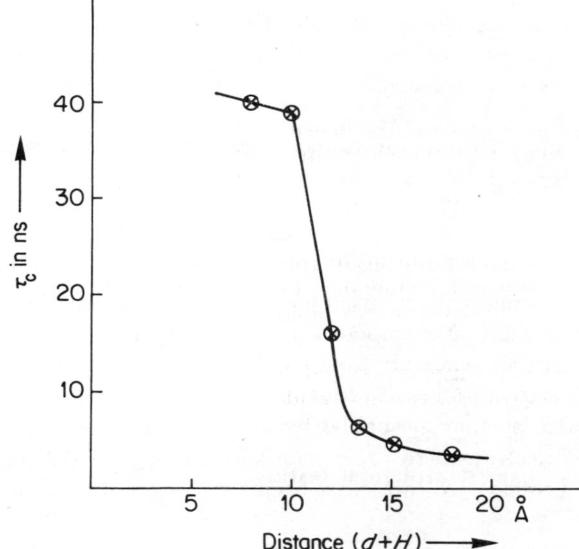

Figure 8.20 Plot of τ_c *vs* hapten length (see Figure 8.19). (From Hsia and Piette, 1969. Reproduced by permission of Academic Press, Inc.)

Electron microscope studies of antibody–hapten complexes indicate that the active site on the antibody is located in a crevice at a distance of about 12 Å from the surface. Hsia and Piette (1969) have used spin-labelled haptens of different chain lengths to measure this distance (Figure 8.19). When the length of hapten chain is less than the crevice depth, the label will be immobilized. Figure 8.20 shows the plot of chain length *vs* the correlation time, τ_c, determined by comparison of the observed spectra with those from the simple spin label TEMPO in solutions of different viscosity and application of equation (6.18). An abrupt change in τ_c occurs at a chain length of approximately 13 Å providing confirmation for the estimates of the crevice depth by electron microscopy. The above approach has obvious extensions to the study of enzyme active sites.

This conclusion is supported by a more quantitative spin labelling investigation on purified Fv fragment from a homogeneous immunoglobin A (Dwek *et al.*, 1975) which analyses both anisotropic motion and the isotropic splitting factor (Ao) of the spin label. At short chain lengths (see Figure 8.19), the spin label is rigidly immobilized and Ao corresponds to a non-aqueous medium (see Table 6.4). When the total length of the spin-labelled hapten is approximately 10 Å, the amplitude of anisotropic motion about a single bond adjacent to the nitroxide ring is approximately 50° and Ao corresponds to free spin label in aqueous solution. Thus the hapten binding site must be close to 10 Å in depth. Dwek *et al.* (1975) also apply NMR paramagnetic difference spectroscopy (see Section 5.5) to the rigidly immobilized bound hapten and conclude that 20 aliphatic and 30 aromatic protons lie within a sphere of radius 12–16 Å centred on the nitroxide grouping. On the basis of pH titrations, two histidines with pKs of 6.1 and 6.9 are amongst the perturbed aromatic resonances; comparison with the results of protein sequencing and X-ray diffraction studies indicates that these are probably at positions 97 of the light chain and 102 of the heavy chain. The prospects for mapping antibody–hapten binding sites using magnetic resonance methods seems as promising as those described in Section 5.5 for the active site of lysozyme.

8.4 Membranes

One of the more complex problems of contemporary molecular biology is to relate the structure of biological membranes to their function. There is considerable evidence to support the structure for biological membranes shown in Figure 8.21. Thus X-ray diffraction studies (Wilkins *et al.*, 1971; Levine, 1973) are consistent with a major part of the phospholipid having a bimolecular lamellar structure. Biochemical and electron-microscopic evidence (Bretscher, 1973) favours the view that membrane proteins are located at both the polar surface and integrated into the membrane.

It is necessary that the structural features shown in Figure 8.21 should have mobility in order to account for biological processes associated with membranes such as pinocytosis, phagocytosis and permeability to both polar and non-polar molecules. This mobility, which is associated with the liquid crystalline phase of the phospholipids, means that X-ray diffraction cannot be used to locate the individual atoms in a membrane. Spectroscopy particularly magnetic resonance spectroscopy, has great potential for the study of membrane structure and mobility.

Membranes however have no inherent paramagnetism. In order to apply ESR to the study of membranes, a suitable spin-labelled probe molecule must be incorporated into the membrane. The spin label may be attached to a membrane protein (e.g. Kirkpatrick and Sandberg, 1973) or to a lipid (McConnell and McFarland,

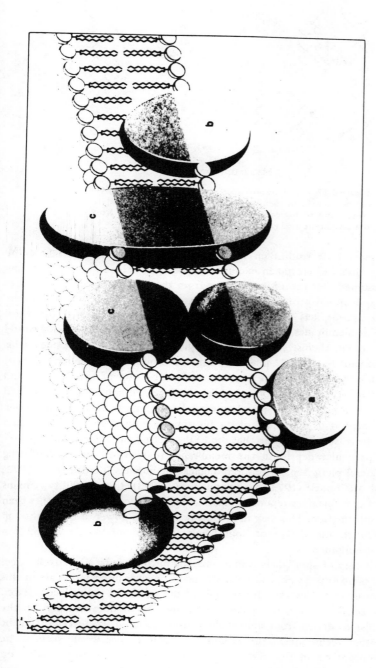

Figure 8.21 Proposed model for cell membranes; a matrix of phospholipid molecules with their hydrophilic heads at the surfaces and hydrophobic tails meeting at the bilayer centre which has proteins embedded to varying depths. (From Capaldi, 1974. Reproduced by permission of W. H. Freeman and Company)

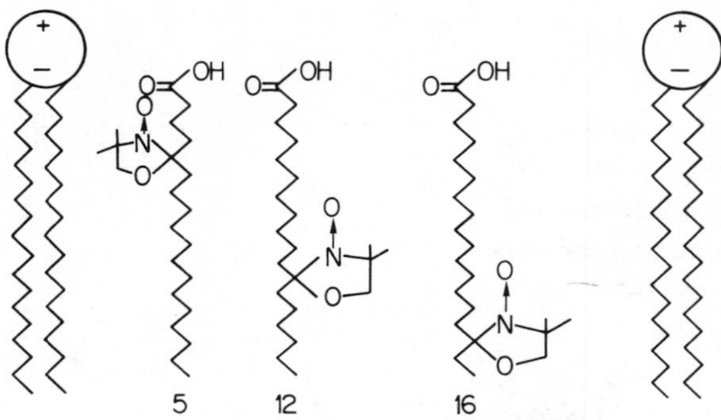

Figure 8.22 Orientation of various nitroxide derivatives of stearic acid in membranes. The numbers 5, 12 and 16 correspond to increasing separation of the nitroxide from the carboxylic acid grouping

1970). Since most ESR studies on membranes have used lipid spin labels, the examples to be discussed are taken exclusively from this field. In all spin-labelling studies, it is assumed that the ESR spectrum from the probe faithfully reproduces the structure and mobility of the biological system. This is most likely to be the case when the probe has close structural resemblance to normal biological components. For membranes, therefore, nitroxide derivatives of fatty acids would be expected to orient themselves with their alkyl chains adjacent to the side chains of the phospholipid; Figure 8.22 illustrates this for various nitroxide derivatives of stearic acid. However it is possible that the carboxyl group of these stearic acid derivatives is not located at the polar/apolar interface and consequently the lipid spin labels of choice for many membrane studies are those in which nitroxide derivatives of fatty acids form part of the phospholipid molecule. With such spin labels one can be reasonably certain that the ESR spectra from the nitroxide relates to events at particular depths in the membrane. In view of the accumulating evidence for lateral phase separations in biological membranes (Linden *et al.*, 1973; Shimshick and McConnell, 1973; Sackmann *et al.*, 1973), the possibility remains that these lipid spin labels are reporting on select areas in the membrane rather than giving general information. This may in fact prove to be the power of the method in the future through the design of spin labels which more closely resemble a particular phospholipid class.

Another criticism of spin labels is that since the nitroxide ring is relatively large, it perturbs the biological system and the ESR spectrum gives information about this perturbed environment. However the amount of the spin-label probe incorporated (~1%) is very small and it is reasonable to assume that it does not perturb the bilayer. Conclusions drawn from spin-labelling studies should wherever possible be checked by other techniques. ^{1}H, ^{2}H and ^{13}C NMR studies would seem to be particularly appropriate in this respect. In justification of spin-label studies on membranes, the sensitivity of the technique and the comprehensive information which can be obtained, particularly concerning various modes of motion, allow problems to be studied which would be beyond the scope of other techniques. The power of the technique will be illustrated by some examples.

Flexibility gradients

A series of spin-labelled phospholipids can be synthesized with the nitroxide grouping at different positions down one of the fatty acid chains of phosphatidyl choline (also named 'lecithin')

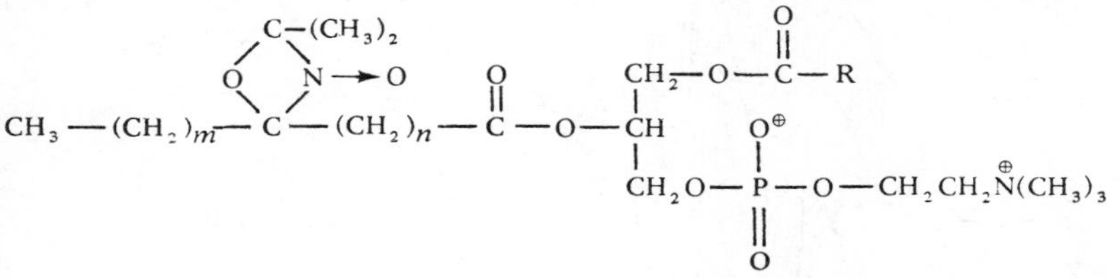

```
                     C—(CH3)2                                      O
                    /   \                                          ||
                   O     N→O          O             CH2—O—C—R
                    \   /             ||             |
CH3—(CH2)m—C—(CH2)n—C—O—CH          O⊕
                                                     |             |           ⊕
                                                    CH2O—P—O—CH2CH2N(CH3)3
                                                                   ||
                                                                   O
```

where R is a long chain alkyl grouping and *m*, *n* are 10,3; 8,5; 5,8; 3,10. Incorporation of these spin labels into phospholipid membranes therefore allows different parts of the bilayer to be monitored by ESR. Figure 8.23 shows the ESR spectra obtained from incorporation into egg lethicin aqueous dispersions which spontaneously form bilayer structures. (See Figure 4.20.)

The spectra indicate anisotropic motion for the nitroxide of the type discussed in Chapter 6. Hyperfine splittings $A_{\parallel}$ and $A_{\perp}$ can be measured as described more fully in Figures 6.14 and 6.16. The order parameters (defined in equation 6.20) and isotropic splitting constants (defined in equation 6.10) calculated from these spectra are given in Table 8.5.

Table 8.5
Order parameters and isotropic splitting constants for spin-labelled phospholipids incorporated into egg lecithin aqueous dispersions

Spin label (*m*, *n*)	Order parameters	Isotropic splitting constant (gauss)
10, 3	0.547	15.0
8, 5	0.468	14.9
5, 8	0.343	14.1
3, 10	<0.3	~13.5

Two important conclusions can be drawn from this data.

(i) The order parameters decreases towards the centre of the bilayer. This shows that the amplitude of motion which averages out the anisotropy increases towards the centre of the bilayer, i.e. the centre of the bilayer is fluid.

(ii) The isotropic splitting constant decreases towards the centre of the bilayer. This corresponds to a more hydrophobic environment.

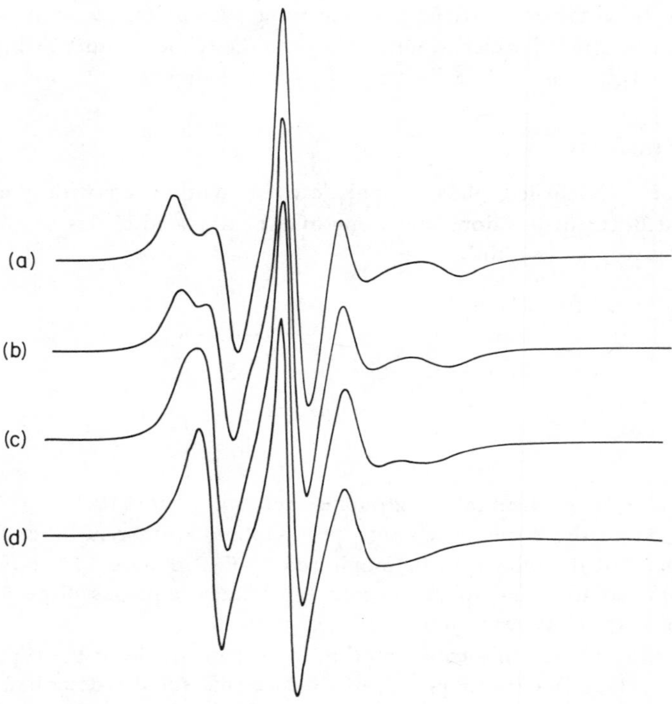

Figure 8.23 ESR spectra from various phospholipid spin labels incorporated into egg lecithin aqueous dispersions. Spectra (a), (b), (c) and (d) refer to incorporation of phospholipid probes with $m, n = 10,3$; 8,5; 5,8 and 3,10 respectively. Values for $A_{\parallel}$ and $A_{\perp}$ can be obtained from these spectra as shown in Figures 6.14 and 6.16

Hubbell and McConnell (1971) discuss these results in terms of the different motions which the fatty acid side chains can undergo. Firstly they consider the segmental motion within the fatty acid chains through rapid isomerizations between gauche and trans conformations about carbon–carbon single bonds in the chain. This motion would be cumulative down the chain, i.e. the methyl terminal section would have greater mobility than the methylenes close to the glycerol backbone. These chain isomerizations are the molecular basis for the fluidity of the bilayer. Secondly, Hubbell and McConnell (1971) consider the chain as a whole precessing as a 'rigid stick' about the perpendicular to the bilayer surface with an anchor point at the surface; this mode of motion is similar to that illustrated in Figure 6.22. An expression for the measured order parameter in terms of these two modes of motion is given by equation (8.4)

$$\log S_n = n \log P_t + \log S_o \tag{8.4}$$

where S_n is the measured order parameter, n is the number of methylene carbons separating the nitroxide from the carboxyl head, P_t is the probability of the energetically favoured trans conformation and S_o approximates to the 'rigid stick' order parameter.

Applications of this analysis to the data of Table 8.4 for egg lecithin gives $S_o = 0.73$ and $P_t = 0.91$. Thus there is an approximately 10% probability of gauche conformations in the lipid chains; this corresponds to between one and two gauche conformations per chain.

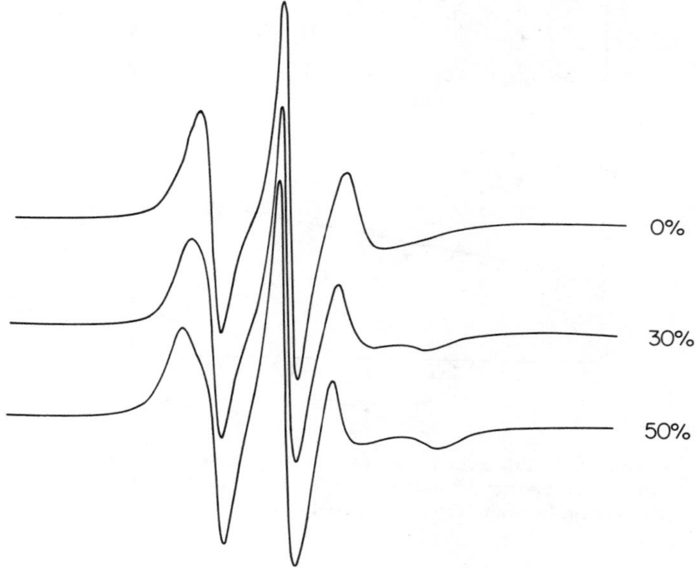

Figure 8.24 ESR spectra from phospholipid spin label ($m, n = 3,10$) incorporated into egg lecithin aqueous dispersions containing 0, 30 and 50 mole% cholesterol

The effect of adding cholesterol, an important component of many biological membranes, to egg lecithin dispersions incorporating a phospholipid spin label is shown in Figure 8.24. Addition of cholesterol is seen to increase the anisotropy of the spin-label spectra, corresponding to an inhibition of the motion of the lipid chains by the rigid cholesterol molecule. Values for P_t at various cholesterol concentrations can be calculated from the measured order parameters using equation (8.4) and are shown in Figure 8.25. It can be seen that the probability of the trans conformation increases with increasing cholesterol. Thus one effect of cholesterol on egg lecithin membranes is to extend and rigidify the fatty acid chains of the phospholipid.

By contrast, when dipalmitoyl lecithin is used instead of egg lecithin, increasing cholesterol causes a decrease in S_o (see equation 8.4) and P_g changes from zero to a finite value (Schreier-Muccillo *et al.*, 1973). In other words the system is fluidized by the formation of gauche isomers in the fatty acid chains. A reasonable explanation for this is the following: dipalmitoyl lecithin, unlike egg lecithin, is

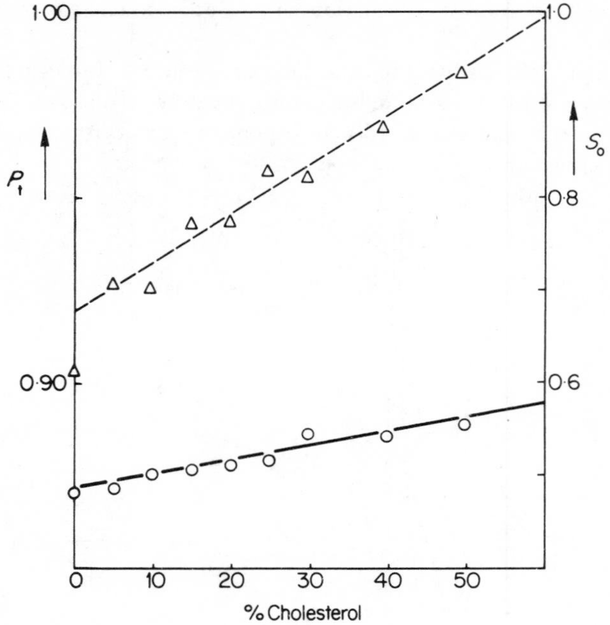

Figure 8.25 Effect of cholesterol on the probability of the trans conformation (P_t-upper curve) in the fatty acid side chains of egg lecithin. (From Schreier-Muccillo *et al.*, 1973)

present in the gel phase at ambient temperatures; the saturated fatty acid chains are present in the all-trans conformation which allows good packing; addition of cholesterol weakens the strong interchain interactions and promotes transition to the liquid-crystalline phase.

The conclusions drawn above about flexibility gradients in the fatty acid side chains of egg lecithin apply equally to functioning biological membranes. ESR spectra from phospholipid spin labels incorporated into the membranes of electron transfer particles prepared from yeast mitochondria are shown in Figure 8.26. The similarity to Figure 8.23 is immediately apparent; a flexibility gradient is again seen, but in this case the profile of the order parameter gradient is modified by the presence of membrane protein.

This is perhaps an appropriate point to discuss briefly how lipid spin labels are incorporated into membranes. For model membranes, incorporation is easy since the spin label and phospholipid can be dissolved together in chloroform. For biological membranes, treatment with chloroform would disrupt the lipid–protein organization. Direct addition of spin label has been surprisingly successful (Rottem *et al.*, 1970; Barnett and Grisham, 1972). Protein mediated exchange (Landsberger *et al.*, 1971; Kamp *et al.*, 1973) and fusion between spin-labelled model membrane vesicles and the biological membrane (Grant and McConnell, 1973) have consider-

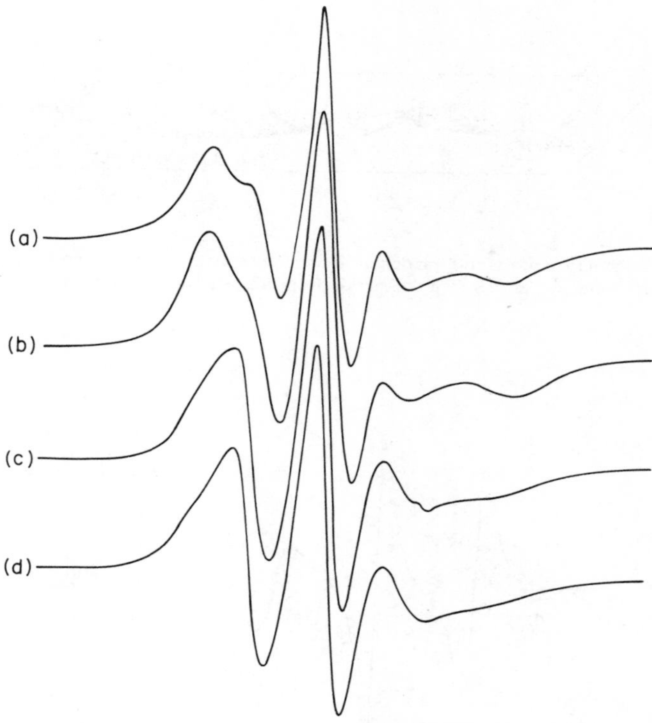

Figure 8.26 ESR spectra from various phospholipid spin labels incorporated into the membranes of electron transfer particles isolated from yeast mitochondria. Spectra (a), (b), (c) and (d) refer to incorporation of phospholipid probes with m, n = 10,3; 8,5; 5,8 and 3,10 respectively

able promise. For microorganisms, perhaps the method of choice is biosynthetic incorporation (Tourtellotte *et al.*, 1970).

Motion of rigid steroids

As an alternative to observing the effect of cholesterol on the behaviour of membranes incorporating phospholipid spin label, steroid spin labels (for example 4′, 4′-Dimethylspiro (5α-cholestane-3,2′-oxazolidin)-3′-yloxyl which is abbreviated to 'cholestane spin label') can be used. Cholestane spin label is a long rigid molecule which would align parallel to the fatty acid side chain in membranes. From Figure 8.27 it can be seen that the largest hyperfine splitting, A_{zz}, would be obtained for the orientation perpendicular to the long axis which is the opposite to that which pertains with fatty acid and related phospholipid spin labels (c.f. Figure 6.20).

ESR spectra obtained from cholestane spin label incorporated into oriented

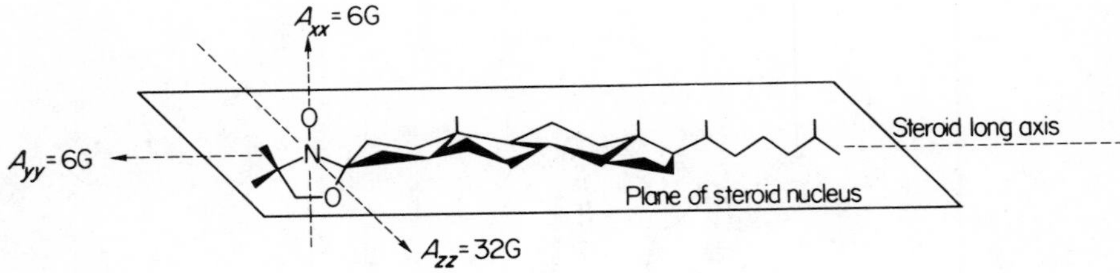

Figure 8.27 Principal axes and principal hyperfine splittings of the cholestane spin label. (From Schreier-Muccillo and Smith, in press. Reproduced by permission of Academic Press, Inc.)

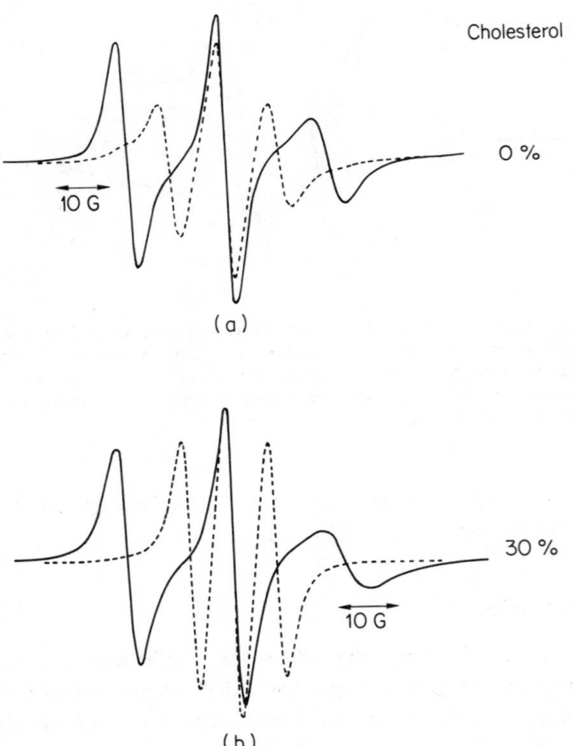

Figure 8.28 ESR spectra of egg lecithin/cholesterol multibilayer films incorporating cholestane spin label. Spectra (a) = 0 mole% cholesterol; Spectra (b) = 30 mole% cholesterol. The solid and dashed lines refer to the magnetic field applied parallel and perpendicular to the film surface respectively. (From Schreier-Muccillo *et al.*, 1973)

multibilayers of egg lecithin plus 0 and 30% cholesterol are shown in Figure 8.28. The advantage of multibilayer films over dispersions is that values for $A_{\parallel}$ and $A_{\perp}$ can more readily be determined. From spectra (a), (0% cholesterol) three conclusions can be drawn. Firstly, the spin label is oriented preferentially parallel to the bilayer normal; this is shown by the smaller splitting when the magnetic field is applied in this direction. Secondly, the spin label must be rotating rapidly about its long axis, otherwise the spectrum recorded with the applied magnetic field parallel to the film surface would be a powder spectrum (as in Figure 6.14a) rather than the clear three-line spectrum which results from rapid motional averaging of the A_{zz} (32 gauss) and A_{xx} (6 gauss) hyperfine splittings. Thirdly, the order parameter (equation 6.20) calculated from Figure 8.28(a) is 0.55. The cholestane spin label must be undergoing another type of motion which averages out the anisotropy. This is a conical motion of the cholestane spin-label long axis of the type shown in Figure 6.22. The angle of the cone, γ (which is a measure of the amplitude of this motion) can be obtained from the order parameter using equation (6.21), giving a value of $\gamma = 46^{\circ}$.

The spectra in Figure 8.28(b) (30% cholesterol) are much more highly ordered with a spin-label order parameter of 0.8. As can be seen from Figure 8.29, the

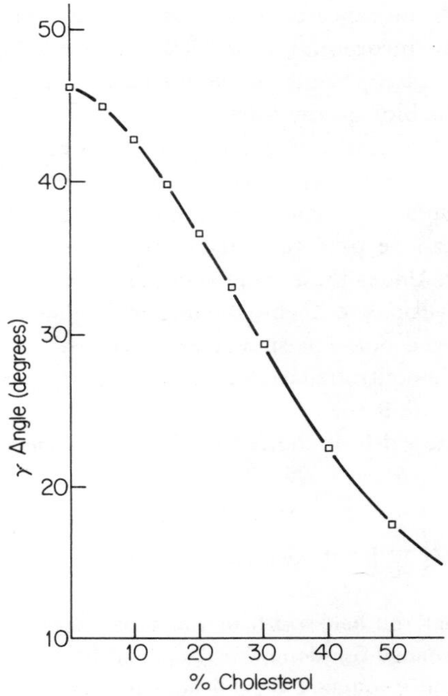

Figure 8.29 The amplitude of conical motion (γ) as a function of cholesterol concentration for cholestane spin label incorporated into egg lecithin multibilayers. (From Schreier-Muccillo *et al.*, 1973)

amplitude of the conical motion decreases with increasing cholesterol until at 50% cholesterol one is approaching almost complete order.

Thus it seems clear that cholesterol can have two effects on egg phosphatidyl choline bilayers. Firstly, it extends and rigidifies the fatty acid chains and secondly, it decreases the amplitude of motion of the fatty acid chains.

Lateral diffusion

Spin labels have been used to study the rates of lateral diffusion in several model and biological membranes (Sackmann and Traüble, 1972; Scandella *et al.*, 1972). Lateral diffusion is an important biological process. The formation of human/mouse hybrid cells leads to complete mixing of surface antigens within 40 minutes of fusion (Frye and Edidin, 1970); a lateral diffusion coefficient of 10^{-10} cm^2/s has been estimated. Again it has been speculated (Adam and Delbrück, 1968) that hormones might reach their target receptors in cells by two-dimensional diffusion along the membrane rather than a less efficient three-dimensional diffusion process.

The method suggested by Sackmann and Traüble (1972) based on analysis of spin—spin exchange interactions has found general acceptance and will therefore be discussed in some detail. Relatively high levels of spin-label incorporation (> 5%) are needed, which might be expected to perturb the membrane; however, Scandella *et al.* (1972) report that incorporation of 2.5% spin-labelled phospholipid does not diminish the ability of sarcoplasmic reticulum to accumulate calcium ions so the perturbation seems to be biologically tolerable.

The spin exchange interaction is quantum mechanical in origin and has a very short range, requiring that the spin labels should virtually be in contact. For situations in which spin-label contacts are controlled by diffusion, the spin exchange interaction can be used to measure the rate of lateral diffusion of the spin-labelled molecules. Under these conditions the diffusion is usually sufficiently rapid that other contributions to linebroadening are negligible; in particular, dipolar contributions are averaged out. For spin-label concentrations up to approximately 30 mole %, the diffusion-controlled exchange interaction leads to broadening of the spin-label spectrum (Figure 8.30).

The peak-to-peak linewidth of the central line in the spectrum (see Figure 8.30) is given by

$$\Delta H_{\text{exchange}} = 2\left(\frac{h}{g\beta}\right) \times W_{\text{exchange}} \tag{8.5}$$

This essentially says that the half-width of the broadening expressed in frequency units is equal to the exchange frequency, W_{exchange}. In this case, the spin-exchange frequency is equal to the frequency of collision between spin labels. The collision frequency clearly depends on the spin-label lateral diffusion coefficient, D_{diff}, and on the fractional mole concentration of spin label, c, together with other geometrical factors. Träuble and Sackmann (1972) utilize the expression

$$W_{\text{exchange}} = 0.17 \times 10^{16} \times D_{\text{diff}} \times c \tag{8.6}$$

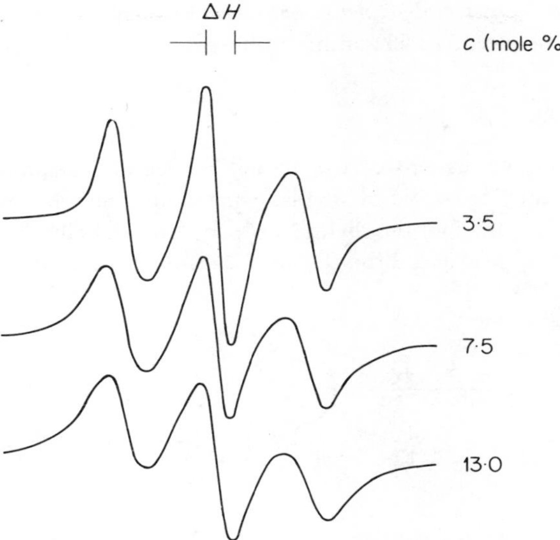

Figure 8.30 Diagram illustrating the exchange broadening of the spin-label spectrum for increasing concentration (*c*) of spin label in phospholipid bilayers. (Reprinted from Sackmann, E., and Traüble, H. (1972). *J. Amer. Chem. Soc.*, **94**, 4482. Copyright by the American Chemical Society)

where the constant (0.17×10^{16}) includes the geometrical factors. Hence the diffusion coefficient can be calculated. It has been found that the lateral mobility of lipids in *E. coli* cytoplasmic membranes ($D_{diff} = 3.25 \times 10^{-8}$ cm^2 s^{-1}; Sackmann *et al.*, 1973) and sarcoplasmic reticulum membranes ($D_{diff} = 6 \times 10^{-8}$ cm^2 s^{-1}; Scandella *et al.*, 1972) is about the same as for dipalmitoyl lecithin aqueous dispersions above the phase transition temperature ($D_{diff} = 3 \times 10^{-8}$ cm^2 s^{-1}; Träuble and Sackmann, 1972). This suggests that the lipids in the two biological membranes providing the diffusion medium are organized as bilayers. In fact fluidity assays using the simple spin label TEMPO (McConnell *et al.*, 1972) suggest that over 80% of sarcoplasmic reticulum membrane is fluid at ambient temperatures and not immobilized by interaction with proteins. Sackmann *et al.* (1973) have calculated from their data on lipid lateral diffusion a value for the lateral diffusion of intercalated proteins; for a protein of molecular weight 100,000 the lateral diffusion coefficient is approximately 3×10^{-10} cm^2 s^{-1} which agrees reasonably with the value obtained for surface antigens by Frye and Edidin (1970). Lateral diffusion of chemically distinct phospholipid species in membranes underlies the phenomenon of lateral phase separations (Linden et al., 1973; Shimshick and McConnell, 1973; Sackmann *et al.*, 1973) which are very important to biological membrane function. However there is reason to believe that not all biological membranes will show high lateral diffusion rates; from the known properties of the purple membrane from *Halobacterium halobium* Scandella *et al.* (1972) speculate that D_{diff} would be several orders of magnitude slower than 10^{-8} cm^2 s^{-1}.

Protein–lipid interactions

From the foregoing discussions of the various modes of phospholipid motion in biological membranes, the value of spin-labelling studies may be appreciated. As a final example, the contributions being made by spin labelling to protein–lipid interactions will be considered. From Figure 8.21 it can be seen that there are many

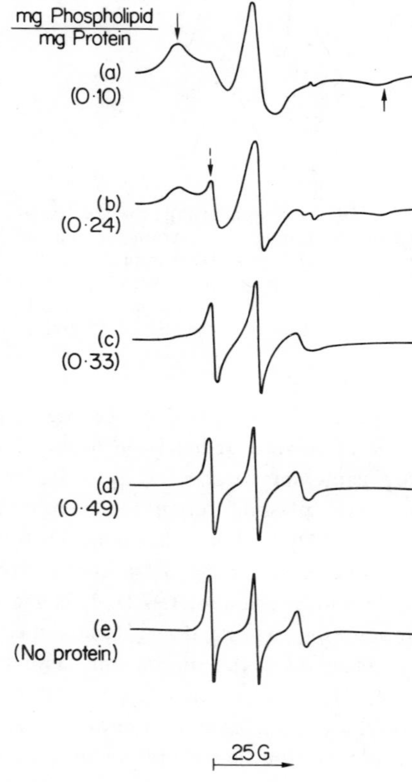

Figure 8.31 ESR spectra of 16-doxyl stearic acid spin label (see Figure 8.22) in buffered aqueous dispersions of membranous cytochrome oxidase with various lipid contents. The lipid-to-protein ratio expressed as mg of lipid per mg of protein is indicated. The spectra have been normalized to the central line height. (From Jost *et al.*, 1973)

different proteins in membranes; even the erythrocyte membrane with its limited biological functions has 10–15 major protein species (Fairbanks *et al.*, 1971). The most promising systems for study of specific protein–lipid interactions are those membranes containing a single protein or a major protein. For direct studies, the purple membrane of *Halobacterium halobium* which contains a single protein resembling rhodopsin, the protein present in retinal rod membranes, is almost unique (Oesterhelt and Stoeckenius, 1971). However, there are several elegant investigations in progress where the biological function of purified protein are reconstituted by reintegration into membranes with defined composition. Rhodopsin (Hong and Hubbell, 1973), the calcium-dependent ATPase from sarcoplasmic reticulum (Warren *et al.*, 1974; Seelig and Hasselbach, 1971) and cytochrome oxidase (Jost *et al.*, 1973) are good examples. The part which spin labelling might play in these reconstitution investigations is well illustrated by the studies on cytochrome oxidase. The purified protein is depleted of bound phospholipid, then reconstituted by titration with an aqueous dispersion of phospholipid containing incorporated fatty acid spin label. The ESR spectra at different lipid–protein ratios are shown in Figure 8.31.

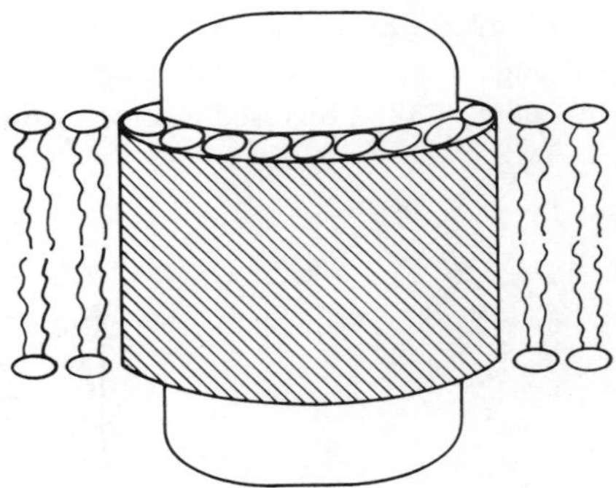

Figure 8.32 Diagrammatic representation of a single protein complex and associated phospholipid in membraneous cytochrome oxidase. (From Jost *et al.*, 1973)

At low lipid–protein ratios, the spectrum consists of a single immobilized component. At higher lipid–protein ratios, both immobilized and mobile components can be seen; these two components can be resolved by computer simulation of the spectra. Calculations show that the immobilized phospholipid provides an immobilized lipid monolayer 'skin' surrounding the protein which is thereby separated from the lipid bilayer (see Figure 8.32); the mobile components in the ESR spectrum corresponds to the spin label in the bilayer.

More detailed spin-label studies on this system should provide information on how the immobilized lipid participates in the function of cytochrome oxidase.

8.5 Application of ESR in biology

Photosynthesis

The biochemical steps in the photosynthesis of sugars have been well characterized through the work of Calvin and others (Calvin and Bassham, 1962). However, our understanding of how light energy is used to generate reduced nicotinamide adenine dinucleotide phosphate (NADPH) is fragmentary. In plant chloroplasts, two different photoreactions are involved each with its own pigment system. One photosystem, designated Photosystem II (PS II), operates efficiently with red light ($\lambda \sim 680$ nm) and produces an oxidant $\overset{+}{P}_{680}$ with an electrode potential (*Em*) $\approx +800$ mV which is sufficiently high to oxidize water to oxygen, together with a reductant (X^-) whose electrode potential is low enough to reduce plastoquinone. Electron transfer through cytochromes and the copper protein plastocyanin then occurs spontaneously and can be coupled to the synthesis of ATP. The second light reaction, designated Photosystem I (PS I), operates with longer-wavelength light ($\lambda \sim 700$ nm) and produces a weak oxidant P^{+}_{700} (*Em* $\approx$ 500 mV) and a strong reductant (A^-) whose *Em* of ~ -500 mV is capable of reducing nicotinamide adenine dinucleotide phosphate ($NADP^+$). These reactions are summarized in Figure 8.33.

The light reactions in photosynthetic bacteria also leads to the production of oxidants and reductants though a recent review (Parsons, 1974) concludes that here the $NADP^+$ is reduced by energy linked reversed electron flow rather than by direct

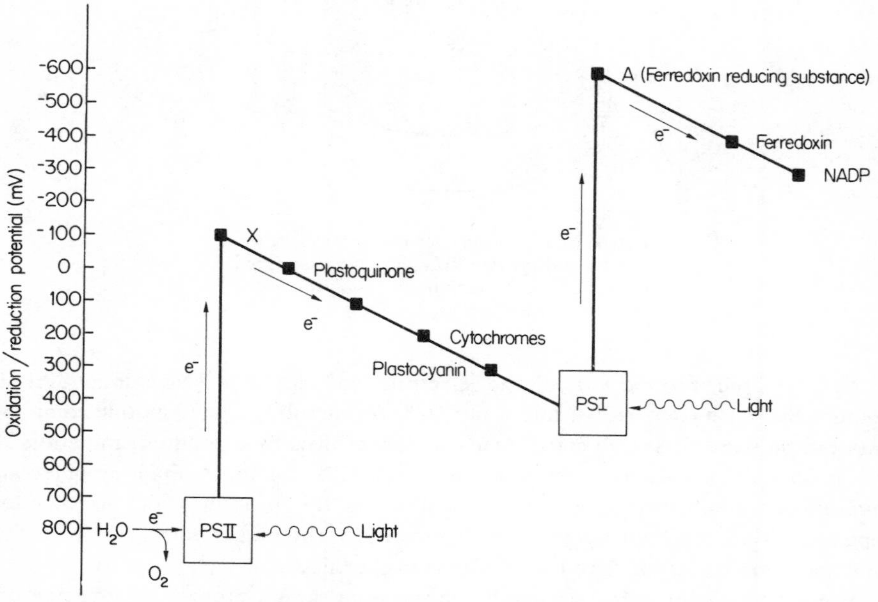

Figure 8.33 Simplified scheme for photosynthetic electron transfer

photoreduction involving a species with a very low *Em*. The identity of the primary oxidants and reductants in chloroplasts (P^{+}_{680}, P^{+}_{700}, A^{-} and X^{-}) and the comparable species in photosynthetic bacteria is still uncertain and it is here that ESR can provide valuable information.

Commoner and his associates (Commoner *et al.*, 1956; 1957) were the first to show that unpaired electrons are generated when suspensions of chloroplasts are irradiated by visible light; two radicals designated signals I and II were detected (see Figure 8.34). Since signal I could also be produced by irradiation of chloroplasts frozen at $-140\,^{\circ}$C (Sogo *et al.*, 1957), the hope was raised that one was observing the primary *physical* event in photosynthesis.

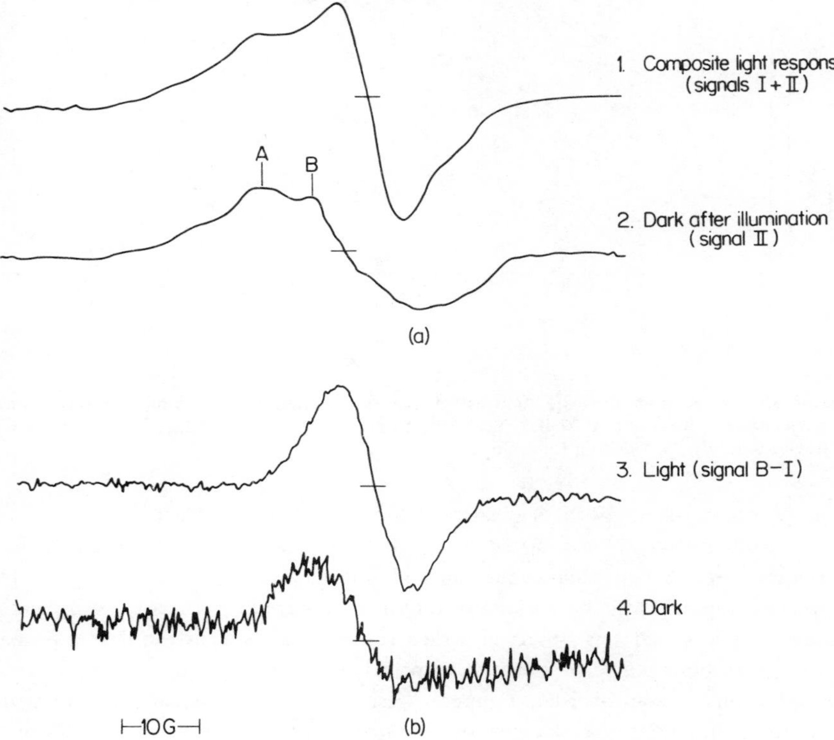

Figure 8.34 Typical ESR signals from chloroplasts (a) and photosynthetic bacteria (b). For chloroplasts, two signals (I and II) are seen during illumination; signal I rapidly decays when illumination ceases leaving only signal II. For photosynthetic bacteria an ESR signal resembling signal I appears on illumination. (From Kohl, 1972)

It is interesting to note that photosynthetic bacteria on illumination give rise to a species resembling signal I only, i.e. no signal II; therefore efforts to identify signal I have been simplified by using 'chromatophores' which are fragments broken from the membranes of photosynthetic bacteria by mechanical shear. There is a good correlation between the light induced optical and ESR changes (Figure 8.35)

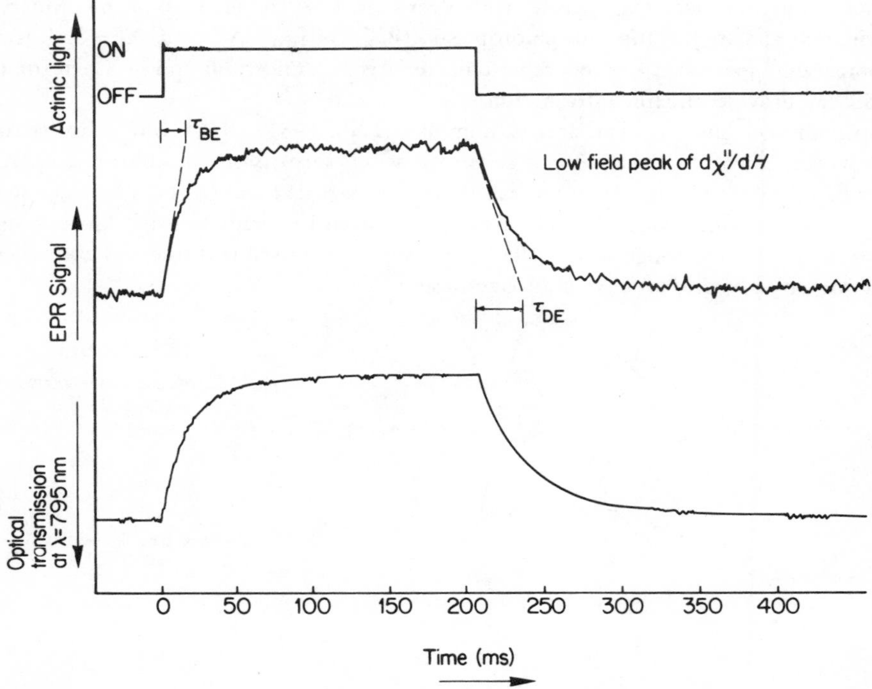

Figure 8.35 ESR and optical kinetics of reaction centres in chromatophores from *Rhodospirillum* spheroides at 77 K. (From McElroy *et al.*, 1969. Reproduced by permission of Elsevier Scientific Publishing Company)

which points to them both originating from bacteriochlorophyll derivatives; the *g*-values and linewidths of signal I are very similar to those obtained from bacteriochlorophyll following oxidation with iodine and it may be concluded that the species responsible is bacteriochlorophyll. In Figure 8.35 there is no indication of a lag before signal I is observed which supports the suggestion that a primary product is responsible; also both the optical and ESR spectral changes can be observed even at liquid-helium temperatures, where no *chemical* reaction would occur, suggesting that the changes are *physical* in origin. Similar kinetic evidence has been presented (Beinert, Kok and Hoch, 1962; Warden and Bolton, 1972) that signal I in chloroplasts is the chlorophyll P^{+}_{700} present in PS I.

The primary electron acceptor in chloroplast PS I (the species A^{-}) has been shown by optical kinetic and low-temperature ESR studies to be a bound iron-sulphur protein (Bearden and Malkin, 1975) which can only be detected by ESR below 40 K (Figure 8.36). In addition to this iron-sulphur protein which functions as the primary electron acceptor, there are probably several other iron-sulphur proteins at PS I. The complexity of the iron-sulphur proteins in chloroplasts could be comparable to that in mitochondria.

Considering now photosystem II, the site in chloroplasts which leads to oxygen

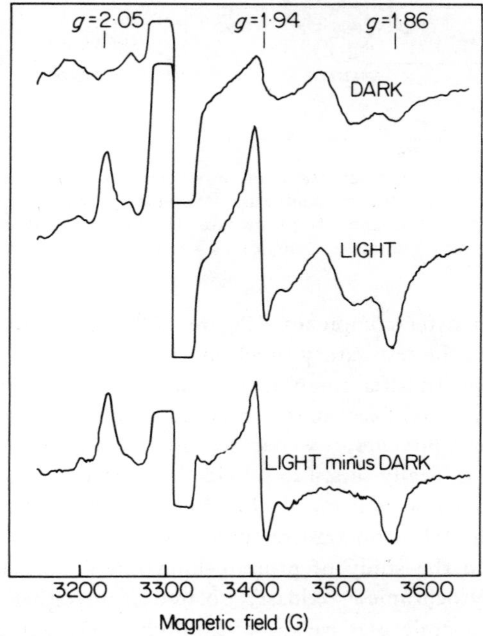

Figure 8.36 Light induced ESR changes of bound iron-sulphur protein in whole chloroplasts after illumination at 25 K with 715 nm actinic light (from Bearden and Malkin, 1972). The light minus dark spectrum should be compared with Figure 9.27 which shows the ESR spectra of iron-sulphur centres in the enzyme xanthine oxidase

production. The ESR properties of signal II are similar to those of P^{+}_{700} and the bacteriochlorophyll radical; it seems reasonable to conclude that it is chlorophyll P^{+}_{680}. Finally the detection by ESR of a species which could be the primary acceptor at PS II has been claimed (Malkin and Bearden, 1973) though it has not yet been identified. There are certainly many other components in the electron-transfer systems of chloroplasts and photosynthetic bacteria which will be detected and identified by ESR.

The mitochondrial respiratory chain

The efficient reoxidation of reduced pyridine nucleotides and flavo proteins through the mitochondrial respiratory chain is a process of fundamental importance in most cells. However, the complexity of the multiprotein mitochondrial membrane is such that, despite intensive effort, the molecular mechanisms involved are essentially unknown. The mitochondrial respiratory chain can be fractionated into

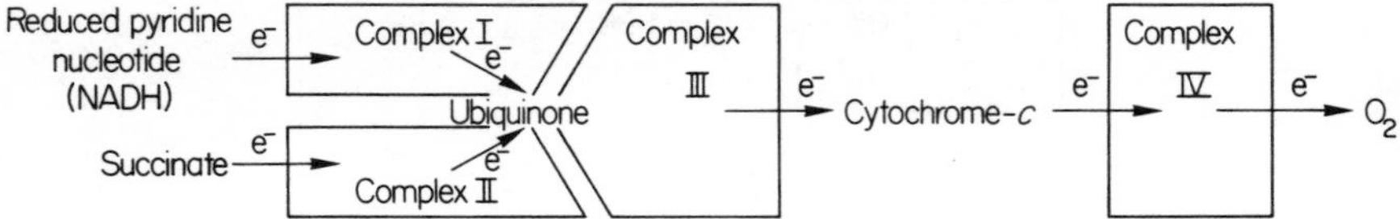

Figure 8.37 Schematic representation of how the four electron transfer complexes reconstitute to produce the mitochondrial respiratory chain. Complex I = NADH–Ubiquinone reductase; Complex II = succinate–Ubiquinone reductase; Complex III = Ubiquinol–cytochrome-*c* reductase; Complex IV = cytochrome-*c* oxidase

simpler 'electron transfer complexes' (Figure 8.37) which, when mixed together, reconstitute some of the respiratory function.

All these electron transfer components contain transition-metal ions which are paramagnetic in their oxidized and/or reduced forms; in addition, several of the electron transfer components give rise to radicals on reduction. It can be seen therefore that ESR is ideally suited to provide information on this problem.

The present discussion will mostly be limited to cytochrome oxidase, the best characterized of the 'electron transfer particles'; the membrane location of cytochrome oxidase and the study of protein–lipid interactions has been considered in Section 8.4. Cytochrome-*c* oxidase, isolated from either beef heart or yeast mitochondria, has a molecular weight of approximately 200,000. The enzyme is composed of seven subunits, three of which are synthesized in the mitochondria and four on cytoplasmic ribosomes (Schatz *et al.*, 1972). The enzyme contains two moles of cytochrome-*a* (cytochrome-*a* and a_3) and two copper ion centres. The cytochromes are present in a variety of high- and low-spin forms (see Chapter 6) according to conditions (Van Gelder and Beinert, 1969; Orme-Johnson *et al.*, 1973). The short electron spin–lattice relaxation times for the cytochromes and copper centres mean that ESR measurements must be made on frozen solutions at 100 K or, better, 10 K; this comment equally applies to paramagnetic centres,found in other electron transfer particles, particularly iron-sulphur proteins. A typical ESR spectru from the *a*-type cytochrome oxidase is shown in Figure 8.38.

The spectrum has contributions from low-spin (*g*-values of 3.0, 2.2 and 1.5) and high-spin (*g*-values of 6 and 2) ferric components. Van Gelder and Beinert (1969) concluded that the high-spin component was due to cytochrome-a_3 (cytochrome-a_3 is the component which, in its reduced state, reacts with oxygen or carbon monoxide and which has a higher electrode potential than cytochrome-*a*). However a more recent investigation (Hartzell, Hansen and Beinert, 1973) concludes that most of the high- and low-spin signals can be attributed to cytochrome-*a* with little contribution from cytochrome $-a_3$. This result will be discussed later in the section.

The ESR spectrum from copper in cytochrome oxidase (see Figure 8.39(has $g_{\perp} = 2.03$, $g_{\parallel} = 2.17$ and an extremely small $A_{\parallel}$ ($<$ 80 MHz) which does not allow the Cu hyperfine structure to be resolved. As has been discussed for type 1 copper in laccase (see Section 8.2), this indicates extensive electron delocalization and is consistent with a redox function for the copper.

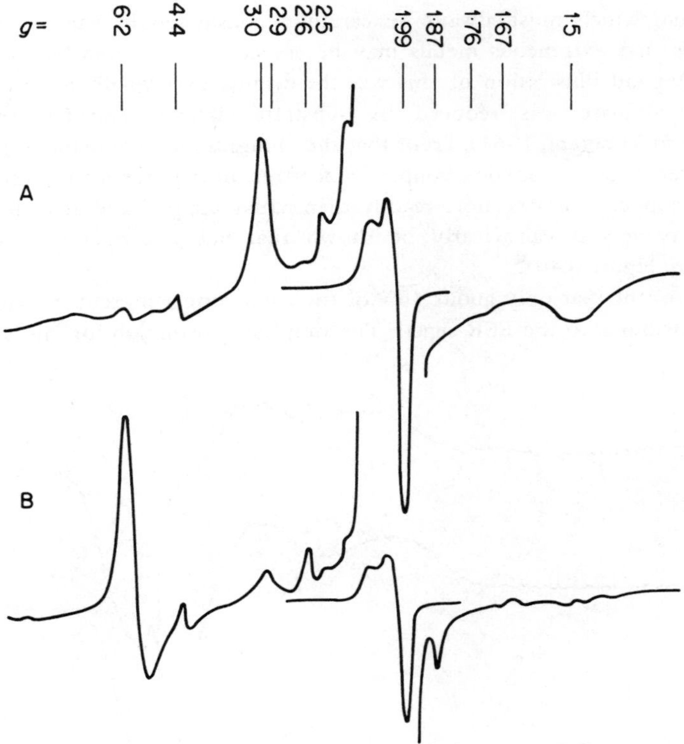

Figure 8.38 ESR spectra from cytochrome oxidase recorded at 81 K. Spectrum A is the native enzyme and spectrum B the enzyme 50% reduced with ascorbate under anaerobic conditions. The copper ESR signal (*g*-value approximately 2.0) had to be recorded with a 20-fold diminished gain.)From Van Gelder and Beinert, 1969. Reproduced by permission of Elsevier Scientific Publishing Company)

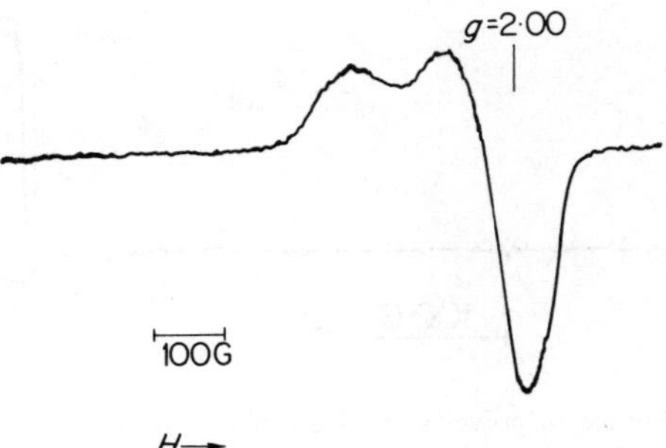

Figure 8.39 Cu^{2+} ESR spectrum of native cytochrome oxidase seen at 100 K. (Modified from Beinert, 1966)

A problem which must always be carefully considered in studies on metalloproteins is that extraneous metals may be associated with even highly purified materials. A good illustration of this was the dispute over whether the copper in cytochrome oxidase was reduced by substrate (Beinert and Palmer, 1964; Ehrenberg and Yonetani, 1961). Proof that the failure to observe reduction was due to the presence of extraneous copper came from microwave saturation studies; extraneous copper saturates more readily than native copper, and at high incident microwave powers it can clearly be shown that native copper *is* reduced by substrate (see Figure 8.40).

It is significant that only about 40% of the total copper present in cytochrome oxidase contributes to the ESR signal. The simplest explanation for this is that the

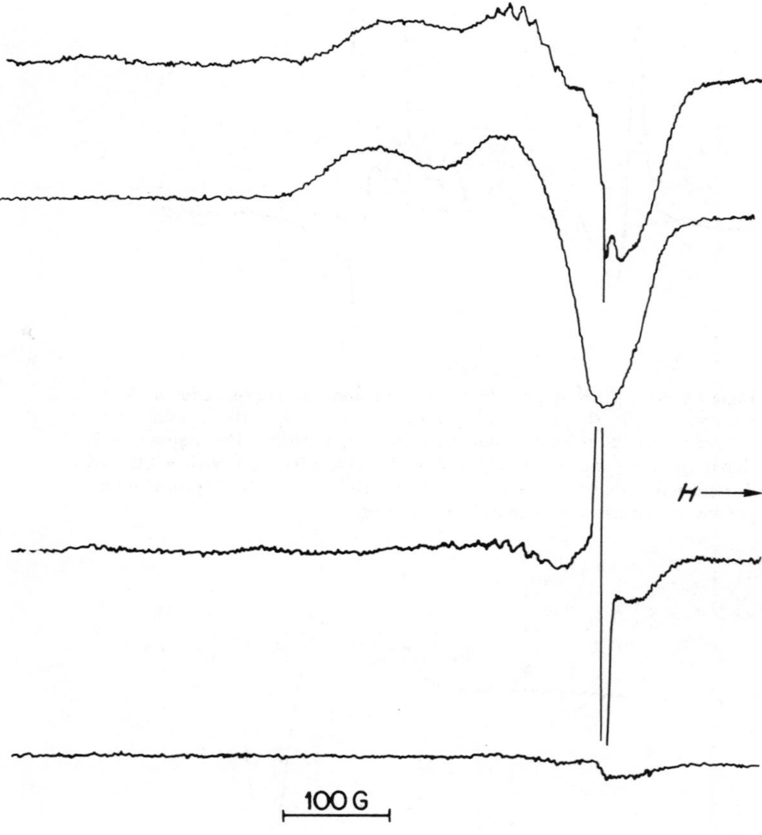

Figure 8.40 Difference in power saturation of two different species of copper present in cytochrome oxidase. The ESR signals from the oxidized enzyme at low and high microwave powers are similar (upper two spectra). Reduction with ascorbate (lower two spectra) plus cytochrome-*c* reveals a residual extraneous Cu^{2+} signal underlying the ascorbate radical. This residual signal disappears at high microwave power. (Modified from Beinert, 1966)

other copper is diamagnetic cuprous. However, this would not be consistent with the results of reductive titration experiments (Hartzell, Hansen and Beinert, 1973) performed under anaerobic conditions which show that electrons from four reduced cytochrome-*c* molecules can be accomodated on the enzyme; since there are only four known redox components (cytochromes-*a*, -a_3 and the two coppers), both coppers in the oxidized enzyme would need to be cupric. An alternative explanation for the low intensity of the copper ESR signal is that interaction occurs between one or both of these coppers and a neighbouring rapidly relaxing species. The iron in the cytochromes has a short electron spin relaxation time and from what has been said earlier about the failure to detect cytochrome-a_3 by ESR, it would seem plausible that one of the coppers and cytochrome-a_3 are spin paired. Certainly adjacent copper and iron centres suggest an efficient electron transfer unit which has been discussed already for laccase (see Section 8.2).

Significant progress is being made through parallel application of electronic absorption spectroscopy and ESR to mitochondria and sonicated submitochondrial particles. Thus although the cytochromes in mitochondria give poorly resolved ESR spectra (Van Gelder and Beinert, 1969), their electronic spectra are clearly resolved with an absorption band for cytochrome-a_3 being particularly marked. The most readily assigned ESR signal observed in mitochondria is that from the cupric centre of cytochrome oxidase. During aerobic reduction of mitochondria with reduced pyridine nucleotide, the copper signal remains essentially unreduced which is consistent with the position of cytochrome oxidase as the terminal electron acceptor. Recently, resolution of the ESR signals from the iron-sulphur proteins in reduced submitochondrial particles has been achieved The experimental approach has been found to feed in electrons selectively to particular sections of the respiratory chain by controlled anaerobic reduction or from artifical electron-reduction mediators of known redox potential. (Orme-Johnson *et al.*, 1971; Ohnishi *et al.*, 1972). From these studies, the redox potentials of several iron-sulphur centres have been determined and the way is cleared for more detailed studies, using rapid-freeze methods (Chapter 9) for example, on the electron transfer sequence and mechanism. Into this sequences it will be necessary to accomodate new carriers whose presence has been indicated by ESR (Orme-Johnson *et al.*, 1971 and 1973) and 'well-established' carriers (for example coenzyme Q) whose behaviour during respiration can be monitored by ESR (Bäckström *et al.*, 1970). It would appear that ESR is a powerful tool for detecting new mitochondrial elementary particles.

8.6 Applications of ESR in medicine

Free radicals are known to be generated in biological material by irradiation or by contact with pyrrolysed hydrocarbons. It is of great medical importance to know how these physical and chemical effectors act and whether the changes are important in carcinogenesis. ESR studies on irradiated amino acids and nucleotides provides a sound basis from which an interpretation of the results of more ambitious studies on proteins, nucleic acids and biological tissue might be possible.

Many hormones and drugs produce free radical derivatives through chemical or metabolic reactions. The importance of these radicals to the biological function can be studied by ESR.

Irradiated amino acids and proteins

When single crystals of cystine are exposed to γ-irradiation, a characteristic ESR spectrum results (Figure 8.41). It can be seen that the splitting in each doublet is independent of microwave frequency and is therefore produced by hyperfine interactions, not by g-value anisotropy (see Chapter 9). By contrast the separation between the two sets of doublets is both frequency and orientation dependent, which shows that the radical has large g-value anisotropy: the magnitude of this anisotropy suggests that a sulphur radical is involved. An explanation for these results is that γ-irradiation has caused rupture of the S–S bond to produce two differently oriented radicals

$$^{3}CH_2{-}S{-}S{-}CH_2$$
$$H_2N{-}^{2}CH{-}CO_2H \quad H_2N{-}CH{-}CO_2H \xrightarrow{\text{irradiation}} \begin{matrix} CH_2 \quad S^{\ominus} \\ | \\ H_2N{-}\underset{H}{C}{-}CO_2H \end{matrix} + \begin{matrix} {}^{\ominus}S \quad CH_2 \\ | \\ H_2N{-}\underset{H}{C}{-}C_2H \end{matrix}$$

Each doublet arises from delocalization of unpaired electron density from the sulphur to an adjacent carbon-bound hydrogen. The reason for interaction with a

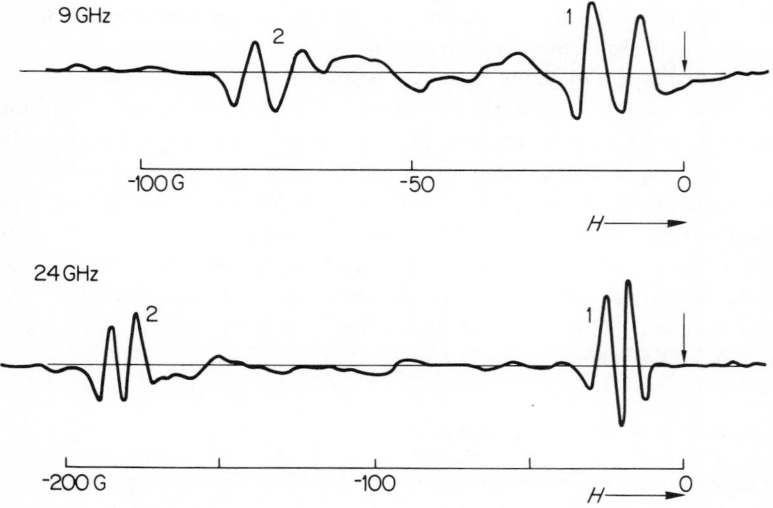

Figure 8.41 ESR spectrum from γ-irradiated cystine hydrochloride. The spectra are plotted for an orientation at which the applied magnetic field makes an angle of 30° to the b-axis and hence both doublets are seen. The spectra here are displayed as the second derivative of the absorption, thus the major peaks correspond to the centres of the lines. (From Gordy and Kurita, 1960)

single proton (to produce a doublet) is not immediately obvious. One explanation is that bond orientation brings the single C_2 proton close to the sulphur. The lability of the S—S bond to irradiation may be noted since cystine linkages are important in maintaining the tertiary structure of proteins.

Similar irradiation of other amino acid single crystals produces radicals of general formula

$$H_2N-\underset{\odot}{\overset{\overset{\displaystyle R}{|}}{C}}-CO_2H$$

Hyperfine splitting in the ESR signal by protons from the side grouping R is observed, e.g. the three methyl protons in alanine produce a 1:3:3:1 intensity quartet. A similar spectrum is observed from irradiated poly-L-alanine (Figure 8.42). However when polypeptides consisting of several amino acids are irradiated, the ESR spectra can be complex. For proteins, a detailed analysis becomes virtually impossible though certain dominating species, for example the doublet resulting from cystine cleavage, can be distinguished. It has been shown that whatever primary amino acid radical is formed from irradiation of a protein, continued irradiation leads to localization of the unpaired spins at the cystine bridge; this can readily be detected by the increase in *g*-value.

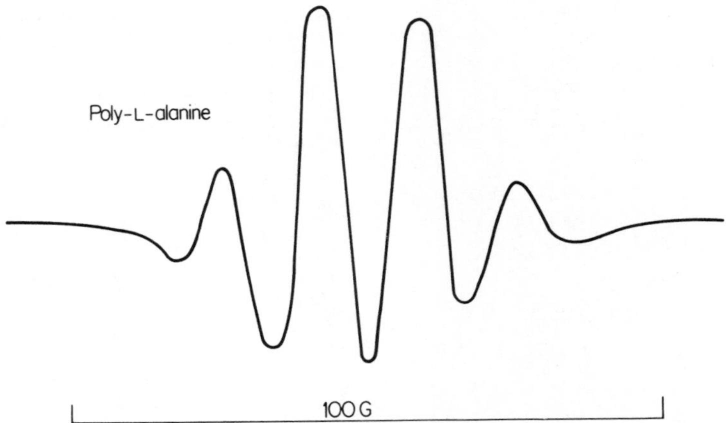

Figure 8.42 Radical generated by X-irradiation of poly-L-alanine showing quartet hyperfine structure. The spectra here are displayed as the second derivative of the ESR absorption. (From Patten and Gordy, 1964)

The mechanism whereby the electron migrates from its primary to its secondary site is of considerable interest since it could provide information on how electron transfer between transition-metal sites in redox proteins occurs. Blumenfeld and Kalmanson (1961) have speculated that conduction of the electron between sites might occur through the hydrogen-bonded secondary structure of the protein (Figure 8.43). Whilst this mechanism might occur in redox proteins, there is no

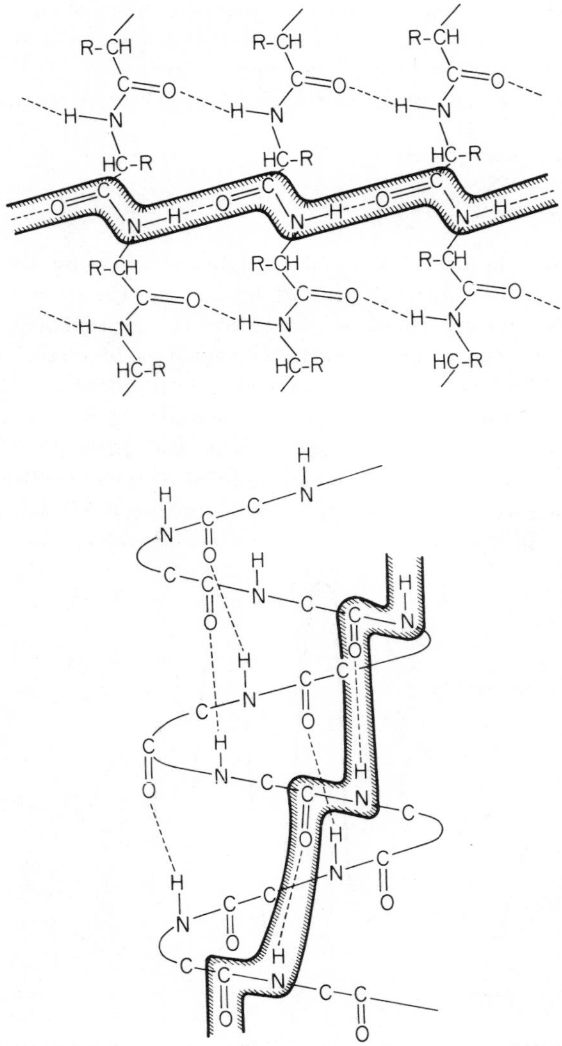

Figure 8.43 Schematic representation of the hydrogen-bonded conduction channels in proteins. The upper part of the figure shows the *inter*-chain hydrogen bonding in the β sheet structure and the lower part shows the *Intra*-chain hydrogen bonding in α helical structure. (Henriksen, 1969. Reproduced by permission of McGraw–Hill Book Company from *Solid State Biophysics*, S. J. Wyard, copyright © 1969 by McGraw–Hill, Inc.)

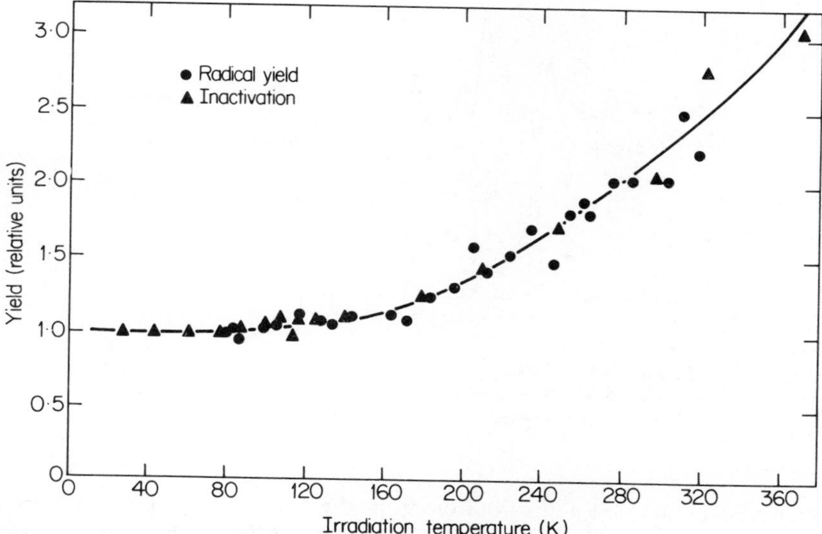

Figure 8.44 Effect of the irradiation temperature on both the production of secondary radicals and the loss of enzymic activities for trypsin. (From Henriksen, 1969. Reproduced by permission of McGraw–Hill Book Company from *Solid State Biophysics*, S. J. Wyard, copyright © 1969 by McGraw–Hill, Inc.)

necessity to invoke it for irradiated proteins since no more radicals are produced in the protein than in an equimolar mixture of the component amino acids. Henriksen (1969) has suggested that direct interaction between the primary radical and the secondary site would give an adequate explanation of the results.

These studies were extended to establish correlations between secondary radicals and biological damage. Solid trypsin was irradiated *in vacuo* at different temperatures and left for 20 minutes to allow secondary reactions to proceed to completion. Figure 8.44 shows clearly that there is a good correlation between radical yield and inactivation of the enzyme.

Irradiated nucleotides and nucleic acids

Detailed studies have been made of the radicals arising from the irradiation of single crystals of thymidine and cytosine. The ESR spectrum for irradiated thymidine is shown in Figure 8.45.

There is an intensity distribution 1:3:5:7:7:5:3:1. The radical responsible for such an intensity distribution is probably

```
          O
          ‖
        ⁄ C ⁀
H — N        ⊙C — CH₃
    |         |  ⁄H
O = C         C
      ⁀ N ⁄     ⁀H
        |
        R
```

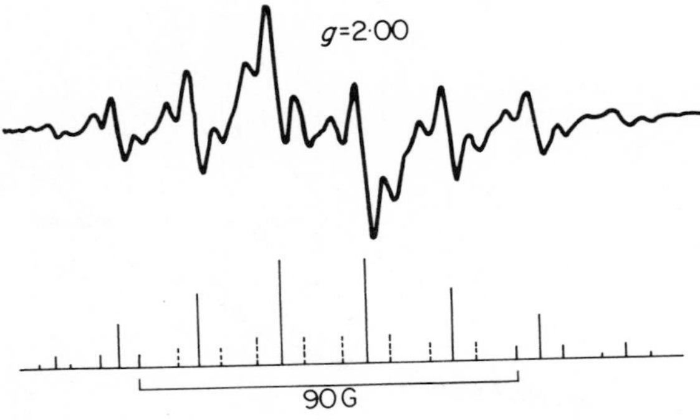

Figure 8.45 ESR spectrum of a γ-irradiated single crystal of thymidine. The magnetic field is applied parallel to the b'-axis of the crystal. (From Pruden, Snipes and Gordy, 1965)

There would be a 1:3:3:1 distribution from the three methyl protons (assumed equivalent if the methyl group is free to rotate); each line of the quartet would be further split by the two methylene protons to give either

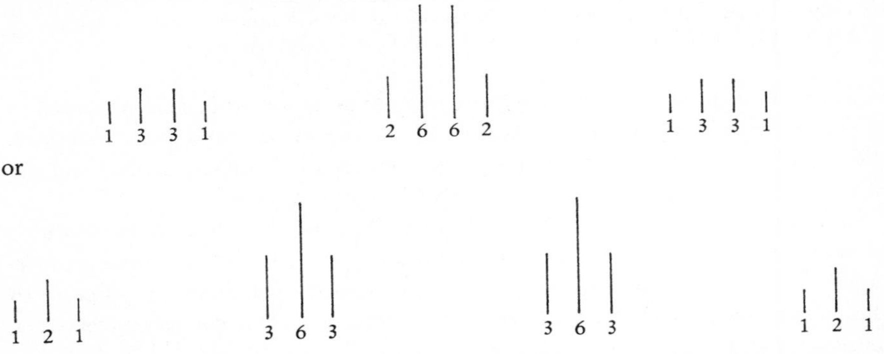

depending upon whether the hyperfine splitting constants for the methylene protons are greater than for the methyl protons and vice versa. In fact

Methyl protons = 20.5 gauss

Methylene protons = 40.5 gauss

The high degree of overlap in the observed spectrum results from one hyperfine splitting being almost an exact multiple of the other.

The ESR spectrum from an irradiated single crystal of cytosine monohydrate is shown in Figure 8.46 and corresponds to the magnetic field being applied along the a-axis. A broad central absorption with satellite structure is clearly seen. When the microwave power incident on the sample is increased, the central and satellite absorption bands saturate differently showing that at least two different radicals have been produced. It is possible to study these separately; the procedure will be

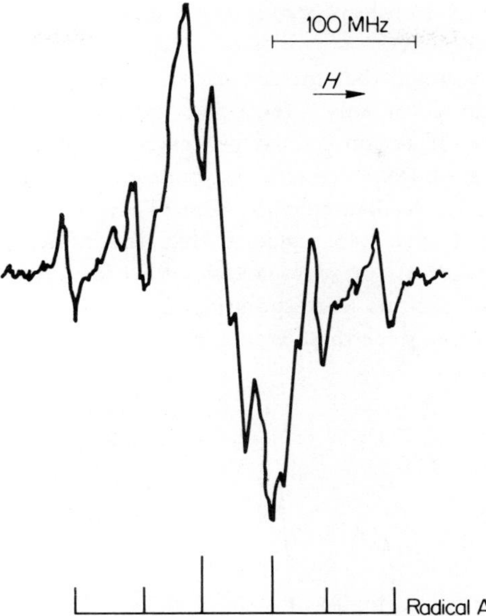

Figure 8.46 ESR spectrum of a γ-irradiated single crystal of cytosine monohydrate. The magnetic field is applied parallel to the *a*-axis of the crystal. The 1:1:2:2:1:1 intensity distribution from one of the radical species present is shown at the bottom. (From Cook and Wyard, 1969. Reproduced by permission of McGraw–Hill Book Company from *Solid State Biophysics*, S. J. Wyard, copyright © 1969 by McGraw–Hill, Inc.)

illustrated for one of the species (Radical A) only. Some of the satellite absorption lines shown in Figure 8.46 correspond to a 1:1:2:2:1:1 intensity distribution which suggests interactions of the unpaired electron with one α-proton and two equivalent β-protons. The satellite spectrum does not change when D_2O replaces H_2O as the medium showing that these hydrogens are not bonded to nitrogen. On the basis of this evidence, the probable structure for the radical is

NH_2
N C H
H
O=C ⊙C—H
N
H

Detailed confirmation for this structure comes from analysis of the splitting by the α-proton as a function of crystal orientation in each plane of rotation. From this data, the isotropic and anisotropic components of the splitting can be obtained together with the relationship between the principal axes (determined by ESR) and the crystallographic axes.

It is generally assumed that the sensitivity of living cells to irradiation is due to DNA damage. Cleavage of only a few bonds in the long DNA polymer chain would have extensive side effects on cellular processes. In agreement with this suggestion, irradiation of isolated DNA reduces the molecular weight dramatically (McGrath and Williams, 1966). A characteristic 8-line ESR spectrum results (Figure 8.47). Comparison with Figure 8.45 suggests that the radical responsible is that of thymidine. Other radicals present have not thus far been identified. Of particular interest would be radicals corresponding to cleavage of the amino groups in adenosine and cytosine since these would greatly influence base pair recognition.

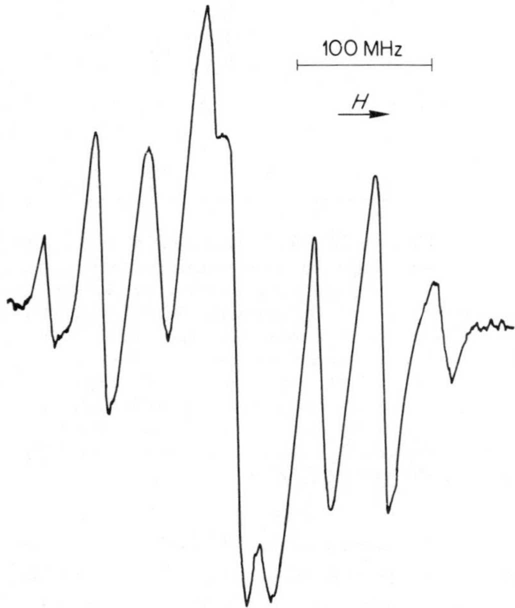

Figure 8.47 ESR spectrum of irradiated DNA. (From Cook and Wyard, 1966. Reproduced by permission of Macmillan (Journals) Ltd)

ESR studies of animal tissue

This is a field which should be left to research workers with extensive experience of both ESR and biology. In a recent review (Heckley, 1972), it was concluded that although there have been numerous investigations of lyophilized tissue, the free radical content of these preparations does not reflect the level of free radicals in the original material. To some extent this is due to reaction of the radicals with oxygen during the lyophilization process. Although there is diagnostic potential in the use of lyophilized samples from biopsy, great caution must be exercised to avoid the many experimental pitfalls.

As has been discussed in Section 7.7, a major problem of working with tissue slices or homogenates at room temperature is the non-resonant absorption by the water; rapid freezing of the sample overcomes this problem though the ESR spectrum becomes more complex due to the detection at low temperatures of both paramagnetic transition ions and radicals, some of which may be artefacts of the freezing process.

With these cautionary points in mind, a brief survey of this field can be attempted. Comparisons of the ESR signals from different organs have been made. The following pattern for radical content has emerged (Swartz, 1972).

$$\text{Liver} > \text{Kidney} > \text{Heart} > \text{Spleen} > \text{Lung} = \text{Muscle}$$

Most of the signals originate from the microsomes and mitochondria where oxidative processes are occurring. However, there does not appear to be a correlation between the free radical and mitochondrial contents. Thus the mitochondrial content of muscle is high but the radical content is low. Again ACTH stimulated adrenals show a small *decrease* in free radical concentrations whilst adrenals from cortisone suppressed animals showed no change from normal.

Mason *et al.* (1965) have fractionated liver cells into mitochondrial, microsomal and supernatant components and shown that qualitatively all the features of the original ESR spectrum can be demonstrated on remixing these components. It is reasonable to believe that as our knowledge of mitochondrial and microsomal oxidative processes advances, so will our understanding of the ESR signals detected from whole cells. At present, identification of individual radical species from the envelope of signals in the $g = 2.0$ region is impossible.

Carcinogenesis

The observations that carcinogenesis can be induced by irradiation of normal tissues or by contact of normal tissue and pyrrolysed hydrocarbons suggests a possible link between free radicals and cancer. A well confirmed finding is that the free radical content of neoplastic tissue is *less* than that of normal. The biological reason for this has been the subject of speculation; for example, radicals normally produced by metabolism might 'scavenge' the carcinogenic free radicals as a defence mechanism or alternatively radical concentration might regulate cell division which is uncontrolled in the neoplastic condition. Reports that addition of free radical scavengers (such as cystine and butylated hydroxytoluene) to the diet of mice increased their life span (Harman 1961, 1962) make fascinating reading but require further substantiation.

ESR signals from transition-metal ions, unlike those from free radicals, are stronger in neoplastic than in normal tissue. Vithayathil *et al.* (1965) have detected a characteristic $g = 2.035$ signal in rat liver following feeding with various carcinogens, notably *p*-dimethylaminoazobenzene (butter yellow), which are known to cause hepatomas (Figure 8.48). This signal precedes by several weeks the usual

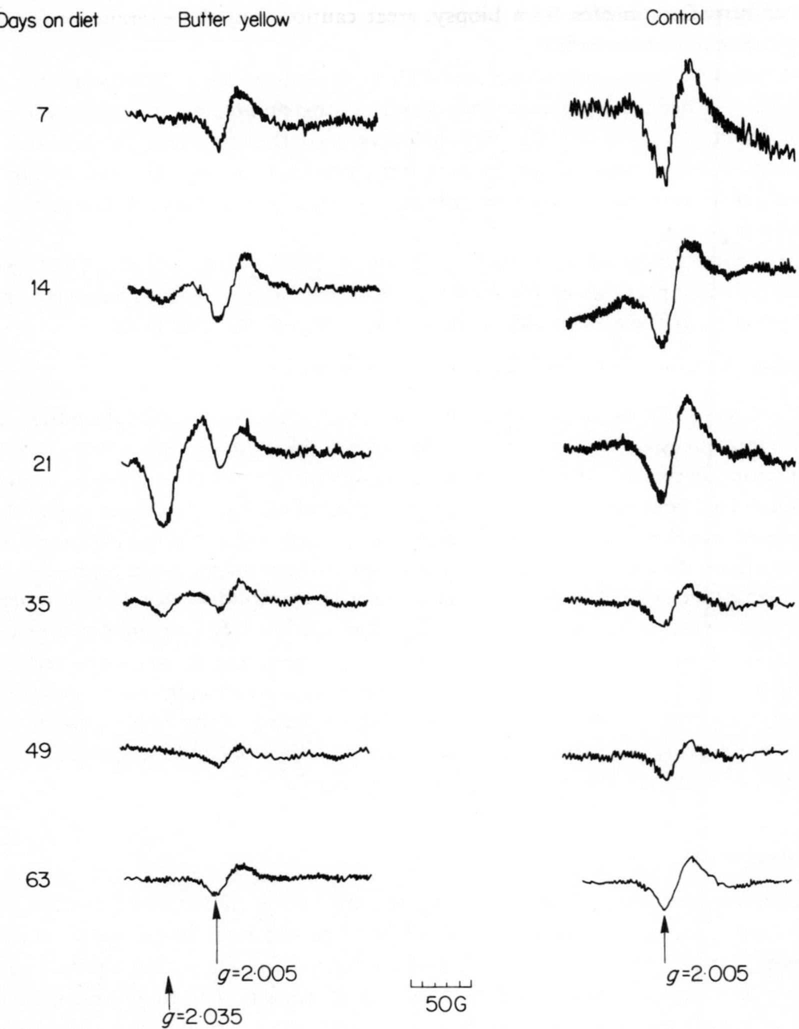

Figure 8.48 ESR signals from liver slices of rats fed on a diet containing 0.06% *p*-dimethylaminoazobenzene and of rats fed on a control diet lacking the carcinogen. (From Vithayathil *et al.*, 1965. Reproduced by permission of Macmillan (Journals) Ltd)

biochemical and histological manifestations of the disease and in fact has disappeared before the tumour transformation has occurred. Obviously this could be important in diagnosis.

The structure of polycyclic carcinogens is compatible with their ready conversion to stable free radical derivatives. However the ability to form free radicals does not immediately allow assignment of a particular hydrocarbon as a carcinogen.

L Region

K Region

Figure 8.49 Regions of polycyclic hydrocarbon structure essential for carcinogenic activity

Pullman and Pullman (1963) have applied molecular orbital calculations to show what features of a polycyclic aromatic ring system are essential to carcinogens. They considered the exchange integrals (β) of the K- and L-regions of the hydrocarbon (see Figure 8.49) and made the predictions that

(i) The K-region must have an index less than 3.31 β.

(ii) If there is both a K- and L-region, then a compound will not be a carcinogen unless the index for the L-region is greater than 5.66 β.

Thus anthracene with indices of 5.38 (L-region) and 3.43 (K-region) fails on both counts. 1,2 benzanthracene with indices of 5.53 (L-region) and 3.29 (K-region) meets condition (i) but not condition (ii). It is thus a borderline carcinogen. 1,2,5,6 dibenzanthracene with indices of 3.30 (K-region) and 5.69 (L-region) fulfils both conditions and has been found to be carcinogenic.

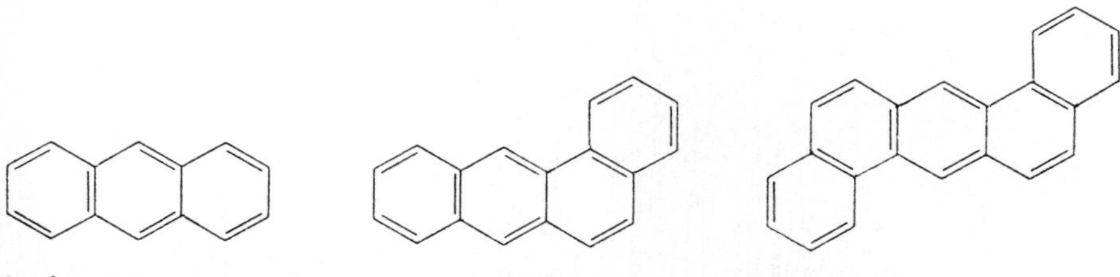

Anthracene 1,2 Benzanthracene 1,2,5,6 Dibenzanthracene

It should be emphasized here that the indices are not unpaired spin densities (the carcinogens are not themselves paramagnetic). However there should be a correlation between the calculated indices and the unpaired spin densities at these sites of radicals formed from the carcinogens. The calculations of spin density would be made as briefly described in Chapter 6. A reasonable correlation between carcinogenicity and unpaired spin density on charge transfer complexes between polycyclic hydrocarbons and the strong electron acceptor tetracyanoethylene (Allison and Nash, 1963) has been found. In this context, it is pertinent to point out that chemical linkages can be formed between 3,4 benzpyrene (a carcinogen) and DNA. Incubation with dilute hydrogen peroxide induces this reaction which probably occurs through radical intermediates. A free radical mechanism for attachment of the carcinogen to DNA may be a common link between different groups of carcinogens; certainly the importance of this linkage in carcinogenesis merits further investigation.

Hormones and drugs

Hormones. Many hormones readily undergo oxidation and/or reduction. Free radicals may be involved as intermediates and could in some cases be the active forms of the hormone. A major problem here is *in vivo* detection: hormones are effective at such low concentrations that any radical derivatives are likely to be below the detection limits of the ESR technique. Certainly the target *specificity* of the hormone must reside in the molecule itself and not simply be a general property of radicals. However, as already discussed for carcinogenesis, a common free radical mechanism for attachment of hormones to target tissue (probably the cell membrane) is plausible.

As in the study of other small biomolecules (Section 8.1), the detection of radicals from hormones as a result of chemical treatment provides evidence on whether a biological counterpart to this reaction occurs. Thus short-lived semiquinone radicals have been detected using rapid-velocity continuous flow ESR from the chemical oxidation of catecholamines (see Figure 8.50), and also free radicals from indole and thyronine hormones have been detected. The spectra are complex and have not been completely analysed. Similarly the phenol ring of estrogenic hormones can be oxidized to give radicals. The observation that identical ESR

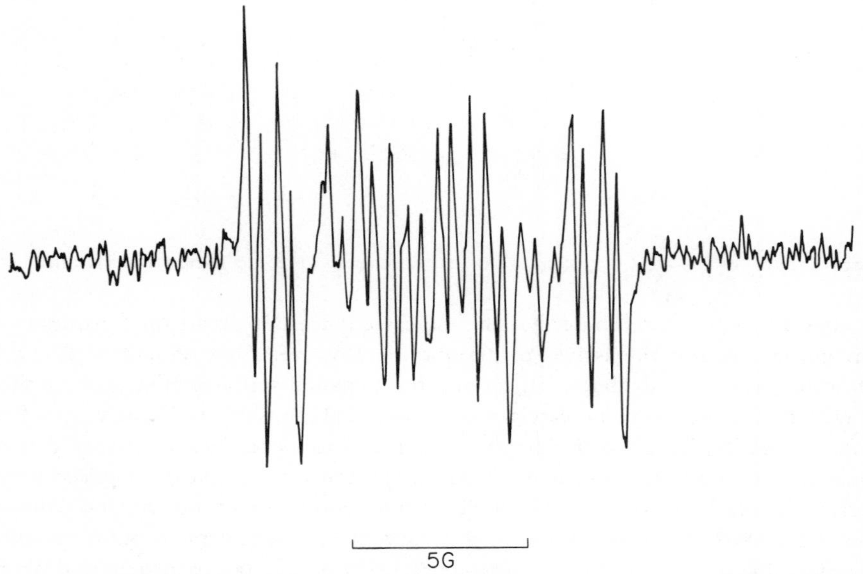

Figure 8.50 ESR spectrum of the transient free radical from dihydroxyphenylalanine (dopa) oxidized by Ce^{4+} at pH 12.7. Spectrum scanned in <3 s. (From Borg, 1972)

spectra are obtained from estradiol, estriol and estrone suggests that some aspects of their action might be through a common radical intermediate.

Drugs. ESR together with other physical techniques, could help in establishing the molecular basis of pharmacological action. The approach may be illustrated by the example of chlorpromazine, a phenothiazine tranquillizer which has had dramatic effects in the treatment of hyperactivity and anxiety conditions (Figure 8.51). ESR signals originating from chlorpromazine have been detected in the urine of patients receiving the drug. The extensive hyperfine structure apparent in the spectrum shows that the unpaired electron is highly delocalized, which accounts for its unusual stability. The stability suggests that perhaps the radical derivative is active in the central nervous system. The radical derivative might be involved in the known inhibition by chlorpromazine of the sodium-potassium ATPase which occurs in nervous tissue.

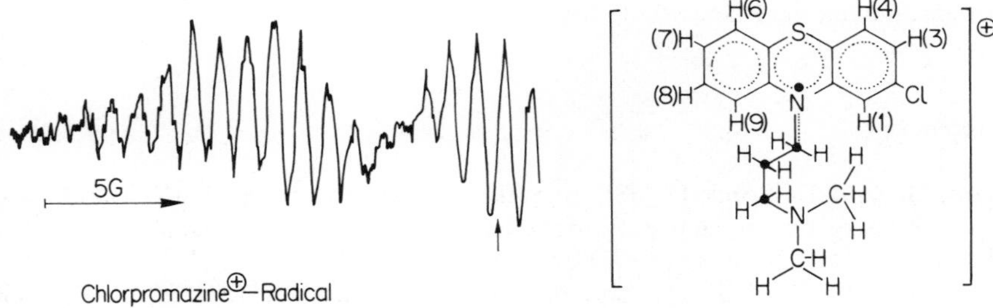

Figure 8.51 ESR spectrum and formula for the cation radical of chlorpromazine. Vertical arrow represents the midpoint of the spectrum. (From Fenner and Möckel, 1969)

Leute *et al.* (1972) have combined spin labelling with the immuno assay technique to produce a procedure for the rapid determination of morphine in urine, saliva and other biological fluids. Morphine coupled to bovine serum albumin was used as antigen to prepare antibodies. When spin-labelled morphine bound to the antibodies, the ESR spectrum of the nitroxide became highly immobilized. Addition of morphine caused the spin-labelled morphine to be displaced from the antibodies and the ESR spectrum reverted to the mobile three-line form. The amplitude of the low field line of this mobile spectrum plotted as a function of added morphine provided a calibration curve from which it was possible to estimate the concentration of morphine in any biological sample. Morphine substitutes such as methadone and propoxyphene and unrelated drugs such as barbiturates and amphetamines were not recognized by the antibody. Thus the technique is well suited for use in heroin treatment programmes.

8.7 Summary

(1) ESR is the method of choice in detecting and identifying radicals generated from enzyme substrates, coenzymes, drugs and hormones by metabolic reactions.

(2) ESR provides information on the structure and function of transition-metal ion centres in metalloproteins.

(3) Spin labelling of selected groupings allows conformational changes in proteins without an inherent paramagnetic centre to be studied by ESR. The distances of various groupings, including substrates and cofactors, from the spin-label reference point can be determined: this information can be derived even though the protein is too complex to study by X-ray diffraction.

(4) The structure and mobility of phospholipid membranes can be studied by ESR if a suitable spin-label probe is added. Detailed information concerning fatty acid side chain flexibility and the lateral diffusion of whole phospholipid molecules can be obtained. ESR is also used to study the nature of protein–lipid interactions in membranes.

(5) Redox components in complex biological systems, for example chloroplasts and mitochondria, can be identified by ESR.

(6) ESR is used to investigate radiation damage and other abnormalities in proteins, nucleic acids and whole tissue.

References

Adam, G., and Delbrück (1968). In *Structural Chemistry and Molecular Biology*, p. 198, Davidson, N., and Rich, A. (Eds.), Freeman, San Fransisco.

Allison, A. C., and Nash, T. (1963). *Nature*, **197**, 758.

Bäckström, D., Norling, B., Ehrenberg, A., and Ernster, L. (1970). *Biochem. Biophys. Acta,* **197**, 108.

Barnett, R. E., and Grisham, C. M. (1972). *Biochem. Biophys. Res. Comms.*, **48**, 1632.

Bearden, A. J., and Malkin, R. (1972). *Biochem. Biophys. Acta.*, **283**, 456.

Bearden, A. J., and Malkin, R. (1975). *Quart. Rev. Biophys.*, **7**, 131.

Beinert, H. (1966). In *The Biochemistry of Copper*, Peisach, J., Aisen, P., and Blumberg, W. E. (Eds.), Academic Press, New York.

Beinert, H., Kok, B., and Hoch, G. (1962). *Biochem. Biophys. Res. Comms.*, **7**, 209.

Beinert, H., and Palmer, G. (1964). *J. Biol. Chem.*, **239**, 1221.

Bennett, J. E., Gibson, J. F., and Ingram, D. J. E. (1957). *Proc. Roy. Soc.*, **A240**, 67.

Berliner, L. J., and McConnell, H. M. (1966). *Proc. Nat. Acad. Sci. USA,* **55**, 708.

Blumenfeld, L. A., and Kalmanson, A. E. (1961). In *The Initial Effects of Ionising Radiation*, p. 59, Harris, R. J. C. (Ed.), Academic Press, London.

Borg, D. C. (1972). In *Biological Applications of Electron Spin Resonance*, p. 265, Swarz, H. M., Bolton, J. R., and Borg, D. C. (Eds.), Wiley–Interscience, New York and London.

Bränden, R., Malmström, B. G., and Vänngård, T. (1971). *Eur. J. Biochem.*, **18**, 238.

Bretscher, M. (1973). *Science,* **181**, 622.

Calvin, M., and Bassham, J. A. (1962). *The Photosynthesis of Carbon Compounds*, Benjamin, New York.

Capaldi, R. A. (1974). *Scientific American*, **230**, 26.

Chance, B. (1952). *Arch. Biochem. Biophys.*, **41**, 416.

Commoner, B., Heise, J. J., and Townsend, J. (1956). *Proc. Nat. Acad. Sci. (US)*, **42**, 710.

Commoner, B., Heise, J. J., Lippincott, B. B., Norberg, R. E., Passonnean, J. V., and Townsend, J. (1956). *Science*, **126**, 57.

Cook, J. B., and Wyard, S. J. (1966). *Nature*, **210**, 526.

Cook, J. B., and Wyard, S. J. (1969). In *Solid State Biophysics*, p. 107, Wyard, S. J. (Ed.), McGraw–Hill, New York.

Dickerson, R. E., Takano, T., Eisenberg, D., Kallai, O. B., Sampson, L., Cooper, A., and Margoliash, E. (1971). *J. Biol. Chem.*, **246**, 1511.

Dwek, R. A., Knott, J. C. A., Marsh, D., McLaughlin, A. C., Press, E. M., Price, N. C., and White, A. I. (1975). *Eur. J. Biochem.*, **53**, 25.

Ehrenberg, A., Müller, F., and Hemmerich, P. (1967). *Eur. J. Biochem.*, **2**, 286.

Ehrenberg, A., and Yonetani, T. (1961). *Acta Chem. Scand.*, **15**, 1071.

Fairbanks, G., Steck, T. L., and Wallach, D. F. H. (1971). *Biochemistry*, **10**, 2606.

Feher, G. (1970). *Electron Paramagnetic Resonance with Application to Selected Problems in Biology*, Gordon and Breach, New York.

Fenner, H., and Möckel, H. (1969). *Tetrahedron Letters*, 2815.

Frye, L. D., and Edidin, M. (1970). *J. Cell. Sci.*, **7** 319.

Gordy, W., and Kurita, Y. (1960). *J. Chem. Phys.*, **34**, 282.

Grant, C. W. M., and McConnell, H. M. (1973). *Proc. Nat. Acad. Sci. USA*, **70**, 1238.

Harman, D. (1961). *Lancet*, 200.

Harman, D. (1962). *Radiation Research*, **16** 753.

Hartzell, C. R., Hansen, R. E., and Beinert, H. (1973). *Proc. Nat. Acad. Sci. USA*, **70**, 2477.

Heckley, R. J. (1972). In *Biological Applications of Electron Spin Resonance*, p. 197, Swartz, H. M., Bolton, J. R., and Borg, D. C. (Eds.), Wiley–Interscience, New York and London.

Henriksen, T. (1969). In *Solid State Biophysics*, p. 203, Wyard, S. J. (Ed.), McGraw–Hill, New York.

Hong, K., and Hubbell, W. L. (1973). *Biochem.*, **12**, 4517.

Hsia, J. C., and Piette, L. H. (1969). *Arch. Biochem. Biophys.*, **129**, 296.

Hubbell, W. L., and McConnell, H. M. (1971). *J. Am. Chem. Soc.*, **93**, 314.

Ingram, D. J. E. (1969). *Biological and Biochemical Applications of ESR*, Adam Hilger, London.

Jones, R., Dwek, R. A., and Walker, I. O. (1972). *FEBS Letters*, **26**, 92.

Jones, R., Dwek, R. A., and Walker, I. O. (1973). *Eur. J. Biochem.*, **34**, 28.

Jost, C. P., Griffith, O. H., Capaldi, R. A., and Vanderkooi, G. (1973). *Proc. Nat. Acad. Sci. USA*, **70**, 480.

Kamp, H. H., Wirtz, K. W. A., and Van Deenan, L. L. M. (1973). *Biochem. Biophys. Acta*, **318**, 313.

Kirkpatrick, F. H., and Sandberg, H. E. (1973). *Biochem. Biophys. Acta*, **298**, 209.

Kohl, D. H. (1972). In *Biological Applications of Electron Spin Resonance*, p. 213, Swartz, H. M., Bolton, J. R., and Borg, D. C. (Eds.), Wiley–Interscience, New York and London.

Landsberger, F. R., Paxton, J., and Lenard, J. (1971). *Biochem. Biophys. Acta*, **266**, 1.

Leute, R. K., Ullman, E. F., Goldstein, A., and Hertzenberg, L. A. (1972). *Nature (New Biol.)*, **236**, 93.

Levine, Y. K. (1973). *Progress in Surface Science*, **3**, 279.

Linden, C. D., Wright, K. L., McConnell, H. M., and Fox, C. F. (1973). *Proc. Nat. Acad. Sci. USA*, **70**, 2271.

McConnell, H. M., and McFarland, B. G. (1970). *Quart. Rev. Biophys.*, **3**, 91.

McConnell, H. M., Wright, K. L., and McFarland, B. G. (1972). *Biochem. Biophys. Res. Comms.*, **47**

McElroy, J., Feher, G., and Manzerall, D. (1969). *Biochim. Biophys. Acta*, **172**, 180.

McGrath, R. A., and Williams, M. W. (1966). *Nature*, **212**, 534.

Malkin, R., and Bearden, A. J. (1973). *Proc. Nat. Acad. Sci. (US)*, **70**, 294.

Malkin, R., Malmström, B. C., and Vängård, T. (1968). *FEBS Letters*, **1**, 50.

Malmström, B. G., Reinhammar, B., and Vänngård, T. (1968). *Biochim. Biophys. Acta*, **156**, 67.

Mason, H. S., Yamano, T., North, J., Hashimoto, Y., and Sakagishi, P. (1965). In *Oxidases and Related Redox Systems*, p. 879, King, T. S., Mason, H. S., and Morrison, M. (Eds.), Wiley, New York and London.

Müller, F., Eriksson, L. E. G., and Ehrenberg, A. (1970). *Eur. J. Biochem.*, **12**, 93.

Oesterhelt, D., and Stoeckenius, W. C. (1971). *Nature*, **233**, 149.

Ohnishi, T., Asakura, T., Wilson, D. F., and Chance, B. (1972). *FEBS Letters*, **21**, 59.

Orme-Johnson, N. R., Orme-Johnson, W. H., Hansen, R. E., Bienert, H., and Hatefi, Y. (1971). *Biochem. Biophys. Res. Comms.*, **44**, 446.

Orme-Johnson, N. R., Orme-Johnson, W. H., Hansen, R. E., Beinert, H., and Hatefi, Y. (1973). In *Oxidases and Related Redox Systems*, King, T. E., Mason, H. S., and Morrison, M. (Eds.), University Park Press, Baltimore.

Parsons, W. W. (1974). *Ann. Rev. Microbiol.*, **28**, 41.

Patten, R. A., and Gordy, W. (1964). *Radiation Research*, **22**, 29.

Pruden, B., Snipes, W., and Gordy, W. (1965). *Proc. Nat. Acad. Sci. USA*, **53**, 917.

Pullman, A., and Pullman, B. (1963). *Nature*, **199**, 467.

Reinhammar, B., and Vänngård, T. (1971). *Eur. J. Biochem.*, **18**, 463.

Rottem, S., Hubbell, W. L., Hayflick, L., and McConnell, H. M. (1970). *Biochem. Biophys. Acta*, **219**, 104.

Sackmann, E., and Träuble, H. (1972). *J. Am. Chem. Soc.*, **94**, 4482.

Sackmann, E., Träuble, H., Galla, H. J., and Overath, P. (1973). *Biochem.*, **12**, 5360.

Scandella, C. J., Devaux, P., and McConnell, H. M. (1972). *Proc. Nat. Acad. Sci. USA*, **69**, 2056.

Schatz, G., Groot, G. S. P., Mason, T., Rouslin, W., Wharton, D. C., and Saltzberger, J. (1972). *Fed. Proc.*, **31**, 21.

Schreier-Muccillo, S., Marsh, D., Dugas, H., Schneider, H., and Smith, I. C. P. (1973). *Chem. Phys. Lipids*, **10**, 11.

Schreier-Muccillo, S., and Smith, I. C. P. (in press). *Spin Labels as Probes of Biological Membranes*, Academic Press.

Seelig, J., and Hasselbach, W. (1971). *Eur. J. Biochem.*, **21**, 17.

Shimshick, E. J., and McConnell, H. M. (1973). *Biochem.*, **12** 2351.

Sogo, P., Pon, N. G., and Calvin, M. (1957). *Proc. Nat. Acad. Sci. (US)*, **43**, 387.

Song, P.-S. (1969). *Ann. N.Y. Acad. Sci.*, **158**, 410.

Stryer, L., and Griffith, O. H. (1965). *Proc. Nat. Acad. Sci. USA*, **54**, 1785.
Swartz, H. M. (1972). In *Biological Applications of Electron Spin Resonance*, p. 155, Swartz, H. M., Bolton, J. R., and Borg, D. C. (Eds.), Wiley–Interscience, New York and London.
Tourtellotte, M. E., Branton, D., and Keith, A. D. (1970). *Proc. Nat. Acad. Sci. USA*, **66**, 909.
Van Gelder, B. F., Beinert, H. (1969). *Biochim. Biophys. Acta*, **189**, 1.
Vithayathil, A., Ternberg, J., and Commoner, B. (1965). *Nature*, **207**, 1246.
Warden, J. T., and Bolton, J. R. (1972). *J. Am. Chem. Soc.*, **94**, 4352.
Warren, G. B., Toon, P. A., Birdsall, N. J. M., Lee, A. G., and Metcalfe, J. C. (1974). *Proc. Nat. Acad. Sci. USA*, **71**, 622.
Wilkins, M. H. F., Blaurock, A. E., and Engelman, D. (1971). *Nature (New Biology)*, **230**, 72.
Yamazaki, I., Mason, H., and Piette, L. H. (1959). *Biochem. Biophys. Res. Comms.*, **1**, 336.
Yamazaki, I., Mason. H., and Piette, L. H. (1960). *J. Biol. Chem.*, **235**, 2444.
Yamazaki, I., and Piette, L. H. (1961). *Biochim. Biophys. Acta*, **50**, 62.

Reading list

Bearden, A. J., and Malkin, R. (1975). 'Primary photochemical reactions in chloroplast photosynthesis', *Quart. Rev. Biophys.*, **7**, 131–177.
Beinert, H., and Palmer, G. (1965). 'Contributions of epr spectroscopy to our knowledge of oxidative enzymes', *Advances in Enzymology*, **27**, 105–198.
Dwek, R. A. (1973). In *NMR in Biochemistry: Applications to Enzyme Systems*, Oxford, Clarendon Press.
Ingram, D. J. E. (1969). *Biological and Biochemical Applications of Electron Spin Resonance*, Hilger, London.
McConnell, H. M., and McFarland, B. G. (1970). 'Physics and chemistry of spin labels', *Quart. Rev. Biophys.*, **3**, 91–136.
Swartz, H. M., Bolton, J. R., and Borg, D. C. (1972). *Biological Applications of Electron Spin Resonance*, Wiley–Interscience.
Wyard, S. J. (1969). *Solid State Biophysics*, McGraw–Hill.

Chapter 9
Advanced ESR Methods

There is a danger that the word 'advanced' will deter any reader approaching magnetic resonance for the first time. However, a more appropriate title for this final chapter, which consists of several unrelated ESR methods, could not be found. The topics covered in this chapter are linked wherever possible to the appropriate sections of earlier chapters to provide coherence.

9.1 Higher-Frequency Instruments

The main advantage of higher-frequency ESR spectrometers is enhanced spectral resolution. Consideration of Equation (6.1) will show how this originates:

$$h\nu = g\beta H \tag{6.1}$$

Differentiating, we obtain

$$\Delta H = -\left(\frac{h\nu}{g\beta}\right)\left(\frac{\Delta g}{g}\right) \tag{9.1}$$

Thus, if we have two species which differ in their g-values by Δg, then the magnetic field separation between them, ΔH, will be proportional to the microwave frequency, ν. This is illustrated in Figure 9.1.

Consideration of equation (6.2) shows that the hyperfine structure in an ESR spectrum is independent of the applied magnetic field. Thus the hyperfine splitting,

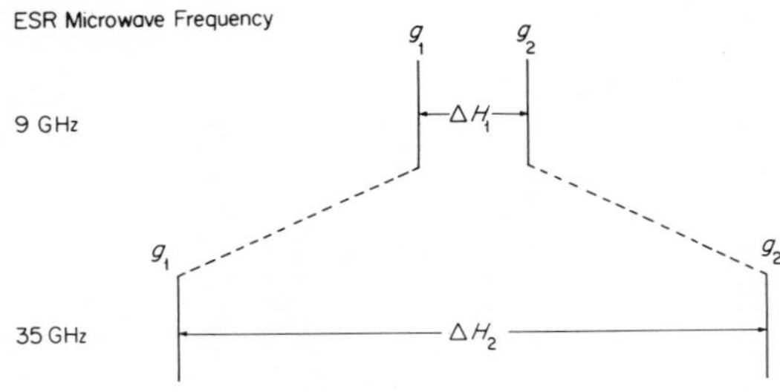

Figure 9.1 Diagram showing increased field separation of g-factors at higher microwave frequencies ($\Delta H_2 = 35/9 \times \Delta H_1$)

A, would be the same at a microwave frequency of 9 GHz as at 35 GHz. Comparison of spectra seen at two different frequencies allows g-value anisotropy, or separate g-values from two chemical species, to be distinguished from hyperfine structure. Examples of this have been discussed in Chapter 8 (see Figure 8.41 and Figures 8.9 and 8.10). Two further examples from the field of metalloenzymes will emphasize the value of higher-frequency instruments.

The enzyme benzylamine oxidase contains two Cu^{2+} ions per mole of enzyme. The ESR spectrum at 9 GHz (Figure 9.2a) is typical of copper complexes having axial symmetry and suggests that both copper sites are identical This conclusion is open to doubt when the 35 GHz spectrum is considered (Figure 9.2b). The splitting of the $g_{\perp}$ peak and the unequal widths of the hyperfine peaks in the $g_{\parallel}$ direction both suggest two different copper species.

The use of 35 GHz spectroscopy by Bray and coworkers (Bray and Vänngård, 1969; Bray and Swann, 1972) to study Mo^{V} species generated by reduction of xanthine oxidase is an even more impressive example. When the enzyme is reduced, the ESR spectrum recorded at 100 K can be composed of seventy-two lines from

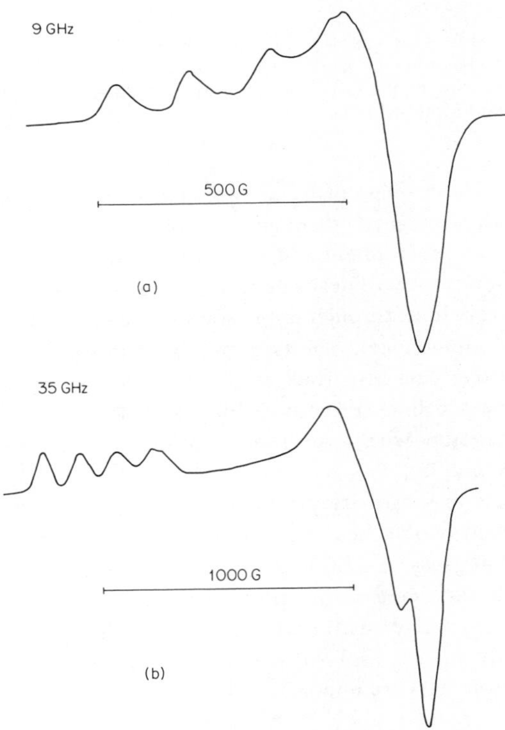

Figure 9.2 (a) 9 GHz, and (b) 35 GHz, spectra of the copper-containing enzyme benzylamine oxidase. The spectra were run at 100 K. (From Charlton, 1972)

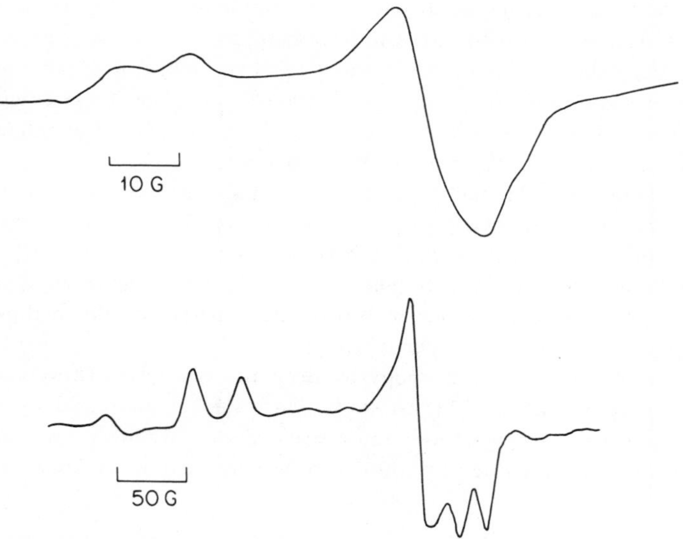

Figure 9.3 Mo^V ESR signals obtained from xanthine oxidase in D_2O reduced with 15 moles of xanthine for 1 minute at 20°C. The upper spectrum was run at 9.1 GHz and the lower at 34.4 GHz. (Adapted from Bray and Swann, 1972)

molybdenum species. These lines, many of which overlap (see Figure 9.3), have now been satisfactorily assigned through use of both 9 and 35 GHz ESR measurements, deuterium replacement and computer simulation of the spectra.

The origin of the seventy-two lines is as follows: each of the three g-values (g_x, g_y and g_z) is split into six lines through hyperfine interaction with Mo^{95} and Mo^{97} isotopes (25% natural abundance). The two molybdenums present in the enzyme operate as separate active sites and thus at any one time are chemically distinct, which results in thirty-six lines therefore. Finally each of these lines yields a doublet through interaction with a proton. Xanthine oxidase will be discussed further in Sections 9.5 and 9.6.

Although an increase in sensitivity proportional to $(H)^2$, or perhaps some even higher power of the field, would be expected when the magnetic field is increased (for example from 3000 gauss to 12,000 gauss), this is not realized in practice. The reason lies partly with the decrease in sample size dictated by the reduced ESR cavity dimensions, and partly with the increase in linewidth at the higher frequency. It is mainly in the area of spectral resolution and assignment that higher-field ESR spectrometers are important.

9.2 Electron–Nuclear Double Resonance (ENDOR)

ENDOR is a technique of growing importance in the study of paramagnetic biological material. The principal application of ENDOR is to the measurement of

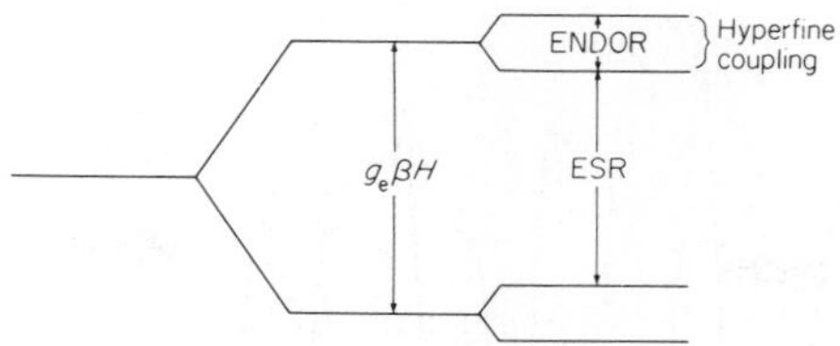

Figure 9.4 Simplified illustration of the relationship between the ESR and ENDOR transitions for a radical interacting with a single proton

hyperfine splittings which are often unresolved by the ESR method. A simplified representation of the relationship between ESR and ENDOR is given in Figure 9.4. Since ENDOR detects radiofrequency-induced NMR transitions by the change in the ESR signal, it combines the sensitivity of ESR detection with the resolution of NMR scanning. This is achieved by using a modified ESR cavity around which the NMR radiofrequency coils are wound.

The major contributions which ENDOR can make in biological systems are well illustrated by the radicals derived from low-molecular-weight flavins (which have been discussed in Section 8.1) and from flavoproteins. The ESR spectrum in Figure 9.5(a) is extremely difficult to interpret. One cannot with any certainty assign hyperfine splitting constants to the various protons in the molecule.

By contrast, the ESR spectrum in Figure 9.5(b) is devoid of structure. This is because the large protein molecule is tumbling slowly in solution – in fact at a rate comparable to the frequency of the hyperfine line separations. Thus anisotropic dipolar interactions are not adequately averaged and broadening results.

ENDOR spectra from flavin radicals associated with low or high molecular weight species are simple (see Figure 9.6). In the case of low molecular weight flavin radicals (Figure 9.6a), one can from this spectrum unambiguously determine hyperfine splittings, whilst with flavoprotein radicals (Figure 9.6b), resolution of the hyperfine structure now becomes possible.

ENDOR of a radical having a single proton

Let us now examine the theoretical basis for an ENDOR experiment. Suppose we have a radical ($S = \frac{1}{2}$) interacting with a single proton ($I = \frac{1}{2}$). In a magnetic field, the energy levels would be split as shown in Figure 9.7. The major splitting comes from the magnetic field interaction with the electron spin; $g\beta H$. Then each of these two levels are split both by the electron–nuclear hyperfine interaction which splits them equally by $\frac{1}{2}A$, and by the interaction of the nuclear spin with the magnetic field (as in NMR) which *decreases* the splitting of the upper level by $g_n\beta_n H$ and *increases* the splitting of the lower level by $g_n\beta_n H$.

In the ENDOR experiment, we saturate the $2 \rightarrow 3$ ESR transition by application of microwave radiation at the appropriate frequency. Further absorption of microwave power is then not possible. If we simultaneously sweep through a range

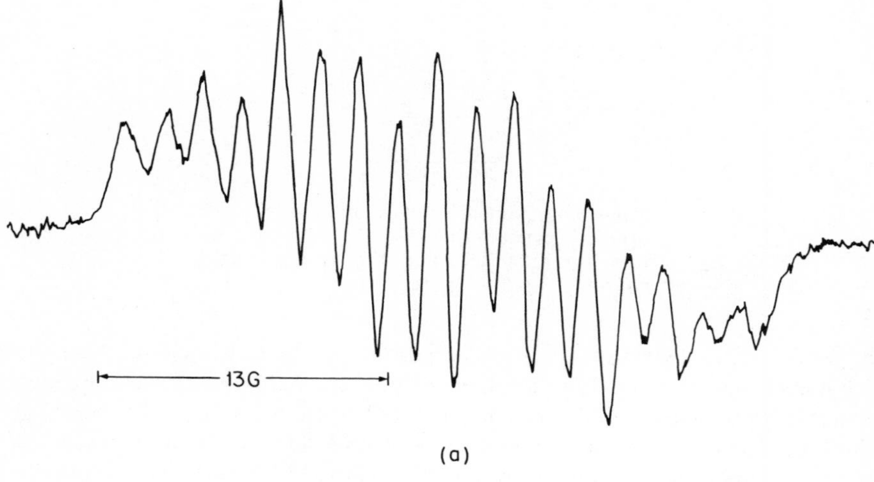

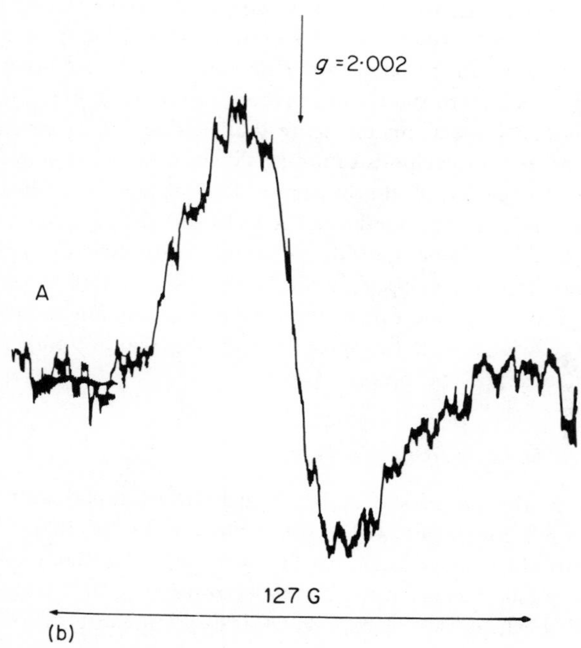

Figure 9.5 (a) ESR spectra of 7,8-dichloro-10-ethyl isoalloxazine in 1 N NaOH. (From Guzzo and Tollin, 1964. Reproduced by permission of Academic Press, Inc.) (b) Room temperature ESR spectrum of 'Old Yellow enzyme' reduced with NADPH at pH 7.0. The signal is broad and has a poor signal-to-noise ratio. (From Ehrenberg and Ludwig, 1958. Reproduced by permission of the American Association for the Advancement of Science).

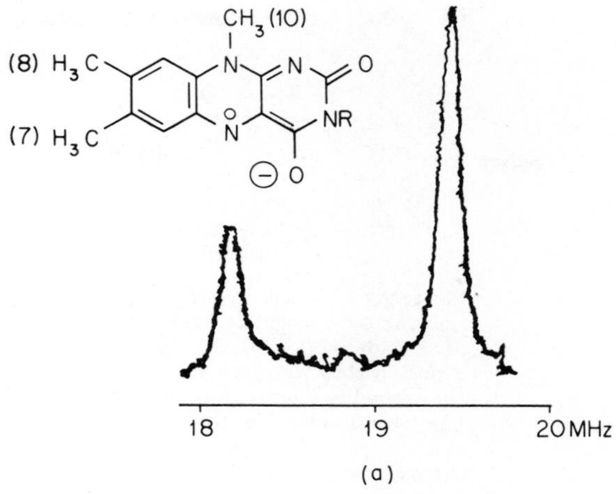

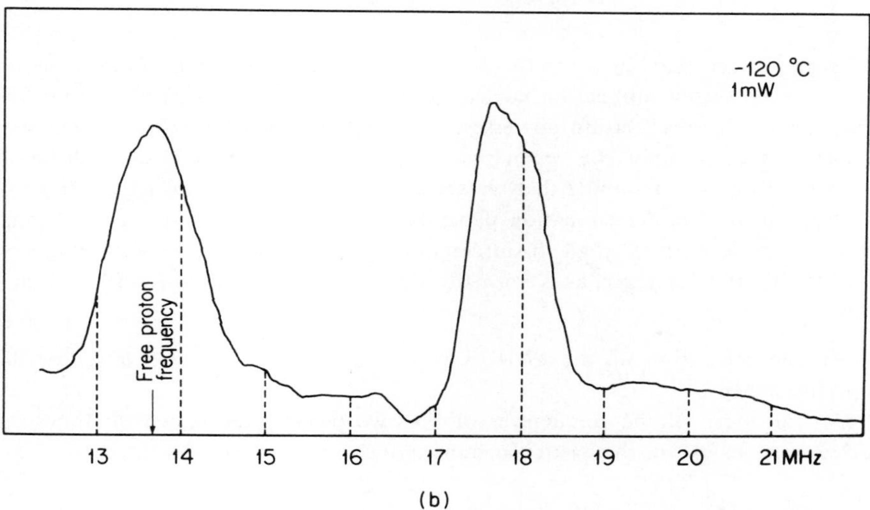

Figure 9.6 (a) Part of the ENDOR spectrum from lumiflavin anion radical in dimethyl formamide at 200 K. (b) Part of the ENDOR spectrum from *Azotobacter* flavoprotein radical. (From Ehrenberg *et al.*, 1971. Reproduced by permission of University Park Press).

of radiofrequencies, the frequency which effects the nuclear spin transition $3 \rightarrow 4$ will relieve the microwave saturation in level 3 and allow further absorption of microwave power. This is the ENDOR signal. At slightly higher radiofrequencies, the nuclear spin transition $1 \rightarrow 2$ will be bridged; this results in a higher population in level 2 than in level 1. Spins will consequently be 'pumped' from $2 \rightarrow 1$ and the resulting unequal populations between levels 2 and 3 again allows absorption of microwave power producing a second ENDOR transition.

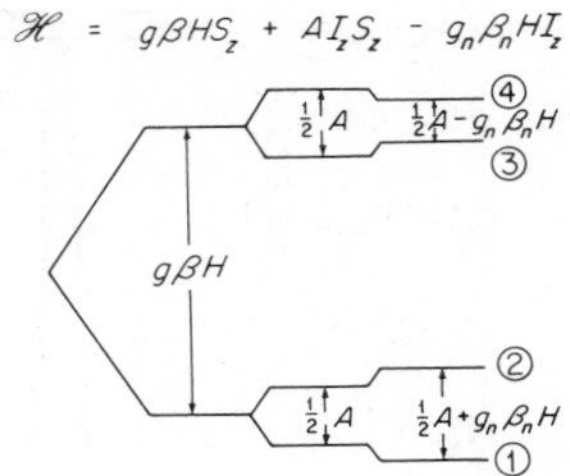

Figure 9.7 Energy-level splitting by a magnetic field of a radical ($S = ½$) interacting with a proton. The corresponding terms in the Spin Hamiltonian are shown at the top of the figure. At thermal equilibrium, the lower $M_S = -½$ levels will be marginally more highly populated

It can be seen that the ENDOR spectrum will depend not only on the electron relaxation processes but also on nuclear relaxation processes. Depending upon the efficiency of these relaxation processes, it is quite possible to observe only the first ENDOR signal or only the second, or with the two ENDOR lines of different intensity. However, assuming that we see both ENDOR lines, two parameters can be determined. The determination depends upon whether the hyperfine splitting, A, is greater than or less than the interaction of the nuclear spin with the magnetic field. If the latter is larger, as is normally the case for proton hyperfine structure, then:

(1) The separation of the ENDOR peaks gives a very accurate value for the hyperfine splitting.

(2) The mean of the frequencies of the two peaks gives g_n which allows the nucleus responsible for the particular transition to be positively identified.

ENDOR of Radicals with several Equivalent Protons

Consider 4 equivalent protons. The ESR spectra would have 5 lines with a 1:4:6:4:1 intensity distribution. Since however the hyperfine splitting between these lines is the same, there would be only 2 lines in the ENDOR spectrum. Consequently ENDOR gives no information on the numbers of protons in a particular chemical environment and it can be seen that complete identification of the radical requires application of both ENDOR and ESR.

ENDOR of Radicals with several non-equivalent protons

There would be an ENDOR doublet corresponding to each set of non-equivalent protons. The hyperfine splittings and g_n values of each set can be determined.

Similar principles apply to radicals interacting with other nuclei, e.g. nitrogen. An example of the application of nitrogen ENDOR will be considered below.

Most ENDOR experiments have been made on frozen solids. The reason for this is that electron spin-relaxation processes in solution are very efficient and very high microwave powers would be required to achieve partial saturation. In the solid, however, relaxation is governed by the spin–lattice relaxation time T_1 which increases with decreasing temperature: at liquid-nitrogen or in some cases liquid-helium temperatures, partial saturation can be achieved at modest microwave powers.

9.3 Examples of ENDOR

Flavin Systems

In Section 8.1, ESR spectra arising from Flavin radicals were discussed. Spectral assignment was achieved through replacement of selected nitrogens and hydrogens in the structure with other isotopes or by replacement of side groups (e.g. chlorines replacing methyls at positions 7 and 8) and observing the effects on the ESR spectra. Even though the spectrum has been assigned, it is not possible to accurately measure the various hyperfine splittings by ESR; this is however possible by ENDOR. Ehrenberg, Eriksson and Hyde (1971) have made detailed ENDOR studies on flavin radicals. A typical spectrum from lumiflavin anion radical in dimethyl formamide (DMF) at 200 K is shown in Figure 9.6. Even though this temperature is below the melting point of the solvent, only two lines are observed for protons in the methyl groups at positions 8 and 10. This is clear evidence that, at this temperature, free rotation still occurs about the carbon–carbon bonds joining the methyl groups to the ring, which makes the methyl hydrogens equivalent. The weaker signal has been assigned to $CH_3(10)$ and the stronger signal to $CH_3(8)$. Other coupled protons, including those from $CH_3(7)$, have not been detected.

Another ENDOR signal close to that for the free proton has been observed from frozen solutions of a flavoprotein radical from *Azotobacter Vinelandii* (see Figure 9.6b) and from NADH dehydrogenase. This 'free proton' signal is thought to come from protons in the immediate vicinity of the flavin radical – either directly bound to protein or as part of the solvation sphere. Addition of D_2O decreases the ratio: Area (free proton peak)/Area (methyl peak) to zero for the *Azotobacter* protein but to only 40% for NADH dehydrogenase. This suggests a more hydrophilic environment for the partially reduced flavin site in the *Azotobacter* protein since the free-proton site can obviously exchange freely with the D_2O solvent, a result which could be confirmed by comparison of the relaxation enhancements by the radical for water protons in the two cases.

Haem Systems

The ESR spectrum of laccase (see Figure 8.9) shows only hyperfine structure due to interaction between the unpaired electron and the Cu nucleus. There is no ESR

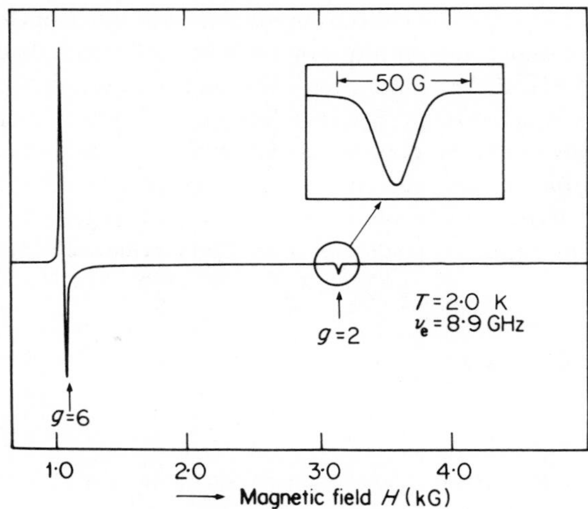

Figure 9.8 The ESR spectrum from a frozen solution of metmyoglobin. No ligand hyperfine structure is visible on either $g_{\|}$ or $g_{\perp}$. (From Feher *et al.*, 1973. Reproduced by permission of the New York Academy of Sciences)

evidence suggesting the identity of the ligands bonded to the copper ion. The ability of ENDOR to resolve the proton hyperfine structure from flavin radicals in proteins has been illustrated. Can ENDOR similarly resolve ligand hyperfine structure in metalloproteins? Haem systems have been studied to answer this question.

The ESR spectra of a frozen solution of metmyoglobin is shown in Figure 9.8. There is no indication of nitrogen hyperfine interactions which would arise from the ^{14}N nuclei of the haem ring and the unpaired electrons on the ferric centre. Consider the interactions which can occur between an unpaired electron and a ^{14}N nucleus (Figure 9.9). This is a more complicated situation than for a proton because the nitrogen ligand nucleus has a spin $I = 1$. This means that the energy levels are split into three by the nuclear interactions and, because these are composed of both hyperfine interactions, magnetic field interactions and also quadrupole interactions, these splittings are all unequal. Thus there will be *four* ENDOR transitions. In the case of metmyoglobin there will in fact be *eight* nitrogen ENDOR lines; four corresponding to the equivalent nitrogens in the haem plane and four lines originating from interaction of the unpaired electron with the imidazole nitrogen coordinated at position 5. The results obtained by Feher *et al.* (1973) are shown in Figure 9.10. The line assignment is simplified by comparison with the ENDOR spectrum from haemin which lacks the imidazole nitrogen interaction.

This result tells us little new about myoglobin (other than giving accurate nitrogen hyperfine splittings). However, moving to a different radiofrequency scan, we can study the *proton* interaction with the ferric centre. There will be two components (scalar and dipolar) to these interactions. Provided that firstly we can assign which protons originate from which ligand and secondly resolve the scalar and dipolar contributions, it might be possible to determine the proton coordinates accurately using the relationship:

$$\tfrac{1}{2}A(\text{dipolar}) = \frac{g_n \beta_n g \beta}{2r^3}(3\cos^2\theta - 1) \qquad (9.2)$$

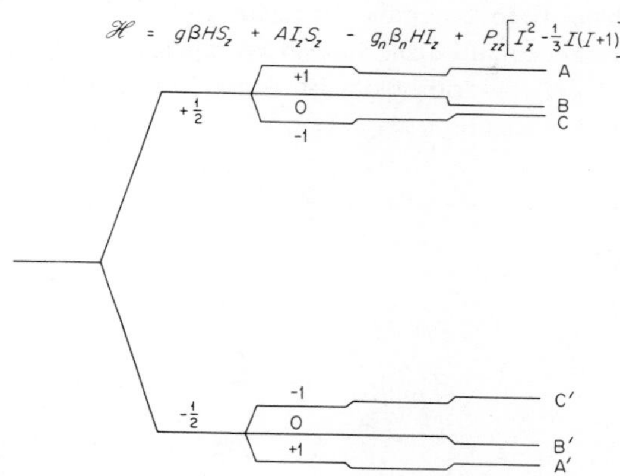

Figure 9.9 Energy-level splitting by a magnetic field of a system with *effective* electron spin $S = \tfrac{1}{2}$ (e.g. high-spin ferric), interacting with nuclear spin $I = 1$ (e.g. ^{14}N). The corresponding terms of the spin Hamiltonian are shown at the top. The last term in the Hamiltonian is the quadrupolar term present for all nuclei with $I > \tfrac{1}{2}$

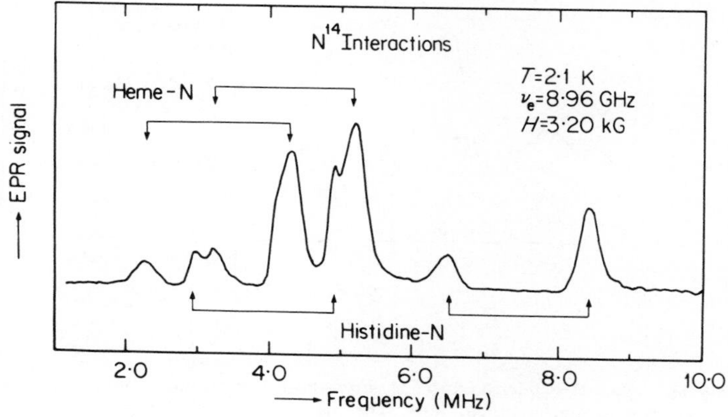

Figure 9.10 ^{14}N ENDOR spectrum from a frozen solution of metmyoglobin. The assignment is based on a comparison with haemin which lacks the histidine nitrogen interaction and therefore shows only the four haem nitrogen ENDOR lines. (From Feher *et al.*, 1973. Reproduced by permission of The New York Academy of Sciences)

where r and θ are the proton coordinates relative to the iron. The placing of the hydrogens adjacent to iron in myoglobin has not been forthcoming from either X-ray diffraction or from NMR measurements. Feher *et al.* (1973) report assignment of the different protons through deuterium exchange and progress towards resolution of the scalar and dipolar contributions through use of single crystals.

These studies have been extended to haemoglobin. Mutant forms of haemoglobin in which certain amino acids have been replaced are well characterized. A comparison of the ^{14}N spectrum from Hb-A and Hb-Hyde Park present in intact erythrocytes is shown in Figure 9.11.

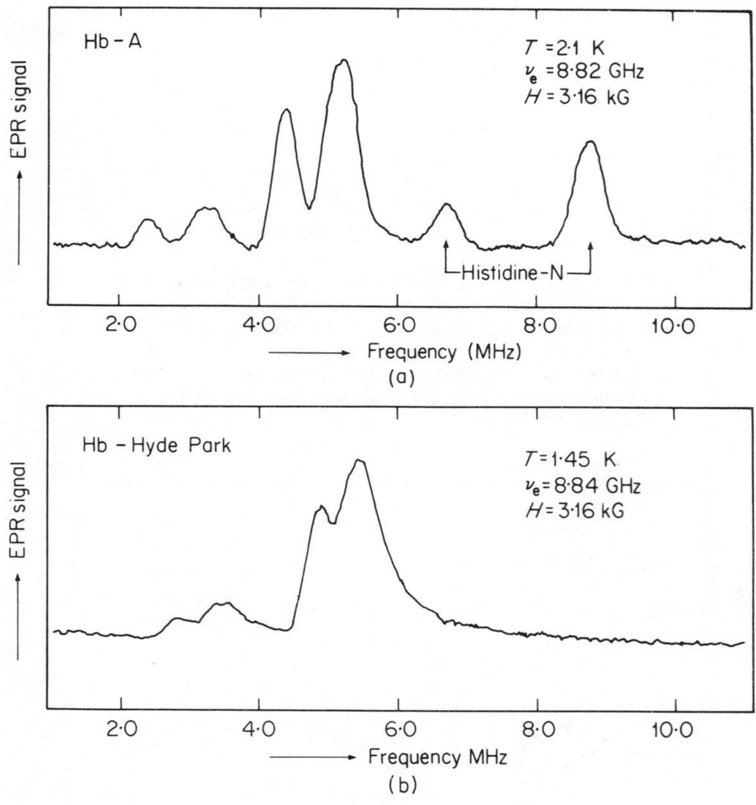

Figure 9.11 ENDOR spectra from ^{14}N interactions in haemoglobin.
(a) Normal human methaemoglobin-A. The main features of the spectrum are similar to those obtained from metmyoglobin (Figure 9.10).
(b) Haemoglobin – Hyde Park which has the histidine coordinated to iron in the β subunit replaced by tyrosine. Note the absence of high-frequency peaks. These spectra were obtained on whole oxygenated red blood cells. (From Feher *et al.*, 1973. Reproduced by permission of the New York Academy of Sciences)

The absence of two high field peaks in the Hb-Hyde Park spectrum correlates with the known replacement of histidine-92 by tyrosine and shows that it is this histidine which is coordinated to the 5-position of haem.

Perhaps the most important aspect of haemoglobin structure and function upon which ENDOR might provide information is that of oxygen binding. The advantage of ENDOR over other magnetic techniques in this respect is that:

(a) No perturbation to the system is necessary (*cf.* spin-labelling studies by McConnell, 1971).

(b) We are looking directly at the haem where bonding of oxygen is occurring.

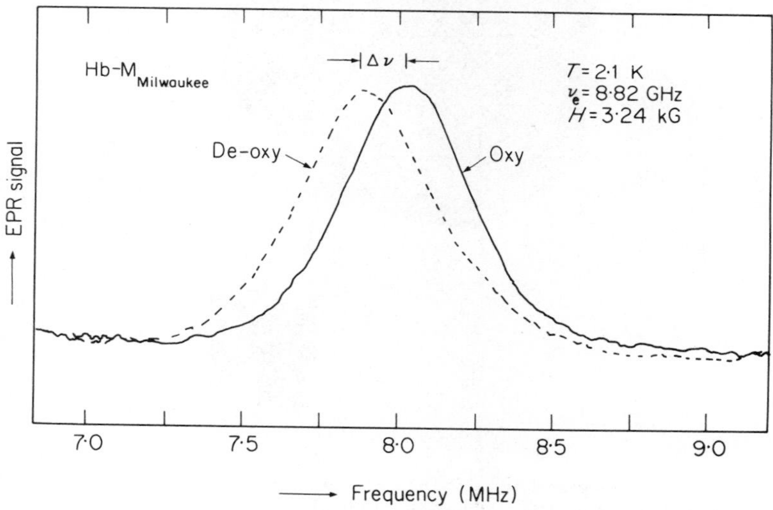

Figure 9.12 Effect of oxygenation of haemoglobin on one of the histidine ^{14}N ENDOR lines. Wa shed whole red blood cells were used. (From Feher *et al.*, 1973. Reproduced by permission of the New York Academy of Sciences)

As shown in Figure 9.12, there is a shift in one of the histidine ^{14}N ENDOR lines on oxygenation.

By a procedure similar to that described for proton interactions (see equation 9.2), it should be possible to calculate how far the histidine nitrogen and also the haem plane nitrogens have moved on oxygenation. As can be seen in Figures 9.10 and 9.11, these groupings in the ^{14}N ENDOR spectrum have been assigned; the remaining problem is to separate the scalar and dipolar contributions to the electron–nuclear interactions. In principle, this can be done by orientation studies with single crystals, but in practice the strong spin–spin interactions between the paramagnetic iron centres in the crystal broaden out the ENDOR lines.

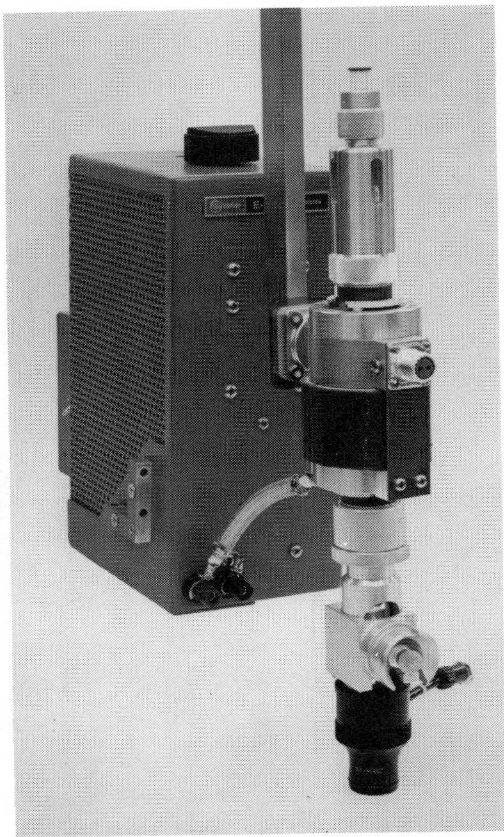

Figure 9.13 ENDOR cavity and RF generator compatible with the VARIAN E-line ESR spectrometer. The cavity is cooled by circulating cold gases (nitrogen or helium) through the inlet at the bottom

Practical aspects of ENDOR

An ENDOR experiment is undertaken as follows: The sample is placed in a special ESR cavity shown in Figure 9.13 and schematically represented in Figure 9.14. The cavity is connected to a radiofrequency generator. With the radiofrequency switched off, the ESR spectrum is scanned (magnetic field scan at low microwave power) until the field appropriate to a particular hyperfine line is reached. The magnetic field is then locked at this position and the microwave power increased to saturate the signal. The radiofrequency field (H_{RF}) is then swept and the ENDOR signals recorded by monitoring changes in the ESR signal level. In addition to modulating the static magnetic field as in normal ESR, it is also usual to modulate the radiofrequency field at a low frequency (6 kHz) and to employ phase-sensitive

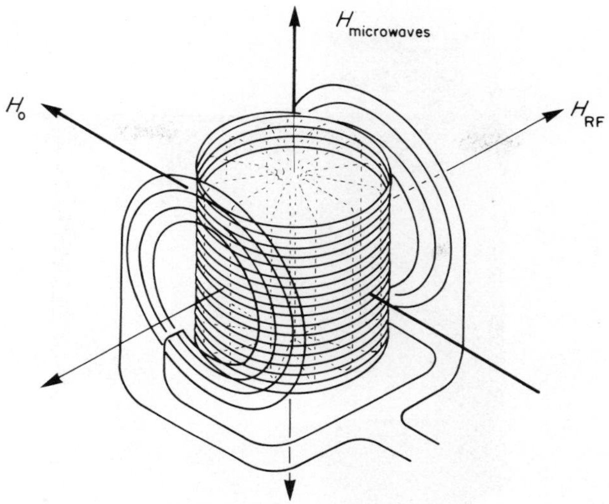

Figure 9.14 Schematic representation of a cylindrical cavity designed for ENDOR studies. The directions of the applied magnetic field (H_0) the radiofrequency field (H_{RF}) and microwave field ($H_{microwaves}$) are shown. The sample is placed parallel to the microwave field direction. (Modified from Wertz and Bolton, 1972. Reproduced by permission of McGraw–Hill Book Company from *Electron Spin Resonance; Elementary Theory and Practical Applications*, J. E. Wertz and J. R. Bolton, copyright © 1972 by McGraw–Hill, Inc.)

detection (see Chapter 7); since this modulation is at low frequency, the ENDOR signal appears in an absorption rather than derivative mode.

9.4 Electron–Electron Double Resonance (ELDOR)

ELDOR, like ENDOR, is useful for measurement of hyperfine splitting. In systems where the electron–nuclear coupling is strong, the hyperfine splittings will be large and perhaps beyond the range of RF sweep used in ENDOR. However, the higher frequency range can be attained if a microwave source replaces the radiofrequency source. This is achieved using a bimodal microwave cavity (see Figure 9.15), one arm of which is the normal ESR system whilst the other connects to a tunable klystron for sweeping through the hyperfine frequency region of the spectrum.

To understand the principle of ELDOR, let us consider the energy levels for an $S = ½$, $I = 1$ system (Figure 9.16) as would occur in a spin-labelled biomolecule. In ELDOR, the effect on one ESR transition (say $M_I = 0$) is observed whilst simultaneously pumping microwave power into another transition ($M_I = +1$ or -1); the relationship relating pumping and observation frequencies is

$$\nu_{(p)} = \nu_{(o)} \pm A$$

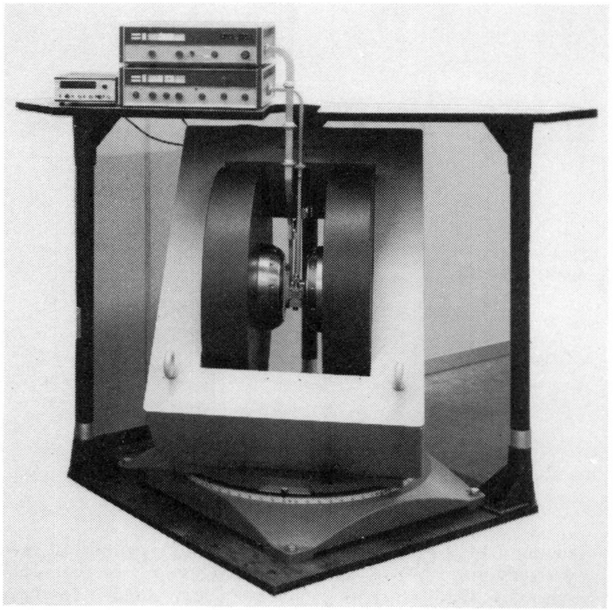

Figure 9.15 Varian Associates ELDOR system showing the bimodal cavity

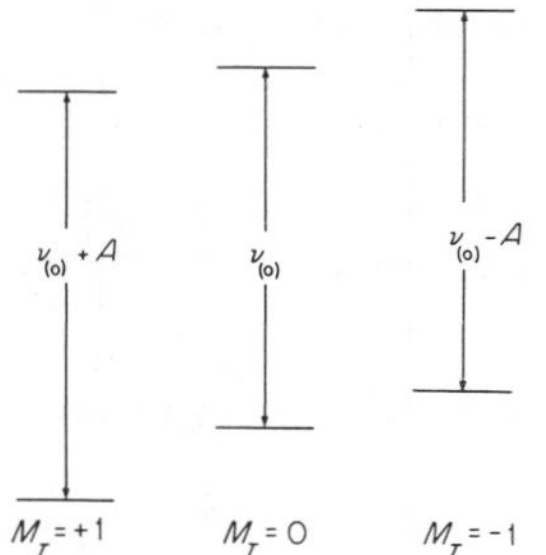

Figure 9.16 ESR and ELDOR transitions for $S = \frac{1}{2}, I = 1$. (*cf.* Figure 6.4)

where $\nu_{(p)}$ and $\nu_{(o)}$ are the pumping and observation frequencies respectively and A is the hyperfine coupling constant. It can be seen that, unlike ENDOR, the observed transition does not have a common energy level with the pumped one.

Practically, the observation frequency is set to a particular resonance whilst the pump frequency is swept using a tunable klystron. The microwave power used to pump heavily saturates the pump frequency transition; saturation can be relieved by relaxation through modulation at frequencies including that of the observation transition; this results in a changed population at the observation frequency and an unbalance in the detecting microwave bridge detector.

In addition to its application in measuring large hyperfine splittings, ELDOR can also be used to study very slow tumbling of paramagnetic species (Smirgel *et al.*, 1974). As will be discussed further in Section 9.5, this could be an important application to biological systems.

9.5 Kinetic Studies

Chapters 7 and 8 covered the applications of ESR to provide structural information about various biomolecules. In certain cases, for example metalloenzymes which are paramagnetic in their native state, and spin-labelled material, samples suitable for ESR can be prepared without special ancilliary apparatus. In other cases, for example metalloenzymes which are only transiently paramagnetic during the catalytic cycle, and unstable free radicals generated from enzyme substrates or from drugs, apparatus involving rapid scanning or flow becomes necessary to observe ESR signals. A complete kinetic analysis of how the concentrations of paramagnetic species change in a particular biological process can provide valuable information on the mechanism.

Flow techniques

Changes in the concentrations of paramagnetic species in biochemical reactions may be studied by flow techniques. Several types of flow system are commonly used.

Continuous flow (see Figure 9.17). This is the simplest procedure requiring only a special aqueous flow cell and, for faster reaction studies, a ram assembly for forcing the two reactants together. Under steady-state flow conditions the time course of the reaction can be sampled at various positions down the reaction tube by varying the distance (d) of the ESR cavity from the mixing chamber (M). The disadvantage of this system is that it consumes large quantities of material. It seems particularly suited for studies on radicals produced from small biomolecules which are available in plentiful amount; for example, drugs, cofactors and enzyme substrates. The time of observation after mixing (the 'dead' time) can be as short as 10 milliseconds. Economy of material and smaller dead times can in principle be realized by continuous-flow studies at 35 GHz instead of 9 GHz; the additional advantage of greater resolution at 35 GHz would significantly assist in spectral interpretation. The studies on peroxidase described in Section 8.1 are a good example of the application of continuous flow.

Stopped flow. The principal advantage of stopped flow over continuous flow is economy of material, which is an important consideration in the study of enzymes. However, a major problem arises when ESR detection is used since the region of detection within the microwave cavity is relatively large (approximately 1 cm at 9 GHz frequencies); as a result, the time coherence of the paramagnetic

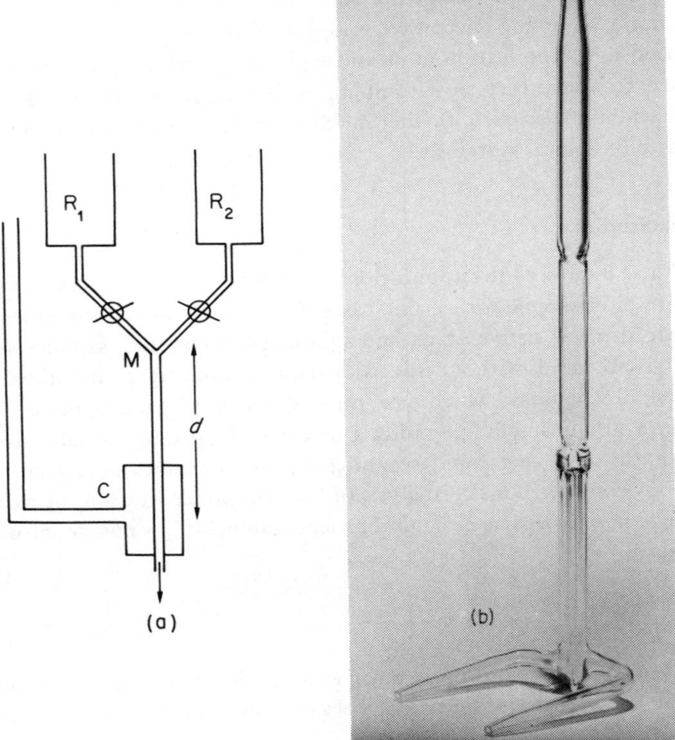

Figure 9.17 (a) Schematic representation of a continuous-flow ESR assembly. The reactants are contained in reservoirs (R_1 and R_2) from which they flow to a mixing chamber M. The reaction mixture is sampled after a distance *d* (which corresponds to a certain reaction time) in the ESR cavity (C). (b) An ESR flow cell; the mixing chamber with inlets from the reservoirs is at the bottom of the flat cell region. (Courtesy of Varian Associates). Similar criteria apply to aqueous flow cells as were discussed in Chapter 7 for aqueous cells.

population giving rise to the ESR signal is smeared out. At 35 GHz, with the decrease in cavity size, these problems would not be so severe, though reverberations caused in the small detection zone at the time when flow is stopped introduce new problems.

Rapid-freeze quenched flow (see Figure 9.18). The technique introduced by Bray (1961) of cooling reaction solutions down to low temperatures which effectively halts their progress has found several biological applications, particularly to the study of electron transfer processes in metalloenzymes. The enzyme and substrate are brought together in a mixing chamber M, allowed to react for a certain time which can be varied by changing the ram velocity or the distance *d* then extruded at high velocity into isopentane maintained at −140 °C. There is efficient

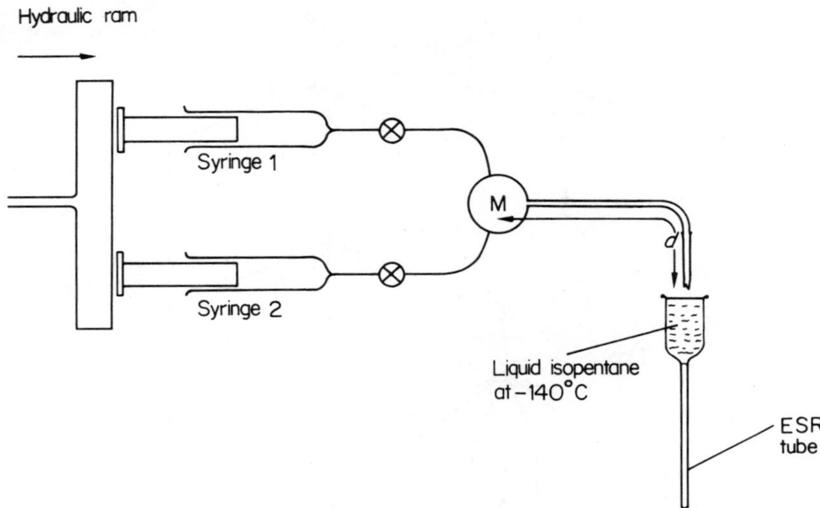

Figure 9.18 Schematic representation of a quench-flow assembly. Reactants (for example enzyme and substrate) contained in syringes 1 and 2 are forced together by the hydraulic ram. After a certain reaction time, the mixture is rapidly cooled by squirting into cold isopentane contained in a modified ESR tube and the frozen sample analysed by low-temperature ESR

heat transfer from the extruded fine droplets to the isopentane; isopentane has the property of remaining fluid at low temperatures yet is not so volatile that it forms an insulating gas blanket as would liquid nitrogen. The frozen solution can then be transferred to the ESR cavity (also at low temperature) and the spectrum examined at leisure; for ESR studies on metalloenzymes, low temperatures are essential due to the short electron spin–lattice relaxation times.

The elegance of this technique is well illustrated by the studies of Bray and coworkers (see Bray and Swann, 1972), on the enzyme xanthine oxidase. Xanthine oxidase isolated from milk contains 2 molybdenum atoms, 8 iron atoms and 2 flavin adenine dinucleotide molecules per mole of enzyme. All these components give rise to paramagnetic species on reduction and the system is ideal for study by ESR. The reaction catalysed by xanthine oxidase is

Xanthine $\xrightarrow{-H^{\ominus}}$ [intermediate, $\oplus$] $\xrightarrow{OH^{\ominus}}$ Uric acid

The ESR studies have been directed towards answering the question of how the reducing equivalents ($H^{\ominus}$) from the 8-position of xanthine are transferred by the

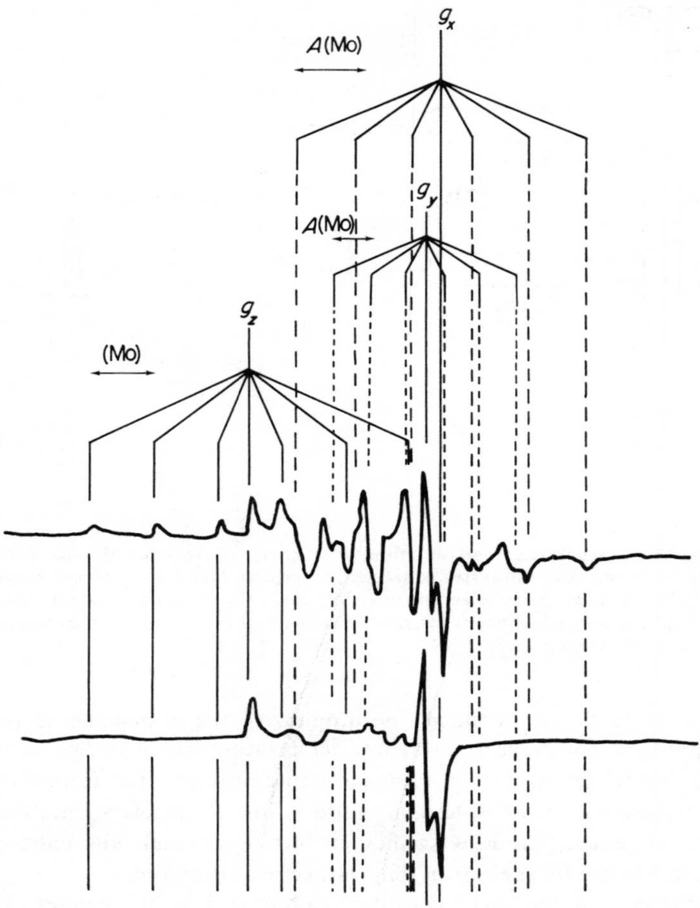

Figure 9.19 'Very rapid' ESR signal from xanthine oxidase reduced with xanthine for 10 milliseconds at pH 10.0 using the rapid-quench technique. The lower trace refers to the normal enzyme; the upper trace refers to the enzyme enriched with ^{95}Mo. Assignment of the signal in terms of ^{95}Mo splitting of three *g*-values (g_x, g_y and g_z) is shown. (From Bray *et al.*, 1967)

enzyme to oxygen. This property is shared by many other enzymes including the multi-protein complexes found in the mitochondrial respiratory chain (see Section 8.5). Detailed knowledge of the mechanism by which xanthine oxidase carries out this transfer would facilitate our understanding of the more complex mitochondrial system.

At the shortest reaction time available by the rapid-quench technique (~10 milliseconds) the ESR spectrum from xanthine oxidase reduced with xanthine at pH 10.0 was as shown in Figure 9.19. The spectrum was assigned through similar

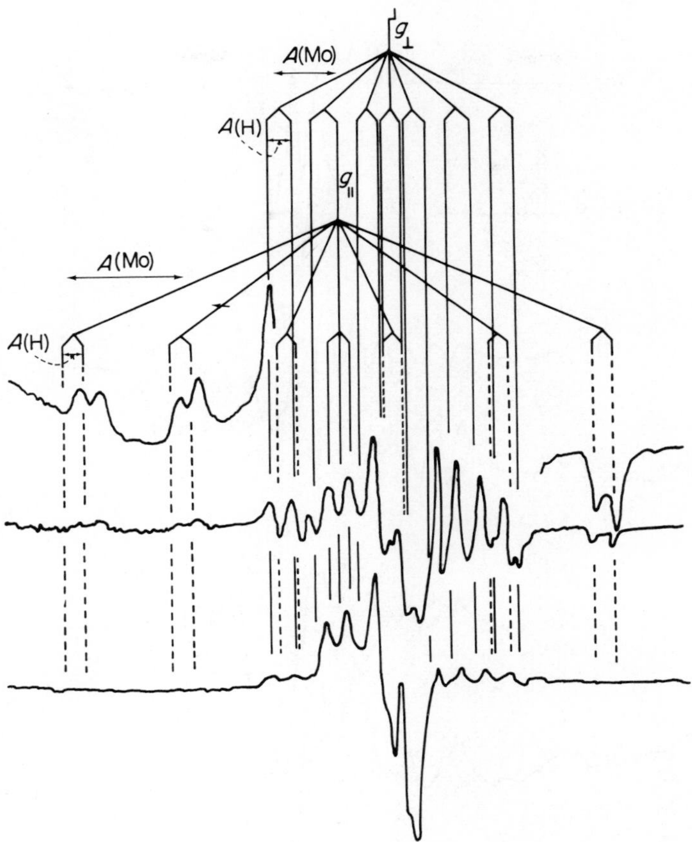

Figure 9.20 'Rapid' ESR signal from xanthine oxidase at pH 10.0 reduced with formaldehyde for 1 minute; similar spectra are obtained using the rapid-freeze technique. *Bottom trace*, normal enzyme; *centre trace*, ^{95}Mo enriched enzyme; *upper trace*, ^{95}Mo enzyme run at higher gain and modulation. Spectral assignment in terms of ^{95}Mo splitting on $g_\parallel$ and $g_\perp$ is shown together with protons splittings. (From Bray *et al.*, 1967)

reduction studies on enzyme enriched with the ^{95}Mo isotope which has $I = \frac{5}{2}$; these studies suggested that the spectrum arose from a Mo^{V} species located at a site of close to axial symmetry.

According to different reaction conditions (time of reaction, pH of the medium, nature of reducing agent), two main types of molybdenum ESR signal could be distinguished. The first of these, termed 'very rapid' was favoured by high pH and short reaction times with xanthine as substrate; this is the signal illustrated in Figure 9.19. The second type was obtained with many reducing substrates at lower pHs for reaction times from milliseconds to hours and was designated 'rapid'. A feature of the rapid signal, clearly visible in Figure 9.20, was the doublet splitting of the outer hyperfine peaks; doublet splitting occurs throughout the spectrum but

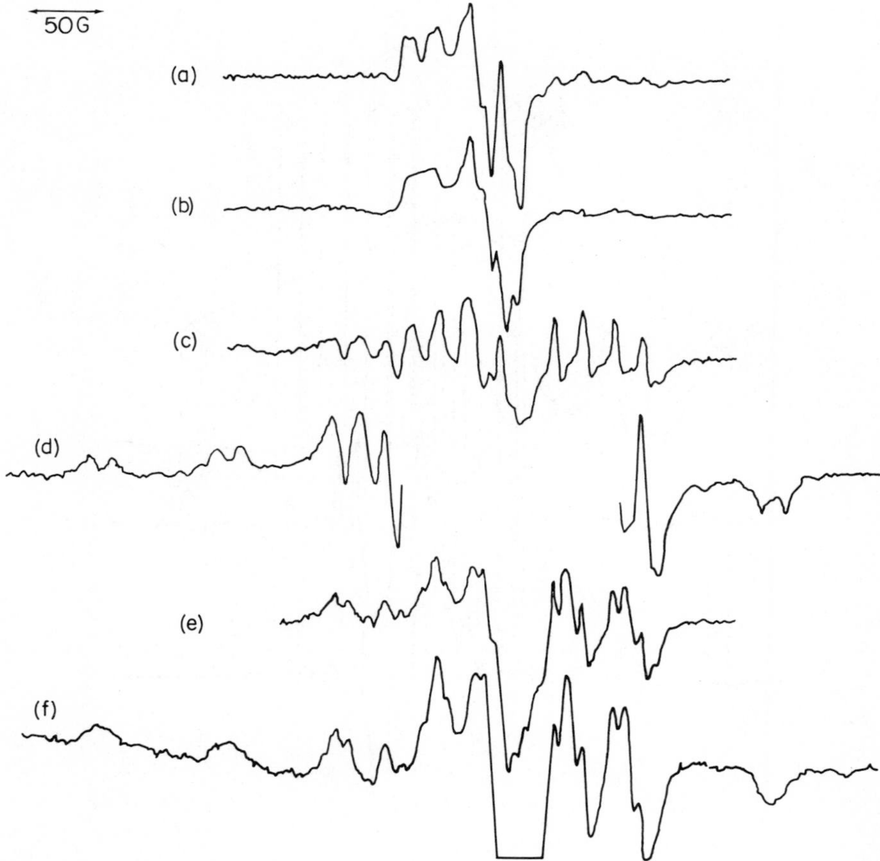

Figure 9.21 'Rapid' ESR signal from xanthine oxidase in H_2O and D_2O. The enzyme at pH 10.0 in water or 70% D_2O was reduced with purine for 1 minute. (a) Enzyme in H_2O; (b) enzyme in D_2O; (c) ^{95}Mo enzyme in H_2O; (d) ^{95}Mo enzyme in H_2O (higher) modulation, centre of trace omitted); (e) ^{95}Mo enzyme in D_2O; (f) ^{95}Mo enzyme in D_2O (at higher modulation). (From Bray *et al.*, 1967. Reproduced by permission of Pergamon Press Ltd)

overlapping signals obscure this fact. The most obvious nucleus to cause such a splitting would be a proton and this was proved by experiments in which the enzyme was dissolved in D_2O instead of H_2O (Figure 9.21). The collapse of the doublets can be seen particularly clearly when the spectra from the ^{95}Mo enriched enzyme dissolved in H_2O and D_2O (spectra d and f) are compared. A plausible explanation for the 'rapid' and 'very rapid' molybdenum species is that the former is the protonated form of the latter. Rapid-freeze experiments using 8-deutero xanthine as substrate showed that the exchangeable proton located at the molybdenum originated from substrate (see Figure 9.22). Thus we have direct evidence for transfer of reducing equivalents from substrate to molybdenum. Extension of these

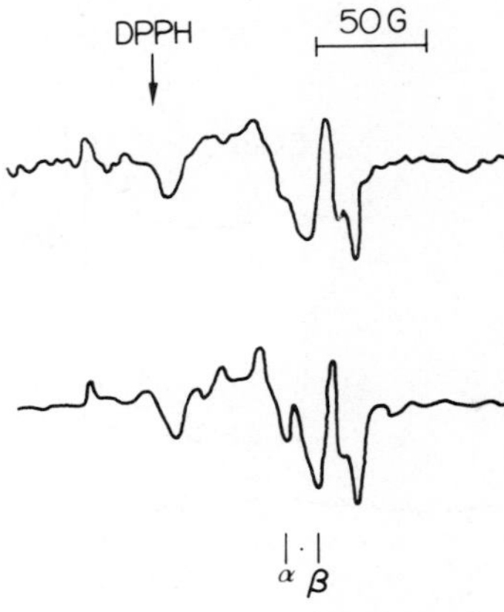

Figure 9.22 ESR signals obtained on treating xanthine oxidase for 130 milliseconds at pH 8.2 with: *top*, 8-deutero xanthine; *bottom*, xanthine. The doublet (α,β) has been almost replaced by a single broad line for the deuterated substrate. (From Bray and Knowles, 1968. Reproduced by permission of the Royal Society)

ESR studies (see Bray and Swann, 1972) have led to a reasonable understanding, not only of changes at the molybdenum centres but also of electron transfer from molybdenum to other enzyme components.

Electron transfer between the molybdenum and iron centres in xanthine oxidase will be discussed in Section 9.6. As a final example of applications of the rapid-freeze technique, we can consider the final steps in the overall chemical reaction catalysed by xanthine oxidase where oxygen is reduced to hydrogen peroxide. The one electron reduction product of oxygen (superoxide radical, O_2^-) is formed as an intermediate. The first direct evidence for this radical in biological systems came from rapid freezing ESR studies with the enzyme xanthine oxidase (Knowles *et al.*, 1969). The dependence of O_2^+ yields on the concentration of oxygen but not enzyme, and the marked asymmetry of the ESR signal (Figure 9.23) clearly distinguish it from flavin semiquinone which is also generated during the catalytic cycle of this enzyme.

Clear evidence for the identity of the species responsible for the asymmetric ESR signal as O_2^- was provided by rapid-freeze ESR studies on oxygenated alkaline solutions reduced by hydrated electrons (Nilsson *et al.*, 1969).

A final word of caution on the interpretation of results obtained by rapid-freeze ESR. One should always be aware of the possibility that the species observed by the quenched-flow technique are not the same as those present in solution before quenching. This has particular relevance to haem systems where the equilibrium between high- and low-spin forms can be perturbed by changes in temperature.

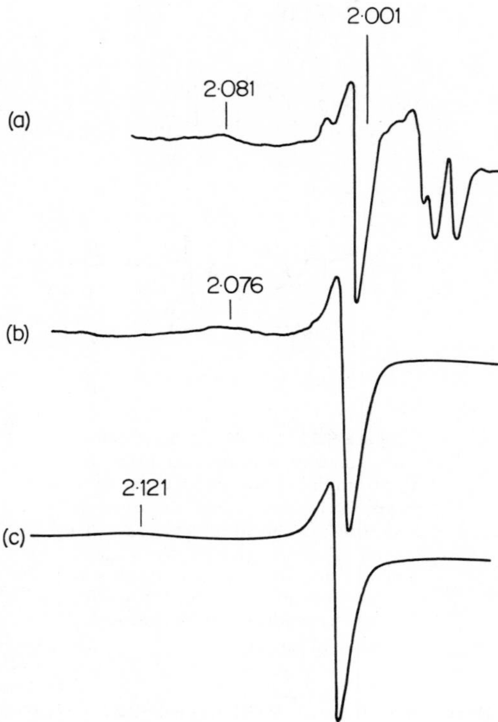

Figure 9.23 ESR signals from O_2^- obtained enzymically and non-enzymically using the rapid-freeze technique. (a) Reaction between xanthine (2.0 mM) and oxygen (0.7 mM) catalysed by xanthine oxidase (0.2 mM) at pH 10.0 after a reaction time of 150 milliseconds. Mo^V and reduced iron signals also contribute to the spectrum. (b) Reaction between H_2O_2 (140 mM) and $NaIO_4$ (70 mM) at pH 9.9 after a reaction time of 600 milliseconds. (c) As for (b) but at pH 13.2 (Knowles *et al.*, 1969. Reproduced by permission of The Biochemical Society).

Rapid Scanning

The recording of transient ESR spectra is limited by the magnetic field sweep rate, which is normally slow. Faster sweep rates can be achieved by having sweep coils mounted on the sides of the cavity which permit sweeping through the magnetic field in times from 100 milliseconds to 1000 seconds, the spectra being stored in a computer after each scan. This rapid sweep capability is potentially useful in biological systems for recording ESR signals which decay rapidly and for obtaining a reaction profile over a broad time range.

Microsecond response ESR spectrometers

A method has been described by Atkins *et al.* (1970) for observation of ESR spectra from transient free radicals formed photolytically. A fast-response ESR spectrometer system enables measurements to be made within 1μs of the photolysis flash. The fastest response time of an ESR spectrometer is approximately equal to 1/Modulation frequency; thus with the 100 kHz modulation provided on most commercial instruments, the fastest response time would be 10 microseconds. This can be reduced to less than 1 microsecond if 2 MHz modulation is used.

In the first mode of operation, the spectrometer is set to observe a particular resonance line. Radicals are generated by a 10 microsecond flash from a pulsed ultraviolet laser and the decay monitored at 5 microsecond intervals using a computer data store; repeated flashes allow an acceptable signal-to-noise level in the decay to be accumulated. The spectrometer is then set to a different position in the spectrum and the procedure repeated. If small enough increments of the magnetic field are taken, a complete analysis of how the ESR spectrum changes with time can be obtained. From this the identity and kinetics of appearance and disappearance of transient species may readily be determined. The spectrum of the $Ph_2\dot{C}{-}OH$ radical 100 microseconds after the laser flash is shown in Figure 9.24(a). In an alternative mode of operation, the magnetic field is scanned slowly and the absorption sampled at a set time (say 100 μs) after the flash. A spectrum accumulated in this way is shown in Figure 9.24(b). Spectra in (a) and (b) are virtually identical.

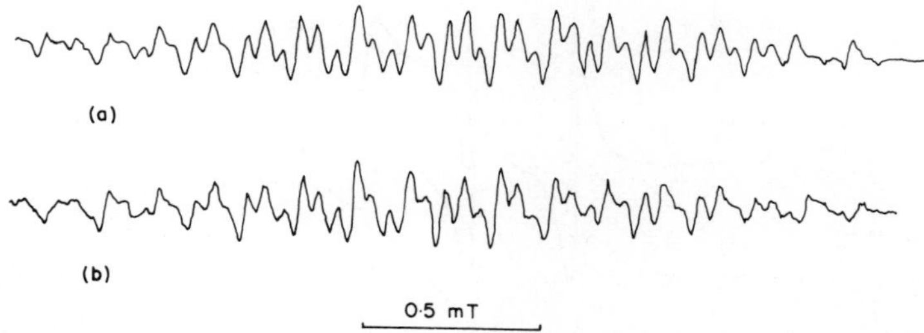

Figure 9.24 ESR spectra of Ph_2COH radical generated by ultraviolet radiation and recorded on a microsecond response ESR spectromoter. Spectrum (a) was obtained by recording the rate of decay of the radical at set field increments, then replotting the signal height at 100 μs against magnetic field. Spectrum (b) was obtained by slowly scanning the field and directly recording the signal height against magnetic field. (From Atkins *et al.*, 1970. Reproduced by permission of The Institute of Physics.)

Alternative ways for generating radicals other than photolysis would be compatible with the fast-response spectrometer. Pulsed radiolysis is finding increasing applications as a source of hydrated electrons for reducing redox enzymes and cofactors (see Fielden *et al.*, 1974; Van Buuren *et al.*, 1974; Land and Swallow, 1969). These studies have so far used ultraviolet/visible absorption spectroscopic detection but ESR detection would have the advantage of higher structural information content.

ESR study of slow motion

There is at present no spectroscopic technique which covers the time range from $10^{-6}-1$ second. It is in this time range that conformational changes in proteins and rotational motion of large macromolecules occur. Development of both the ESR and NMR techniques are needed before they can be applied to the study of slow biological processes.

For the time range in which the rate of molecular tumbling is close to the frequency of the hyperfine separation, the ESR spectrum is a good monitor of motion. Thus as the viscosity of a spin label is raised, the spectrum is appreciably affected (see Figure 9.25).

However, for tumbling or translational times longer than 10^{-8} seconds up to the limit of complete immobilization, changes in the spectrum are minimal. ESR developments which would overcome this '10^{-8} second time barrier' have been suggested from the results of ESR studies on flavin radicals dissolved in supercooled toluene at various microwave powers; the rate of tumbling of the radicals was slower than 10^{-8} seconds and could be altered by varying the viscosity.

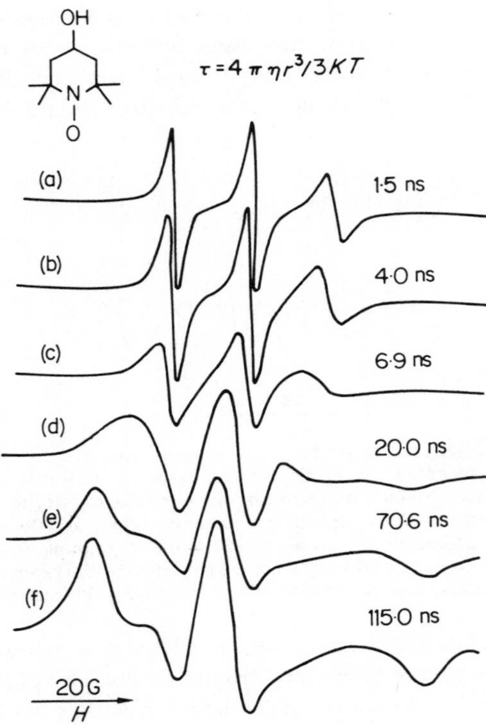

Figure 9.25 The effect of viscosity on the ESR spectrum of a spin label dissolved in glycerol. Spectra (a) → (f) refer to increasing viscosity. (From Smith, 1972)

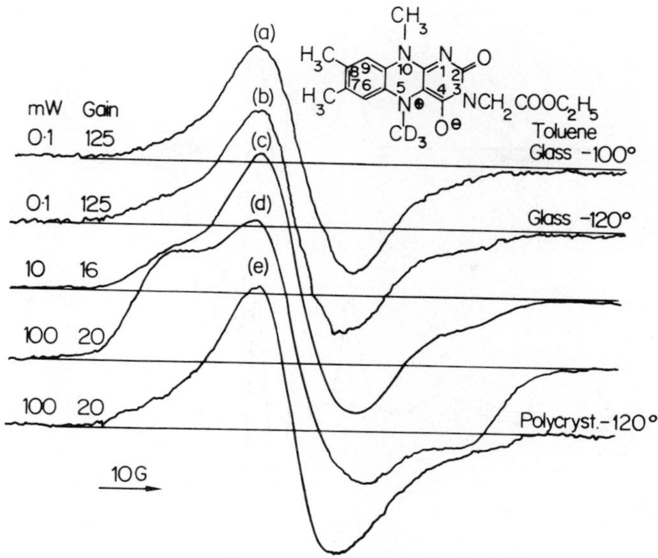

Figure 9.26 ESR spectra of substituted neutral lumiflavin radical in supercooled or polycrystalline toluene at various microwave powers. Spectra (b), (c) and (d) demonstrate clearly anomalous saturation behaviour. (From Hyde *et al.*, 1970. Reproduced by permission of Elsevier Scientific Publishing Company)

The ESR spectra (Figure 9.26) showed anomalous saturation behaviour which suggests that slow motion affects relaxation processes. Hyde and Dalton (1972) have presented evidence that the relaxation times which are dominant in this situation are the electron spin–lattice relaxation time (T_{1e}) and the spin diffusion time (T_D), the latter being a measure of molecular motion. Thus, if experimental conditions can be devised to allow T_D to be distinguished from other relaxation times, a solution to the problem of measuring slow radical motion becomes possible. There are still experimental and theoretical problems outstanding; however, promising preliminary results have been obtained (Hyde and Thomas, 1973), on spin-labelled haemoglobin dissolved in glycerol. From the known dimensions of haemoglobin, it can be calculated (equation 6.18) that T_D would be between 10^{-4} and 10^{-5} seconds. In all probability these measurements of T_D will be possible with only minor modifications to existing 9 GHz ESR spectrometers which can operate in the dispersion mode, have an additional modulation frequency for second derivative presentation and can operate with the phase-sensitive detector 90° out of phase with respect to the field modulation. Alternatively ELDOR (see Section 9.4) may be used as described by Smirgel *et al.* (1974).

9.6 Electron Spin Relaxation

Mention has been made in Section 8.5 of how microwave power saturation studies distinguished different types of copper in the enzyme cytochrome oxidase. The

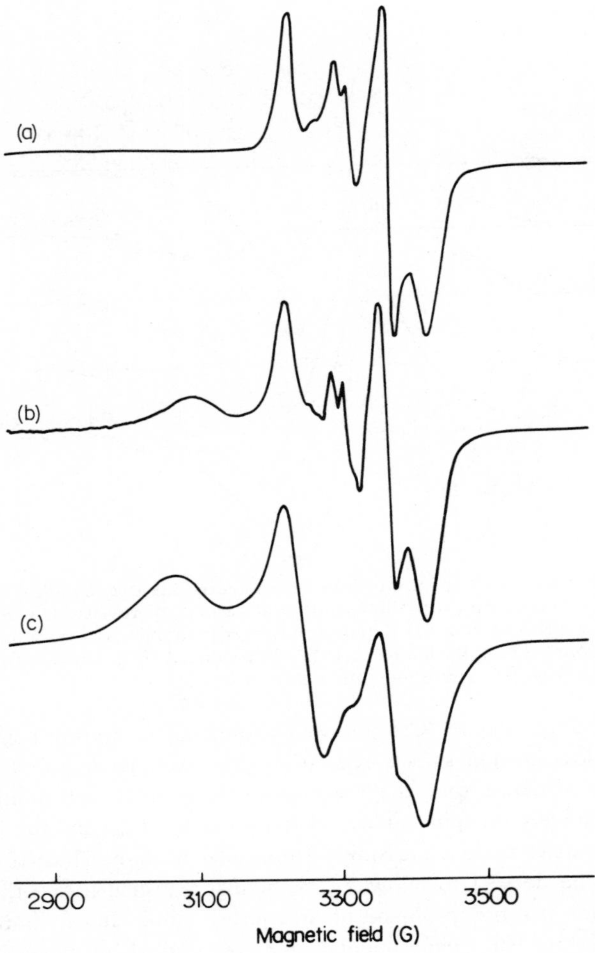

Figure 9.27 Iron-sulphur ESR signals from a sample of xanthine oxidase reduced with sodium dithionite. Signals were recorded under the following conditions: (a) 55 K, 100 mW microwave power; (b) 150 K, 0.1 mW; (c) 15 K, 100 mW. (From Lowe *et al.*, 1972. Reproduced by permission of The Biochemical Society)

studies depend on the different coppers having different relaxation times. Studies on the enzyme xanthine oxidase (Lowe *et al.*, 1972) suggest that more detailed studies of electron spin relaxation processes could provide valuable information on pathways of electron transfer in enzyme systems possessing several paramagnetic centres, and on the spatial separation between these centres. Reduced xanthine oxidase gives two ESR signals which originate from its iron-sulphur centres. The first, detectable at 80 K, sharpens up at helium temperatures (see Figure 9.27) and has g (average) = 1.95. The second signal can only be observed below 35 K and has

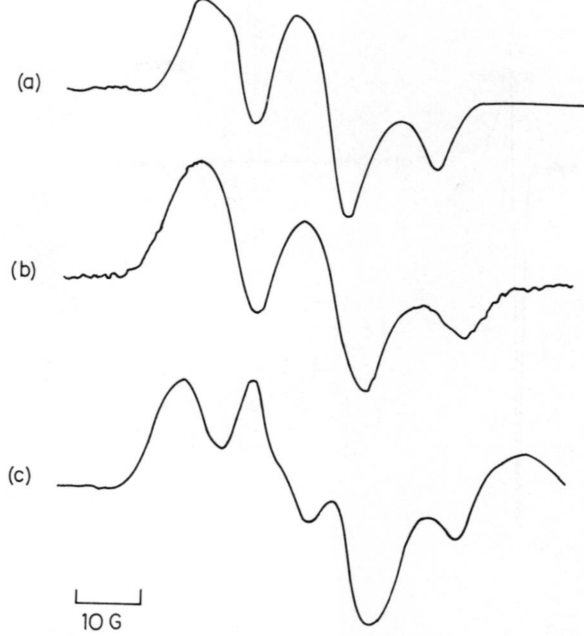

Figure 9.28 High- and low-temperature forms of Mo^V ESR signals from xanthine oxidase. (a) 95 K with both molybdenum and iron-sulphur species reduced. (b) 28 K with only molybdenum reduced; (c) 40 K with both molybdenum and iron-sulphur species reduced. (From Lowe *et al.*, 1972. Reproduced by permission of The Biochemical Society)

g = 2.01. These two iron-sulphur species obviously have different electron spin–lattice relaxation times; adjustment of the temperature and microwave power allows each of these iron-sulphur signals to be observed free from the other.

Interactions between reduced molybdenum and the g_{av} = 1.95 iron-sulphur centre is indicated from further temperature variation studies on fully or partially reduced enzyme. As shown in Figure 9.28, the reduced molybdenum signal does not change with temperature unless the g_{av} = 1.95 iron-sulphur species is also reduced. Assuming dipolar coupling between the reduced molybdenum and iron centres to be responsible for these spectral changes, a separation distance of 4 nm can be calculated.

From the above example, it can be seen that detailed study of electron relaxation times T_{1e} and T_{2e} could provide valuable information. Electron spin echo spectroscopy provides a method for measuring T_{1e} and T_{2e} directly. Most of these measurements are made at liquid-helium temperatures and on magnetically dilute samples. Under these conditions, the electron spin–lattice relaxation time is increased and electron spin–spin interactions are minimized, respectively. Many of the advantages of pulsed NMR over continuous-wave methods apply equally to

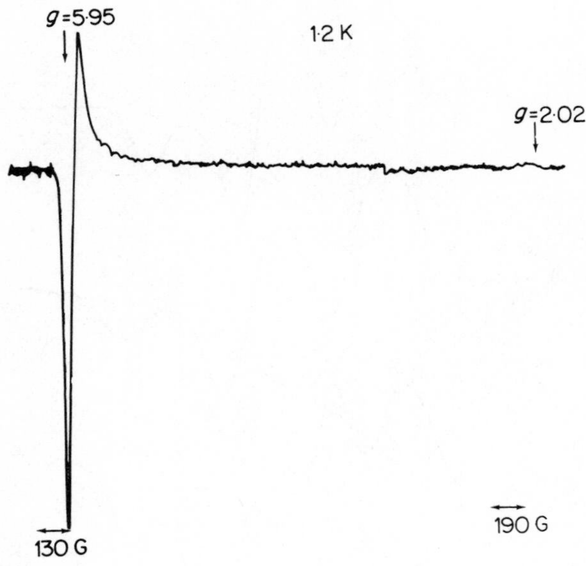

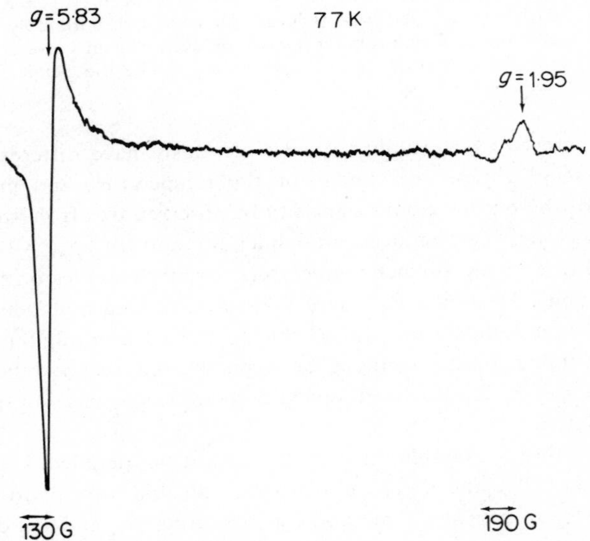

Figure 9.29 ESR spectra of horse heart myoglobin at 77 K (upper) and 1.2 K (lower). (From Bozanic *et al.*, 1969. Reproduced by permission of the American Institute of Physics)

pulsed ESR. Thus some phenomena, for example relaxation, are most conveniently studied in the time domain; one can move into the frequency domain by Fourier transformation of the magnetization decays. Comparable sensitivity has been achieved in spectra obtained from free induction decays at set increments of the Zeeman field followed by Fourier transformation to that obtained by continuous-wave operations.

As an example of electron spin echo applications to biological systems, the studies of Bozanic *et al.* (1969) on metmyoglobin may be cited. The ESR signals at 77 and 1.2 °K are shown in Figure 9.29 and indicate that essentially all the iron is

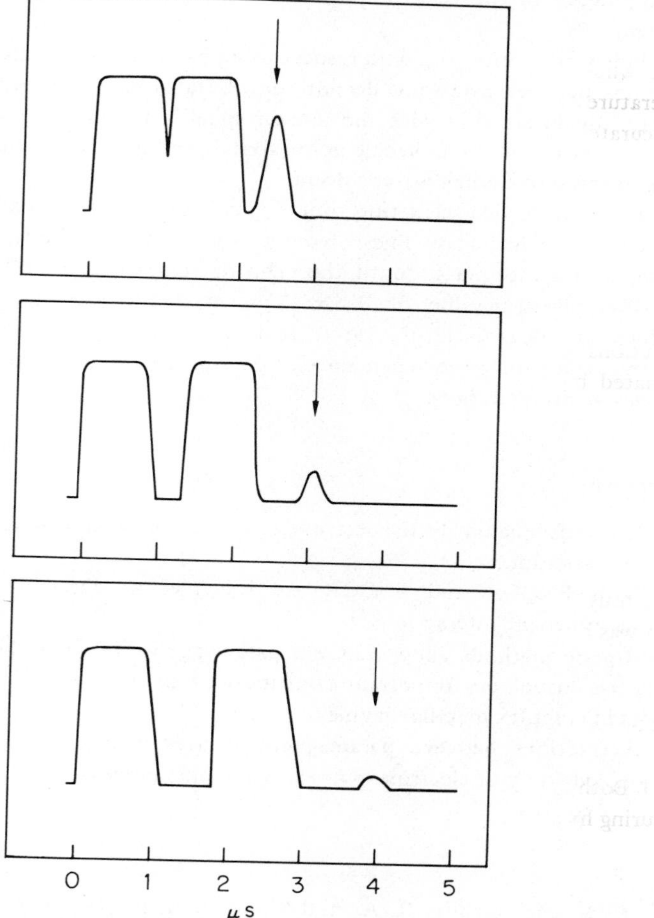

Figure 9.30 Electron spin echoes (arrowed) near $g = 2$ for horse myoglobin solutions at 1.2 K. The upper, centre and lower traces refer to increasing pulse spacings. (From Bozanic *et al.*, 1969. Reproduced by permission of the American Institute of Physics)

in the high spin ferric forms. The decrease in linewidth of both the $g = 6$ and $g = 2$ signals when the temperature is lowered indicates that the linewidth at the higher temperature is determined by the spin–lattice relaxation time.

Accurate values for the electron relaxation times can be obtained in the following way:

(a) Two microwave pulses of short duration applied in a manner similar to NMR spin echo experiments ($120°–\tau–120°$) produce an echo after a further time 2τ (see Figure 9.30) the magnitude of which decreases exponentially with increasing τ. From the decay of the echo amplitude a value for T_{2e} (0.5 μs at 1.2 K) can be calculated.

The independence of T_{2e} with respect to myoglobin concentration suggests that interactions between iron spins do not contribute to relaxation which is probably dominated by interaction with the nuclear spins of the iron ligands, in particular the protons of the water molecule in the sixth ligand position and possibly also the protons of the surrounding water solvent.

(b) The spin–lattice relaxation time T_{1e} can also be measured by a pulse-echo technique. The echo delay time is fixed at 5 μs relative to the first pulse and the pulse repetition rate varied until the echo decreases to $(1 - 1/e)$ of its original value. This gives a value of $T_1 = 3.5$ ms at 1.2 K for the $g = 2$ region of metmyoglobin (Bozanic *et al.*, 1969), and this value decreases rapidly to 2 μs at 4.2 K, thus confirming the dependence of linewidth on spin–lattice relaxation time which was mentioned above.

9.7 Summary

(1) Higher-frequency ESR spectrometers give increased spectral resolution and aid spectral assignment.

(2) Both ENDOR and ELDOR are valuable for detecting and accurately measuring hyperfine interactions.

(3) Kinetic methods allow transient paramagnetic species to be studied. Rapid freezing has made very important contributions to the study of electron transfer processes in complex metalloenzymes.

(4) Interactions between paramagnetic centres in biological material require more detailed study of electron spin relaxation phenomena.

References

Atkins, P. W., McLauchlin, R. A., and Simpson, A. F. (1970), *J. of Physics E.*, **3**, 547.

Bozanic, D., Krikorian, K. C., Mergerian, D., and Minarik, R. W. (1969). *J. Chem. Phys.*, **50**, 3606.

Bray, R. C. (1961). *Biochem. J.*, **81**, 196.

Bray, R. C., and Knowles, P. F. (1968). *Proc. Roy. Soc. A*, **302**, 351.

Bray, R. C., Knowles, P. F., and Meriwether, L. S. (1967). In *Magnetic Resonance in Biological Systems*, p. 249, Ehrenberg, A., Malmström, B. G., and Vänngård, T. (Eds), Pergamon Press, Oxford.

Bray, R. C., and Swann, J. C. (1972). *Structure and Bonding*, **11**, 107.

Bray, R. C., and Vänngård, T. (1969). *Biochem. J.*, **114**, 725.

Charlton, S. C. (1972). PhD Thesis, University of Leeds.

Ehrenberg, A., and Ludwig, G. D. (1958). *Science*, **127**, 1177.

Ehrenberg, A., Eriksson, L., and Hyde, J. (1971). In *Third International Symposium on Flavin and Flavo Proteins*, p. 141, Kamin, H. (Ed.), University Park Press, Baltimore.

Feher, G., Isaacson, R. A., Scholes, C. P., and Nagel, R. (1973). *Annals N.Y. Acad. Sci.*, **222**, 86.

Fielden, E. M., Roberts, P. B., Bray, R. C., Lowe, D. J., Mauntner, G. N., Rotilio, G., and Calabrese, L. (1974). *Biochem. J.*, **139**, 49.

Guzzo, A. V., and Tollin, G. (1964). *Arch. Biochem. and Biophys.*, **105**, 380.

Hyde, J. S., and Dalton, L. (2972). *Chem. Phys. Letters*, **16**, 568.

Hyde, J. S., Eriksson, L. E. G., and Ehrenberg, A. (1970). *Biochem. Biophys. Acta*, **222**, 688.

Hyde, J. S., and Thomas, D. D. (1973). *Annals N.Y. Acad. Sci.*, **222**, 680.

Knowles, P. F., Gibson, J. F., Pick, F. M., and Bray, R. C. (1969). *Biochem. J.*, **111**, 53.

Land, E. J., and Swallow, A. J. (1969). *Biochemistry*, **8**, 2117.

Lowe, D. J., Lynden-Bell, R. M., and Bray, R. C. (1972). *Biochem. J.*, **130**, 239.

McConnell, H. M. (1971). *Ann. Rev. Biochem.*, **40**, 227.

Nilsson, R., Pick, F. M., Bray, R. C., and Fielden, M. (1969). *Acta Chem. Scand.*, **23**, 2554.

Smirgel, M. D., Dalton, L. R. and Hyde, J. S. (1974). *Proc. Nat. Acad. Sci. USA*, **71**, 1925.

Smith, I. C. P. (1972). In *Biological Applications of Electron Spin Resonance*, p. 483, Swartz, H. M., Bolton, J. R., Borg, D. C. (Eds.), Wiley–Interscience, New York.

Van Buuren, K. J. H., Van Gelder, B. F., Wilting, J., and Braams, R. (1974). *Biochem. Biophys. Acta*, **333**, 42, .

Wertz, J. E., and Bolton, J. R. (1972). *Electron Spin Resonance in Elementary Theory and Practical Applications*, McGraw-Hill, New York.

Glossary

AC (alternating current). Current or voltage whose direction (or polarity) varies with time in a wavelike manner.

Algae. Primitive plants lacking roots and leaves but which are still able to photosynthesise.

Allosteric. Macromolecule system in which the binding of a ligand effector produces a cooperative change enhancing further binding of this or other ligands. Normally occurring between protein subunits, e.g. haemoglobin.

Amino acid. Basic chemical building block of proteins, of general formula: $R.CH(NH_2).COOH$, where the R-group characterizes the particular amino acid.

Anisotropic motion. Implies rotation about one axis in a molecule.

Anisotropy. Variation of a property with direction (of the applied magnetic field). An anisotropic substance has properties (spectra) which vary with direction (of the applied magnetic field).

Antibodies. Serum proteins produced by the body to resist attack by foreign bodies (*antigens*).

Automatic frequency control. Device by which the microwave frequency is kept tuned to the resonance frequency of the ESR cavity.

Axial symmetry. System which has one unique axis (the axis of symmetry) and two perpendicular equivalent axes.

Bimodular cavity. A microwave cavity which can simultaneously be subjected to two microwave frequencies.

Boltzmann distribution. Population distribution of a system of particles when they are at thermal equilibrium. The number of particles in energy level E_i at temperature T K is $n_i \propto e^{-E_i/kT}$.

Carcinogenisis. The process by which normal tissue is made neoplastic.

CAT (computer of average transients). A signal averaging device (q.v.).

Cavity wavemeter. Device for measuring the microwave frequency.

Chemical shift. Specifies the position of an NMR line relative to a standard reference. It is determined by the amount of 'shielding' of the applied magnetic field by the electrons surrounding the particular nucleus.

Chlorophyll. The green pigment found in chloroplasts which is important in light energy absorption during photosynthesis.

Chloroplasts. Specialized chlorophyll-containing bodies involved in sugar synthesis which are located in the cytoplasm of plant cells.

Chromatophores. Specialized membranes in photosynthetic bacteria which function in a manner similar to chloroplasts.

Conformation. The overall three-dimensional structure of a molecule. This is determined partly by the fixed bond angles in the molecule, but also by the 'conformations', or angles of rotation, about the various bonds. Various conformations of a particular molecule may be in dynamic equilibrium.

Conformational change. Change in the three-dimensional structure of a molecule. This may be a gross change, as in the unfolding of a protein molecule, or may be a small, possibly localized, change resulting from, e.g., ligand binding to a protein. It may also simply involve the displacement of a conformational equilibrium.

Conjugated molecule. Hydrocarbon molecule whose structure is made up of alternating single and double bonds:

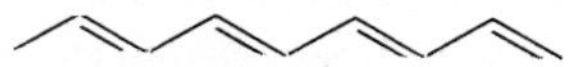

The double bond electrons (π-electrons) are delocalized over the whole of the conjugated system.

Coupling (critical). Introduction of microwave radiation (from a waveguide) into a resonant cavity via an iris, or coupling hole, in the side of the cavity. If the coupling hole is of such a size that all the microwaves are just absorbed by the cavity, then it is 'critically coupled'. If some of the microwaves are reflected it is 'under coupled'.

Coupling iris (hole). See 'coupling'.

Covalent bond. Chemical bond which involves transfer of electrons between the two atoms which are bonded.

Cytochromes. A group of intracellular haemoproteins important in cellular respiration.

DC (direct current). Current or voltage whose direction (or polarity) does not change.

Delocalized. Implies that the unpaired electron density is spread over several atoms.

Denaturation. Process by which a macromolecule (e.g. protein) loses its compact three-dimensional structure, and is unfolded into a random coil. Can be induced by high temperature, extremes of pH, and 'denaturing agents'.

Dewar. Double-wall, evacuated, insulating vessel.

Diamagnetic. Possessing no net electron magnetic moment.

Diamagnetic pair. Two paramagnetic species spin coupled together to produce a diamagnetic dimer.

Dielectric absorption. Strong microwave electric field absorption by polar liquids, particularly water. Such samples are very 'lossy' in ESR, and the sample volume must be strictly limited and kept out of the microwave electric field.

Diode. Device which allows current to flow in only one direction through it. An alternating current is said to be 'rectified' by it.

Dipolar correlation time. The time taken for a spin system to rotate through one radian from its previous orientation due to 'through space' interactions with neighbouring spins.

Dipolar interaction. Magnetic interaction between two magnetic moments by virtue of the effect of the magnetic field of one on the other.

d-Orbital. Electron orbital (or wavefunction, q.v.) which has an orbital angular momentum of 1/2. There are 5 distinct d-orbitals: d_{xy}, d_{xz}, d_{yz}, $d_{x^2-y^2}$, d_{z^2}, with different angular shapes, each of which can accommodate two spin-paired electrons. Electrons in the d-orbitals give rise to the paramagnetism of the transition-metal ions (e.g. the 3d orbitals in iron group metals), since they lie within the valence orbitals.

DSS. 2,2 dimethylsilapentane 5-sulphonic acid. A water-soluble NMR reference compound.

Electron density. Probability density for an electron at a particular nucleus in the molecule.

Electron spin echo spectroscopy. Intense microwave pulses at a frequency which satisfies the resonance condition are applied to a paramagnetic sample in a magnetic field. Phase coherence in the spins is lost through relaxation during time *t* after the pulse is switched off but can be restored by a second 180° pulse. The restoration of phase coherence gives rise to a nuclear induction signal (the echo). The technique gives precise values for electron spin relaxation times.

Electron spin–lattice relaxation time. A measure of the time taken for the spin population to return to its equilibrium value through interaction with fluctuating internal electric fields which surround it ('the lattice').

Electron spin–spin relaxation time. A measure of the time to lose phase coherence, i.e. return to equilibrium through interaction with neighbouring spins during an ESR experiment. It is inversely proportional to the linewidth.

Electron transport chain. Series of electron carriers which are alternately reduced and oxidized in transferring electrons from an initial donating substrate, e.g. NADH, to a terminal accepting substrate, e.g. molecular oxygen.

Energy level. The stable energy states which an atom or molecule can take up. In general the lower, ground state, energy levels are occupied and the higher, excited state, energy levels are not. Quantum mechanics (q.v.) states that only a certain discrete set of energy levels is possible; the energy states of the atom or molecule cannot vary continuously.

Erythrocytes. Red blood cells.

Exchange integral. Represents the energy of interaction between two orbitals.

Filling factor. Fraction of the useful volume of the NMR coil or ESR cavity which is filled by the sample.

Filter. Electronic device which lets through only certain frequencies (as other filters select particle size).

First derivative. The slope of a curve. The normal way of recording an ESR spectrum is as the change in the slope of the absorption line as the spectrometer scans through the spectral line.

Flat cell. Quartz sample cell with flat faces ~0.3 mm apart, commonly used for aqueous samples in ESR.

Flexibility gradients. Imply increasing mobility as one moves along a chain.

Free radical. A molecule which contains an unpaired electron (q.v.), which is often chemically reactive.

Fusion. The process whereby two membranes join together; with enclosed structures, for example cells, a common interior is produced.

Gauche (Trans). Conformation of a hydrocarbon chain has the hydrogens of adjacent methylene groups on the same (opposite) side of the backbone.

Gauss (G). Unit of magnetic field strength (strictly of magnetic induction, though the two are numerically equivalent in air). Formally defined by the fact that unit current flowing in a circular wire loop of radius 1 cm produces a field of 2π gauss at the centre in air (e.m.u. units). 1 kG = 10^3 G and 1 tesla = 10^4 G.

Gaussian lineshape. Shape of a spectral line whose height as a function of frequency ν is given by

$$I(\nu) = I_{max} \exp[-b^2(\nu_0 - \nu)^2]$$

where ν_0 is the frequency of the line centre and the linewidth (q.v.) is $\Delta\nu = 2(\ln 2)^{1/2}/b$. A common approximation for magnetic resonance lineshapes in solids.

Glycolytic pathway. The sequence of enzyme catalysed reactions by which glucose is metabolized.

***g*-Value.** Factor which expresses the size of the magnetic moment of a paramagnetic species. Specifies the position at which the ESR spectrum of the paramagnetic species occurs.

Haem protein. A protein having the iron-containing haem group as its functional centre.

Hall probe. Magnetic field measuring device used for stabilizing the field of electromagnets.

Halobacterium halobium. A bacterium requiring high concentrations of sodium chloride for growth. A 'purple membrane' fragment dissociates from the bacterium when salt is removed.

Haptens. Low molecular weight compounds which, though not antigens themselves, elicit an immune response specific to the hapten when bound to a high molecular weight carrier.

Hepatomas. Cancers of the liver.

Hertz (Hz). Frequency of 1 cycle per s. 1 MHz = 10^6 Hz. 1 GHz = 10^9 Hz.

Heteronuclear decoupling. Elimination of spin–spin interactions between nuclei of different types by irradiation with high RF power at the resonant frequency of one of them. E.g. decoupling of protons from ^{13}C nuclei to simplify the ^{13}C spectrum.

High spin complexes. Complexes of transition-metal ions having a maximal unpaired *d*- or *f*-shell electron arrangement over available orbitals. This electron arrangement occurs when the pairing energy is greater than the crystal field splitting energy.

Histology. The study of the location of substances and groups of substances in cells and in the intercellular material of tissue.

Histones. A group of small basic proteins found in association with DNA in the chromosome.

Homonuclear decoupling. Elimination of spin–spin interactions between nuclei of the same type by irradiation with high RF power at the resonant frequency of one of them. Used in NMR spectral assignment, e.g. by the decoupling of one proton from another adjacent to it in the molecule.

Hormones. Low molecular weight substances involved in the regulation of biological processes.

Hybrids. The fusion of two morphologically distinct cells or model membrane vesicles.

Hydrated electrons. Unpaired electrons having coordinated water molecules; they are highly reactive reducing agents.

Hyperfine splitting. Splittings in the lines of an ESR spectrum arising from the interaction of the unpaired electron with the nuclei in the vicinity. Can be used to determine the structure of a free radical, including the unpaired electron densities on particular nuclei, or to identify the ligands of a paramagnetic ion and to assess the degree of covalent bonding to them.

Interaction broadening. Concentration-dependent broadening of ESR lines resulting from magnetic interactions between paramagnetic molecules.

Isosbestic points. The points of intersection in a spectrum observed when one species is converted to a spectrally distinct species.

Isotopes. Nuclei which have the same atomic number (i.e. the same electrical charge) but different mass numbers (atomic weights). Thus isotopes are all the same element but with different atomic weights, and more importantly *different nuclear spins.*

Isotropic. A property which is the same independent of direction (of the applied magnetic field).

Isotropic motion. Implies random tumbling of a molecule about each of its three axes.

Isotropic spectrum. ESR (or NMR) spectrum in which the overall molecular tumbling is so rapid that all anisotropy in the spectrum is averaged out. Usually the case for small molecules in liquids.

K. Usually kilo (one thousand), this term is used colloquially, often in connection with computers, to denote 1024 (2^{10}) which is the nearest power of 2 to one thousand.

Klystron. Electronic valve which generates microwaves (q.v.).

Lateral diffusion. The two-dimensional motion of membrane components within one half of a bilayer.

Lateral phase separation. Arises when structurally different phospholipids having different phase transition properties occupy discrete domains in a membrane.

Ligand. An atom or small molecular group which binds to an atom or molecule of interest. Can be used either of the covalent bonding of an atom, e.g. nitrogen or oxygen, to a metal ion, or of the non-covalent binding of a small molecule to a macromolecule (e.g. protein or nucleic acid).

Linewidth. The width of a spectral line, normally defined as the distance (in Hz or gauss) between the two points of half-maximum height.

Lorentzian lineshape. Shape of a spectral line whose height as a function of frequency ν is given by

$$I(\nu) = I_{max}/[1 + a^2(\nu_0 - \nu)^2]$$

where ν_0 is the frequency of the line centre, and the linewidth (q.v.) is $\Delta\nu = 2/a$. Commonly the case for magnetic resonance lineshapes in liquids.

Low spin complexes. Complexes of transition-metal ions having maximal pairing of d- or f-shell electrons into the lower energy levels. This arrangement is favoured when the pairing energy is less than the crystal field splitting energy.

Magnetic field. Region of magnetic forces (attraction and repulsion) around a magnet: the stronger the field, the stronger the forces. Normally produced by an electromagnet. For definition of field strength, see Gauss.

Magnetic moment. Elementary directional property of a magnet which endows it with its magnetism. The stronger the magnet, the larger is its magnetic moment. More exactly, the body with the magnetic moment experiences a turning moment (but no translational force) in a magnetic field which tends to align it along the field. Formally the unit of magnetic moment is defined as that which experiences a couple of unit moment (force x distance from axis) when placed perpendicular to a magnetic field of 1 gauss.

Magnetic resonance. Absorption spectroscopy involving transitions between the energy levels corresponding to the different orientations of an (electron or nuclear) magnetic moment in a magnetic field.

Magnetic shielding. The reduction of the applied magnetic field at a nucleus below that applied to the whole sample; the effect is primarily produced by the electron cloud of the molecule.

Magnetic susceptibility. A measure of the intensity of magnetization produced in a substance by an applied magnetic field. Paramagnetic substances have positive susceptibilities; diamagnetic substances have negative susceptibilities.

Metalloproteins. Proteins having a firmly attached metal ion.

Magnetometer. Device for measuring magnetic field strength.

Microwaves. Electromagnetic radiation with frequencies of the order of 10^{10} Hz = 10 GHz (~3 cm wavelength). These frequencies are exclusively used in ESR.

Microwave bridge. The microwave components involved in the detection of ESR spectral absorption.

Modulation. Superimposition of a varying wavelike component onto some steady quantity, e.g. magnetic field modulation: introduction of a small component of the magnetic field whose direction varies with time in a wavelike manner at a particular frequency.

Molecular orbital. Wavefunction (q.v.) of an electron in a molecule. It is usually composed of a linear combination of the electron wavefunctions of the constituent atoms of the molecule.

Multibilayers. Structures composed of many phospholipid bilayers stacked together; multibilayers stacking on a glass slide allows the sample to be oriented in a magnetic field.

Nitroxide. Stable free radical group: $>N{-}O^{\bullet}$

Octahedral (ligand) symmetry. Arrangement of metal ion ligands which has three independent 4-fold axes of symmetry.

Orbital magnetic moment. Magnetic moment of an electron which is associated with its orbiting motion around a nucleus (or nuclei) in an atom or molecule. This magnetic moment is in addition to the spin magnetic moment.

Paramagnetic. Possessing a net electron magnetic moment, i.e. possessing at least one unpaired electron.

π-Electrons. See Conjugated molecule.

Phagocytosis. The ingestion of solid material by cells which is important both for nutrition and defence.

Phase. The phase of a signal is referred to the phase of a wavelike variation of the same frequency. If the peaks of the signal wave directly coincide (in position in time) with those of the reference then the two are exactly in phase. If the peaks of one coincide with the troughs of the other, then the signals are exactly out of phase.

Phase sensitive detector. A filter which allows only those signals modulated at a particular frequency to pass. It does this by comparing the phase (q.v.) of the signal with that of the modulating source.

Photosynthesis. The process by which sugars are synthesized from atmospheric carbon dioxide and water utilizing solar energy.

Photosynthetic bacteria. Specialized bacteria in which some photosynthetic processes can occur.

Pinocytosis. The uptake of fluid vesicles by cells which is important in many absorption processes.

Polypeptide. Amino acid (q.v.) polymer linked by the peptide bond: —CO—NH—. This is the basic chemical structure of proteins.

p-Orbital. Electron orbital (or wavefunction, q.v.) which has an orbital angular momentum of $l = 1$. There are 3 distinct p-orbitals, the p_x, p_y, p_z (directed along the *x*-, *y*-, *z*-axes), each of which can accomodate two electrons of opposite spin. Each p-orbital has two dumbell-shaped lobes.

Potential energy. Energy of a particle by virtue of its position, e.g. orientation within a magnetic field.

Powder spectrum. ESR spectrum in which the molecular axes (and hence principal axes) have completely random orientations with respect to the magnetic field, as in a powder. The powder spectrum consists of the superposition of all the individual spectra from all the different orientations. Usually arises from frozen solutions.

pπ-orbital. π-electron molecular orbital (q.v.) formed from two p atomic orbitals (on adjacent atoms in the molecule, e.g. N—O) which have their axes parallel (e.g. two p_z orbitals).

Principal axes (values). The three independent directions (of the magnetic field) along which the hyperfine interaction, or *g*-value, has its maximum and minimum values. These values are the 'principal values'.

Probe. (a) The part of an NMR spectrometer which contains the sample and radiofrequency coils. (b) Atom or molecule introduced into the sample because it produces a useful perturbing effect or because its own signal is readily detected, e.g. paramagnetic ion introduced for its specific shift effects.

Prosthetic group. Functional group in a (macro)molecule.

Protein sequence (or primary structure). The sequence of particular amino acids in the polypeptide (q.v.) structure of a protein.

Proton magnetometer. Device for measuring the magnetic field by the proton NMR frequency.

Pulsed radiolysis. A technique in which reactive species are generated by ionizing radiation pulses from a linear accelerator. Subsequent reactions of these species are usually followed spectrophotometrically as a function of time.

Pulsed ultraviolet laser. A high-energy short-duration beam of monochromatic ultraviolet light.

Pyrrolysed material. Material produced by heating biological matter; contains a high proportion of condensed aromatics.

Quadrupole interactions. The electric quadrupole moments of nuclei with spins greater than ½ interact with the electric field gradient (arising from surrounding valence electrons and other nuclei) to give a series of quantized energy levels.

Quantization. The situation that the properties of a system, e.g. magnetic moment, energy, cannot have a continuous set of values but must have a set of discrete, discontinuous values.

Quantum. Discrete energy packet. Electromagnetic radiation of frequency ν does not have continuously variable energy, but is made up of packets of energy $h\nu$ where h is Planck's constant.

Quantum mechanics. The set of physical laws which predict quantization (q.v.).

Radiofrequency (RF). Frequencies in the range, approximately 100 KHz to 500 MHz, appropriate to radio transmissions.

Redox reaction. The coupled oxidation and reduction of one substrate by another. Electrons are transferred from the substrate which is oxidized to the one which is reduced.

Reference arm. Device for providing the correct bias (or crystal current) to the microwave detector in an ESR spectrometer.

Relaxation. Process by which an atom or molecule in an excited state falls back into its ground state (see Energy level).

Resonant cavity (ESR). Copper cavity which absorbs the microwave radiation (of a particular frequency) entering it, by setting up standing waves within the cavity. An ESR sample placed in this cavity thus has concentrated microwave power incident on it.

Resonant mode. Standing wave in an ESR cavity in which all the microwaves are absorbed into the cavity.

Sarcoplasmic reticulum. The regular organized membrane structure found in muscle.

Saturation. Situation in which the rates of upward and downward energy-level transitions induced by radiation are equal, so that no net energy is absorbed from the radiation.

Selection rule. Rule which states between which energy levels spectroscopic transitions can take place. For ESR the following changes are necessary in the transition: $\Delta S_z = \pm 1$, $\Delta S = 0$, $\Delta m_I = 0$, and for NMR: $\Delta I_z = \pm 1$.

Shim coils. Flat, often printed-circuit coils used to produce small field gradients of an NMR magnet to cancel out field inhomogeneities.

Shimming. The optimization of magnetic field homogeneity in an NMR spectrometer by adjusting currents through the shim coils.

Signal averaging. Improvement of signal-to-noise ratio of a spectrum by adding up repeated scans through the spectrum. The noise tends to average out whereas the spectral lines reinforce.

Spin. An intrinsic property of an electron or nucleus which determines its magnetic moment. The spin is quantized (q.v.) and may have the value zero (in which case no magnetic moment), or whole or half integer numbers. The spin of an electron or of a proton is ½.

Spin density. The fraction of unpaired electron spin which is in the vicinity of a particular nucleus in the molecule.

Spin diffusion (T_D). The diffusion of a magnetic moment due to translation of the associated molecule and/or chemical exchange processes. *N.B.* The diffusion time used in the context of this application should be distinguished from the time constant for the relaxation of dipolar energy which is commonly denoted in NMR by T_D.

Spin exchange interactions. Occur through the overlap of orbitals on adjacent electrons and lead to exchange of the two spin states.

Spin Hamiltonian. Quantum mechanical (q.v.) formulation used for determining the energy levels of an electron or nuclear spin in ESR or NMR. More commonly used in ESR.

Spin label. Stable free radical (q.v.) used as an environmental probe molecule in ESR. The spin label may be either intercalated or covalently attached.

Spin polarization. Mechanism by which unpaired electron spin on one atom or part of the molecule is transferred to another atom. This is done by interaction between the unpaired electron on the first atom and the paired electrons on the second atom (which has no unpaired electrons). This interaction makes one of the paired electrons have lower energy than the other.

Spin—spin broadening. The increased linewidth caused by interactions between neighbouring dipoles.

Spin—spin splittings. Splittings in the lines of an NMR spectrum arising from the interaction of the nuclear magnetic moment with those of neighbouring nuclei. Can be used to assign the particular nuclear resonances and to determine molecular conformations.

***S*-State ion.** Transition-metal ion having no net orbital angular momentum whatsoever.

Stopped flow. A technique in which the flow of a solution is abruptly stopped a short time after mixing of the reaction components. The time course of the chemical reaction is then followed, usually by absorption spectroscopy.

Strongly (weakly) immobilized. Refers to the mobility of the spin label in a particular environment; strong immobilization produces broadening and distortion of the three-line nitroxide ESR signal.

Submitochondrial particles. Fragmented inner mitochondrial membrane particles prepared by sonication of mitochondria.

Substrate(s). Molecule(s) whose reaction is catalysed by an enzyme. The enzyme ‘acts on’ the substrate.

Superhyperfine structure. Hyperfine splittings in the ESR spectrum of a transition-metal ion, caused by interaction with the ligand nuclei. This is superimposed on the larger hyperfine splitting from the transition-metal ion nucleus itself.

Tertiary structure. The three-dimensional manner in which the polypeptide chain is folded in protein structure.

Tetragonal (ligand) symmetry. Arrangement of metal-ion ligands which has one 4-fold axis of symmetry.

Thermal equilibrium. Condition of a system when there is no tendency of heat to flow within itself or to or from its surroundings, i.e. when all parts of the system and surroundings are at the same temperature.

Time constant. Characteristic response time of a system. The longer the time constant, the longer it takes for the system to respond. (The response is usually exponential in time.)

TMS. Tetramethyl silane. A water-insoluble NMR reference compound.

Transition metals. Group of atoms whose electronic structure is differentiated not by the outer valence shell of electrons but by an inner 'transition' shell of electrons. The most important example is the iron group metals which are characterized by varying numbers of 3D electrons within the 4s valence shell.

Tricarboxylic acid cycle. The sequence of enzyme catalysed processes by which pyruvate is oxidized. The cycle is essential to both energy production in mitochondria and as a link between carbohydrate and protein metabolism.

Triplet states. Energy levels occupied by two unpaired electron spins.

Tuning. Bringing the radiation frequency to match the natural 'resonance' frequency of a particular electronic component, e.g. NMR coil or ESR cavity.

Unit cells. The spaces confined by repeat distances in the x-, y- and z-directions.

Unpaired electron. An electron in an atom or molecule, whose spin is not paired with the oppositely directed spin of another electron in the atom or molecule. Normally in chemical bonding a stable configuration is reached in which all the electrons in the molecule are spin-paired.

Wavefunction. Distribution function which determines the probability that an electron is at a given position in an atom or molecule.

Waveguide. Copper tube which transmits microwaves. Has the same function as wires and coaxial cables have at lower frequencies.

Zero field splitting. Occurs when the degeneracy of energy levels from transition-metal ions with $S > 1/2$ is split by the internal crystalline electric field present in the absence of an applied magnetic field.

Index